David Ip
Orthopedic Rehabilitation,

CW00693067

David Ip

Orthopedic Rehabilitation, Assessment, and Enablement

With 133 Figures

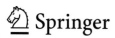 Springer

Dr. David Ip
MBBS (HKU), FRCS (Ed) Orth, FHKCOS,
FHKAM, FIBA (UK), FABI (USA)
Vice-President of the Recognition Board
of World Congress of Arts, Sciences, and Communications
Deputy Governor, American Biographical
Institute Research Association,
Musculoskeletal Rehabilitation Service,
Pamela Youde Nethersole Eastern Hospital, Hong Kong

ISBN 978-3-540-37693-4 Springer Berlin Heidelberg New York

Library of Congress Control Number: 2006931062

Springer is a part of Springer Science+Business Media

springer.com

Editor: Gabriele M. Schröder, Heidelberg, Germany
Desk Editor: Irmela Bohn, Heidelberg, Germany
Production: LE-TeX Jelonek, Schmidt & Vöckler GbR, Leipzig, Germany
Cover: Frido Steinen-Broo, eStudio Calamar, Spain
Typesetting: K + V Fotosatz GmbH, Beerfelden, Germany
Cover illustration: Courtesy of Vicon Motion Systems Ltd.

Printed on acid-free paper   24/3100 Di   5 4 3 2 1 0

Foreword

Medical practitioners involved in the treatment of diseases, disorders, and injuries of the musculoskeletal system will appreciate the very important role of rehabilitation. Following the publication of two books *Orthopedic Principles – A Resident's Guide* and *Orthopedic Traumatology – A Resident's Guide,* Dr. Ip has expended further time and effort to produce a third book, which contains a comprehensive account of orthopaedic rehabilitation. The material is easy to grasp with succinct points.

There are 19 chapters, arranged in a logical sequence. The first chapter gives a holistic view of what the rehabilitation process should include and emphasises that the unique feature of a rehabilitation service is thinking about a patient and his problems, not simply doing something to the patient, and the focus should be on trying to help each patient achieve his own goals.

Chapters 2 to 8 are about the rehabilitation tools for assessing, investigating and treating patients. Chapters 9 to 17 are about rehabilitation for specific types of musculoskeletal disorders, each of which has its own complex problems, requiring practitioners to gain further in-depth training and experience to give effective treatment.

The format is similar to the previous two books, containing brief, yet comprehensive, core information on the subject, which can be enhanced by more detailed literature review if necessary. This unique feature renders the book very readable.

All three books should be available to residents and staff in any orthopaedic department. Therapists and nurses treating patients with musculoskeletal diseases will also find this book useful.

Professor John C. Y. Leong, OBE, FRCS, FHKAM (Orth. Surgery), JP
President, Open University of Hong Kong; Formerly Professor & Head,
Department of Orthopaedic Surgery, University of Hong Kong;
Past President, Société Internationale de Chirurgie Orthopédique
et de Traumatologie (SICOT)

Foreword

Dr. David Ip, author of two extremely successful orthopaedic review texts, has produced yet a third and perhaps his very best, entitled *Orthopedic Rehabilitation, Assessment, and Enablement*. This is a remarkable work of scholarship covering topics that, to date, have rarely received sufficient exposure in the orthopaedic community. I can state with extreme certainty that it will become the standard review text for anyone involved in the rehabilitation aspects of the musculoskeletal system.

Nineteen comprehensive chapters cover not only every aspect of rehabilitation of the musculoskeletal system, but extend further into such topics as alternative medicine, holistic therapies, acupuncture, neurophysiologic testing, overuse injuries, work assessment and outcome measures. Each chapter covers the basic science of the subject, clinical assessments, rehabilitation options and methods, and the outcomes of these. Take for example the chapter on gait analysis. Following the introduction, the subdivisions of information include the nature of gait analysis, key evaluations of the gait cycle, the contributions of ground-reactive force data, kinematic data collection, temporal parameters, dynamic EMG data and gait anomalies. The latter covers gait issues with amputees, prosthetic usage, cerebral palsy, to name but a few issues.

The nineteenth and final chapter is an extremely stimulating one entitled "New Evidence-Based Programme for Preventing and Rehabilitating Hip Fractures". For such a common injury, rarely has such an exhaustive study of all of the issues related to hip fracture rehabilitation been made, and is contained in this thesis written by Dr. Ip to the Hong Kong College of Orthopedic Surgeons. The thesis presents a scientific investigation of the problems regarding not only epidemiology, but also issues as to aetiologic factors in the causation of hip fractures, the science of data analysis, kinematics and joint function, and of equal importance, rehabilitation. There are a number of factors that have been recognised to be important not only in the rehabilitation of the hip, but also in the rehabilitation of the individual back to an independent lifestyle.

The work in this thesis must become part of the general curriculum of all individuals involved in the management of the elderly patient far beyond those that deal primarily with the musculoskeletal system. This should be part of general medical training and knowledge, and in the long run the information presented in this thesis should go far to help our fellow citizens avoid the disastrous effects of a fractured hip and enhance the quality of life for citizens around the world.

While the information throughout the text is presented in bullet points, the subjects are covered in extraordinary detail. I feel for certain that this text will serve a wide community of healthcare professionals and will be part of required reading for any and all disciplines involved in musculoskeletal rehabilitation, neuromuscular disorders, burn rehabilitation, and evaluation of pain and pain management.

Jesse B. Jupiter, M.D.
Director, Orthopaedic Hand Service
Massachusetts General Hospital
Hansjörg Wyss/AO Professor, Harvard Medical School

Preface

It was to the author's delight that the medical and scientific communities have so warmly received his previous two books, also published by Springer, on the subjects of orthopaedic trauma and orthopaedic principles.

The current text summarises the many conceptual and technological advances in the field of orthopaedic rehabilitation that the trainee surgeons will be eager to know. It breaks away from the traditional "cookbook"-like approach detailing "standard protocols" from one or two centres, but rather places stress on a basic understanding of the subject matter, not only in an evidence-based manner, but also by looking at each particular subject from various viewpoints.

The book ends with the description of a thesis originally submitted by the author to the Rehabilitation Sub-Specialty Board of the Hong Kong College of Orthopedic Surgeons detailing a brand new look and new strategies for the rehabilitation of fragility hip fractures. The design of such an evidence-based programme is far from easy, for it requires knowledge of neurophysiology, biomechanics, theoretical physics, physiotherapy, besides orthopaedics and gait analysis.

Overall, the current book represents a distillation of the experiences of the author throughout more than 20 years in medical practice; including his overseas training in rehabilitation in the Scandinavian countries, USA, UK and Canada. The author is now the Hon Director General Asia of the International Biographical Association in Cambridge UK. Besides being a fellow of several orthopaedic societies including the Royal College of Surgeons (orthopaedic sub-specialty) and the Hong Kong College of Orthopedic Surgeons; he is also a member of the AAOS, the Association of Academic Physiatrists in the USA, and an active member of the IASP (International Association for the Study of Pain), the WIP (World Institute of Pain), the ESMAC (European Society of Movement Analysis), and the GCMAS (Gait and Clinical Movement Analysis Society). The author's biography can be found in Marquis Who's Who in Science and

Engineering and Marquis Who's Who in Medicine and Healthcare, among others. Finally, the author wishes to extend his heartfelt gratitude to Professor John Leong and Professor Jesse Jupiter for kindly writing the forewords to this book. Thanks are also due to the many different companies that have kindly provided pictures for illustration purposes, such as Vicon Motion Systems Ltd, Stryker, Bioness, Sigmedics, Ossur, among many others.

David Ip
Hong Kong, November 2006

Contents

| 1 | **The Rehabilitation Process, ICIDH vs ICF** |

Contents

1.1   Introduction and Definition

1.1.1   What is "Rehabilitation"?

▪ Rehabilitation is a problem-solving and educational process aimed at reducing the disability experienced by someone (with physical impairment) as a result of a disease, but always within the limitations imposed by available resources and by the underlying disease (Wade, 1992)

▪ The process normally involves the following key elements viz. assessment, goal setting, intervention, and quality control or evaluation

1.1.2   Two Main Philosophies of Rehabilitation

▪ Rehabilitation is a way of thinking, not a way of doing (Wade, Clin Rehabil 2002)

▪ The special unique feature of a rehabilitation service is that it thinks about the patient and his problems; not simply that it does something to our patient. The service should focus on trying to help each patient achieve his own goals, thinking how each obstacle can be overcome (Wade)

1.1.3   Three Main Aims of the Rehabilitation Process

▪ Maximise the participation of the patient in his/her social setting
▪ Minimise our patient's pain and distress
▪ Minimise the distress of and stress on the patient's family and/or his care-takers

1.1.4   Three Main Features of Effective Rehabilitation

▪ Co-ordinated multidisciplinary teamwork
▪ Involvement of the patient and the family
▪ Members with different expertise with an interest in disability management
▪ Recognises the importance of contextural factors, i.e. personal factors, physical factors, and social factors (such as those set out in the ICF of the WHO)

1.2   Rehabilitative Interventions

1.2.1   Difference Between Medical Intervention and Rehabilitative Intervention

- Medical intervention: interventions aimed at reversing or stopping the underlying disease process
- Rehabilitative intervention: any intervention that reverses, prevents worsening of, or alleviates an impairment and attempts to reduce disability or distress will all be considered part of rehabilitation

1.2.2   Main Types of Rehabilitative Interventions

- Internal interventions
- External interventions
- Interventions that have a positive effect on *another* impairment, which, if improved, can aid the main impairment (e.g. improvement of cardio-pulmonary fitness)

1.2.2.1   Internal Interventions

- Agents that increase function
- Surgery to improve structure
- Patient behaviour and thinking (e.g. biofeedbacks, cognitive behavioural interventions by psychologists, etc.)

1.2.2.1.1 Agents That Increase Function

- An example is the use of botulinium toxin in an attempt to improve function in selected patients with cerebral palsy (CP)

1.2.2.1.2 Surgical Procedures to Improve Function

- Example: surgery (usually at multiple levels) to tackle a crouching gait in CP, this surgery will not reverse the underlying disease process of CP

1.2.2.1.3 Intervention to Change Patient's Behaviour and Thinking

- Example of changing the patient's behaviour is the use of the cognitive behavioural approach in, say, the management of chronic lower back pain (see Chap. 16)
- Changing the way the patient thinks was found to be important in various studies on tackling difficult clinical problems. Examples of the use of this strategy:

- In patients with chronic pain (Arnstein et al., Pain 1999)
- In patients with knee osteoarthritis (Rejeski et al., Arthritis Care Res 1998)

1.2.2.2 External Interventions

▥ Equipment to increase function (e.g. shockwave, neuromuscular electrical stimulation, wheelchair, aids to activities of daily life (ADL), walkers – see Chaps. 2 and 6)

▥ Vocational training (see Chap. 17)

▥ Equipment to replace or support disordered body structure (see Chap. 10)

▥ Arranging carers for the patient

▥ Environmental modifications (be it at home, or in society as a whole, e.g. proper lift access – see Chap. 10)

▥ Social integration (social worker, social services, voluntary agencies, peer groups, etc.) + opportunities (e.g. proper accommodation, transport and job opportunities, and proper respect from members of society)

1.2.2.3 Interventions That Have Positive Effects *Indirectly* on the Main Impairment

▥ Example: a patient was sent to you for rehabilitation after fractured hip surgery – identification and treatment of chronic Dupuytren's contracture of fingers hindering hand function may improve upper limb usage of walking aids.

1.3 Role of Social Context

1.3.1 Importance of the Role of Social Context

▥ There is now increasing evidence that cultural attitudes and expectations can be changed to reduce the burden of disability

▥ Thus, the response of an individual does not depend only on personal context (i.e. his beliefs), but also on social context (i.e. more widespread cultural expectations)

1.3.2 Evidence in Support of the Social Context

▥ Recent evidence, such as an important study on chronic back pain, which focuses on changing the social context, can reduce disability as measured by sick leave or claims of disability (Buchbinder et al., BMJ 2001)

1.4   Forming a Multidisciplinary Rehabilitation Team

1.4.1   Formation of a Rehabilitative Team

■ From the aforesaid, it will be more than obvious that proper rehabilitation of our patients will involve a multi-disciplinary team effort
■ This is particularly important in the rehabilitation of well-known complicated clinical problems in orthopaedics such as:
  – Spinal cord injuries
  – Chronic pain
  – Cerebral palsy
■ This book has separate sections devoted to discussing these three challenging clinical problems in rehabilitation

1.4.2   Key Concept

■ An inter-disciplinary approach to rehabilitation is essential (Davis et al., Clin Rehabil 1992)
■ There is no one intervention that characterises all rehabilitation

1.4.3   Functions and Expectations of the Multi-Disciplinary Team

■ Work together towards common goals for the patient
■ Involve and educate the patient and family
■ Have relevant expertise and experience including knowledge and skills
■ Can resolve most (around 90%) of the clinical problems presented to the service (Clin Rehabil 2000)

1.5   Proper and Smooth Execution of Proposed Internal and External Interventions

1.5.1   Important Steps to Ensure Proper Execution of Planned Interventions

■ Setting up of a multi-disciplinary orthopaedic rehabilitative team (discussed above)
■ Goal setting: short- and long-term goals
■ Proper assessment and identification of patient's problems (not just orthopaedic) and with due attention to contextural factors (personal, physical and social)

■ Possible use of special illness models, especially in more difficult/challenging scenarios or issues (e.g. the Permission to be Sexual, Limited Information, Specific Suggestions, Intensive Therapy [PLISSIT] model)
■ Assess the need for behavioural modification
■ Periodic review of progress
■ Liaison with community service providers for follow-up upon patient's discharge from rehabilitative service

1.5.2 Key Concept
■ Goal setting is central to the process of any systematic rehabilitative process
■ Together with proper and adequate assessment, the two processes form the cornerstone of rehabilitation
■ Members of the rehabilitative team must be competent in the identification and setting up of proper treatment goals

1.6 The Importance and Process of Goal Setting

1.6.1 Definition
■ Goal: a future state that is desired and/or expected. It can include matters involving the patient, his environment, his family or another party. It is a generic term with no implications about timeframe or level
■ Goal setting: the process of agreeing on goals, this agreement is usually between the patient and all interested parties. It may involve setting goals at various levels and in various timeframes (according to Holliday)

1.6.2 Advantages of Goal Setting
■ Increase rehabilitative team collaboration
■ Acts as a reminder of the patient's interest
■ May improve the long-term effectiveness of our interventions
■ Shown to be associated with more behavioural change than in its absence (Theodorakis et al., J Sports Rehabil 1996)

1.6.3   Steps That May Improve the Positive Effects of Goal Setting

- Setting *both* short- and long-term goals is better than setting only long-term goals
- Goal setting is accompanied by specific interventions intended to facilitate positive behaviour changes of the patient
- Significant patient participation is important for a successful outcome (Webb et al., Rehabil Psychol 1994)

1.6.4   Outcome Measure to Assess Our Goal-Sharing Effort

- The author favours the use of measures like goal attainment scaling (Stoole et al., J Am Geriatr Soc 1992)

1.7   Principles of Assessment

1.7.1   Introduction

- As mentioned, careful assessment is one of the cornerstones of the process of rehabilitation
- It should be noted that the use of outcome measures (which have been given lots of emphasis in recent years) forms only a part of the assessment process
- The myths and pitfalls in the use of outcome measures will be discussed in Chap. 18

1.7.2   Essentials of Assessment

- Two key questions:
  - What is the most efficient assessment algorithm for the clinical problem?
  - Which specific assessment is able to give the most information with the least cost in time and effort

1.7.3   Key to Success

- There is evidence that a structured approach to assessment might lead to a better outcome than a simple clinical approach (Wikander et al., Scand J Rehab Med 1998)
- Meta-analysis studies showed that assessment is only effective (especially in the elderly) if it is linked to later management (Rubenstein et al., Aging 1989)

1.8   Use of Models of Illness

1.8.1   Which Model of Illness?
◼ Currently popularly used model of illness = ICF of the WHO
◼ ICF = International Classification of Functioning, Disability, and Health (see next section)
◼ Other models may be useful in other special circumstances

1.8.2   Ways to Overcome Difficult Problems Faced by the Rehabilitation Team
◼ Explore several alternative interventions for difficult problems until the problem is overcome, but always performed in the context of the patient's long-term goal
◼ Special case scenarios may resort to the use of special illness models to tackle problems, e.g. the use of models like PLISSIT when it comes to sexual issues in spinal cord injury (SCI) patients (see Chap. 12)

1.9   World Health Organisation's ICIDH vs ICF

1.9.1   ICIDH
◼ The ICIDH was the attempt by the WHO (World Health Organisation) to better define and classify the impact of chronic illness on the individual. It attempts to classify illness in terms of diagnosis and pathological abnormalities. This concept being based on the theoretical model of disablement (disease → impairment → disability → handicap) originally proposed by Dr. Philip Wood from UK who is a consultant of WHO
◼ The ICIDH presented three levels of classification: "impairment ICIDH", "disability ICIDH", and "handicap ICIDH". In other words, "I" the impairment code best describes the skeletal problem facing the patient; "D" the disability code, reveals problems in functional activity; while "H" stands for the (six) handicap codes. For details, the reader is referred to the ICIDH manual published by WHO in 1980

1.9.2   Criticism of the ICIDH
◼ The classification was made without due consultation with the relevant organisations like disability movement groups whose opinion should have been respected and consulted before the classification was made
◼ The inventors of ICIDH claimed it was not based on the medical model, but the fact that its framework is such that impairment, disability and

handicap, being all determined by a disease or disorder within the person, are manifestations of a direct link to the medical model

■ The ICIDH's framework stresses the role of the person within their own disability; thus, if an impairment causes a person to be unable to achieve certain tasks, they will be said to have a disability, and it has a connotation that a person will be in charge of his own disability and search for the corresponding coping mechanisms

■ Little stress was put on the effect of the environment on the person's level of disability

■ The last point is important and merits clarification. For example, there are now cars designed for paraplegics, and the mere presence of the impairment – in this case paraplegia from, say, spinal cord injury – does not automatically make the person disabled. Similarly, when this patient may well return to his workplace (e.g. supposing he does paper work) provided the design of the building, including the lift and corridors, are designed with the need of persons with an impairment (in this case, mobility impairment) in mind

■ The above serves to illustrate the extreme importance that the environment has on the individual with the impairment

■ Too much stress and concentrating on the individual means that the ICIDH model does not pay enough attention to the social factors and environment. The individual is supposed to develop adequate coping strategies himself

1.9.3   Summarising the Key Drawbacks of ICIDH

■ ICIDH works on the medical model of illness

■ The medical model focuses on the functional capabilities of patients within the scope of their disease and not on considering what patients want to do (i.e. personal context and beliefs in the performance of his or her occupational needs), where they want to perform activities meaningful to them, and what they need to allow them to perform – in other words, importance of environmental needs and social context

1.9.4   Revision of ICIDH

■ After its inception in 1980, it was revised in 1993 to take account of the role of the environment

■ Subsequent revisions occurred in 1996, 1997 and 1999; then was renamed ICIDH-2, which aimed to use more neutral terminology, and attempts were made to focus more on communication among health workers

1.9.5   Revision of ICIDH to ICF
- Despite the inception of ICIDH-2, the pressure groups are of the opinion that WHO still defines disability medically, i.e. regarding a disabled person as abnormal! In view of the criticisms, the ICIDH devised by the WHO was revised in 2001 to become the ICF (The International Classification of Functioning, Disability and Health)

1.9.6   ICF
- The new classification is a component of health classification, as opposed to consequences of disease
- Consists of two parts, and two components within each part
- The two parts are:
    - Functioning and disability
    - Contextual factors
- The two components within each part can be expressed in either positive or negative terms

1.9.7   Aim of ICF
- Aims to change the focus from that of the individual to focus on things that are important to the individual, like the environment and the social factors
- The second aim was to ease communication among different health care professionals

1.9.7.1   What Is Included Under "Functioning and Disability"?
- Includes aspects of body functions (domains) and activities of daily living

1.9.7.2   What Is Included Under "Contextual Factors"?
- Includes personal factors as well as environmental/societal factors

1.9.8   Disadvantages of ICF
- Does not cover disease or diagnosis
- Lacks a more positive terminology with regard to impairment and disease. We should pay due respect to patients with physical impairment in our society (see Fig. 1.1)
- Does not take temporal factors into account, like the patient's stage of life and illness

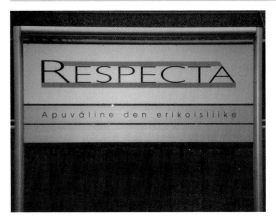

Fig. 1.1. Signpost raised in front of one of the buildings of the Orton Foundation (Finland) for the disabled, acting as a reminder for us to pay due respect to persons with physical impairment

- Does not acknowledge a possible difference between the person's perspective and the perspective of external observers
- Does not have a method of handling the question of "free-will" or freedom of choice
- Does not consider personal values and quality of life

1.9.9   Canadian Occupational Performance Measure
- This is the assessment tool much favoured by the author and will be mentioned throughout the text
- In the author's view, the Canadian Occupational Performance Measure (COPM) is favoured mainly because it has been shown to be sensitive to temporal factors; this is important, e.g. SCI patients may change their neurological status and hence functional abilities. A brief discussion now follows. For details, contact the Canadian Association of Occupational Therapists in Ottawa

1.9.9.1 COPM Categories
- Divided into:
  - Self-care (includes personal care, functional mobility, community management, etc.)

- Productivity (includes paid/unpaid work, household management, play/school)
- Leisure (includes quiet recreation, active recreation, socialisation)

1.9.9.2 COPM Scaling System

▨ The COPM has the clients prioritise the importance of reported tasks or activities into three categories as mentioned, and a scaling system used to assess the priority

▨ The scaling system consists of 1 = highest priority to 10 = lowest priority

1.9.9.3 Reason for Author's Preference for COPM over ICF

▨ It is a client-based semi-structured interview. Recall that the true philosophy of rehabilitation revolves around our client, not a neutral medical model

▨ COPM helps identify the five most important problems facing our client, thereby easing the process of goal setting between the team and client. We will recall that goal setting is another key cornerstone of the rehabilitation process

▨ COPM was validated as an indicator of the client's perception of occupational performance and sensitive to change. Serial ratings with COPM are therefore useful (Law et al., 1998). Notice, as pointed out, that the ICF does not make much allowance for the temporal factor. That said, the ICF can be used as a model to help the therapist to prioritise and make a more comprehensive assessment when using COPM

▨ Recently, COPM was also found to be adaptable to changes in patient's situations and environments as well. COPM will be used throughout the text

1.9.9.4 Useful Adjunct to COPM in Patient's Assessment 1: "Goal Attainment Scaling"

▨ Many chapters of this book deals with more complex problems in rehabilitation including rehabilitation of SCI, and CP patients

▨ Goal attainment scaling (GAS) is a useful tool as goal setting is important in rehabilitation. This measure will be mentioned throughout this book and nicely compliments the COPM. Even in the management of amputees, it has been shown to be a reliable outcome measure relative to, say, the Locomotor Capabilities Index (LCI) (Rushton et al., Arch Phys Med Rehabil 2002)

▪ The GAS will be used throughout this book

1.9.9.5   Useful Adjunct to COPM in Patient's Assessment 2: Functional Independence Measure

▪ COPM is a useful tool to assess client's priorities, but in order to assess client's ADL and instrumental activities of daily living (IADL), both the functional independence measure (FIM) and Barthel's Index (BI) can be used

▪ FIM is preferred to BI and used in this book

▪ For more complex conditions like CP, goal setting is very important and the concomitant use of COPM with goal scaling measures is useful

1.9.9.6   Preference for FIM over BI

▪ FIM is a more comprehensive measure of disability associated with physical impairment compared with BI

▪ It was developed by the Uniform Data System for Medical Rehabilitation (UDSMR) at the University of Buffalo)

▪ It includes assessment of communication and cognitive function, and more detailed assessment of functional mobility and self care

▪ Sometimes, the author uses other tools if deemed appropriate. Example: the Amputee Mobility Index is preferred to FIM for amputees

1.10   Viewpoints and Surveys Concerning "Disability"

1.10.1   Definition of Impairment

▪ Any loss or abnormality in the patient that is psychological, physiological, anatomical or functional in nature

1.10.2   Definition of Disability

▪ Any restriction or lack of ability to perform an activity in a manner or within the range considered normal

1.10.3 Definition of Handicap
▥ The way in which the disability influences the individual's ability to fulfil a role that is normal for that individual

1.10.4 Evidence That Disability is Frequently Missed by Practitioners
▥ There is evidence in the literature to suggest that clinicians sometimes miss some of the disability experienced by patients
  - By general practitioners: (Patrick et al., J R Coll Gen Pract 1982)
  - By physicians: (Calkins et al., Ann Int Med 1991)
  - These two papers provide clear evidence that it is not uncommon for practitioners to miss some of the disability that patients are suffering

1.10.5 Viewpoint of Health-Workers on "Disability": (Room for Improvement)
▥ In a recent survey, it was found that health professional students held less positive attitudes than the norm. Nursing undergraduate students were at greater risk of holding negative attitudes. Specific educational experiences are needed to promote more positive attitudes among health-care workers (Clin Rehabil 2006)

1.10.6 Better Detection of "Disabilities" by a Multi-Disciplinary Team
▥ Workers like Cunningham have shown in fact that detection of "Disabilities" among our patients are much better in the presence of a multi-disciplinary care team (Cunningham et al., Clin Rehabil 1996)

1.11   Community Rehabilitation

1.11.1 Introduction
▥ Rehabilitation services in the community are important, especially as a form of continuous care for the patient post-discharge. Liaison with community service providers by the multi-disciplinary care team for follow-up upon patient's discharge from the rehabilitative service will provide a better and smoother transition

1.11.2 Classification of Community Rehabilitative Services
■ By location of service delivery: e.g. in general hospital, rehabilitation hospital, or nursing home
■ By degree and nature of specialisation
■ By location of the team's management and administrative base

1.11.3 Components of Community Rehabilitation Services
■ Those specialised in specific impairments
■ Those specialised in specific groups of disease (e.g. neurological disability)
■ Those that concern specific interventions (e.g. wheelchairs and seating)
■ General supportive role

1.11.4 Relationship Between Community Services and the Rehabilitation Team
■ Community rehabilitation should be an integral part of a rehabilitation network spanning all aspects of a patient's needs, although there may be huge variations in management and goals amongst these different agencies (Enderby et al., Clin Rehabil 2001)

1.11.5 Key Concept
■ Community rehabilitation service should not be seen as an alternative to existing rehabilitation service. Channels for mutual referrals and liaison are most important for the continuous care of the patient

1.11.6 Concluding Remarks
■ The reader should by now have an idea of what constitutes a "rehabilitation process"
■ The importance of goal setting and proper assessment will be stressed throughout the text in many chapters

General Bibliography

World Health Organization (1980) The International Classification of Impairments, Disabilities and Handicaps. World Health Organization, Geneva
World Health Organization (2001) International Classification of Functioning, Disability and Health. World Health Organization, Geneva
Harder HG (2005) Comprehensive disability management. Elsevier, London

Selected Bibliography of Journal Articles

1. De Kleijn-de Vrankijker MW (2003) The long way from the International Classification of Impairments, Disabilities and Handicaps (ICIDH) to the International Classification of Functioning, Disability, and Health (ICF). Disabil Rehabil 25:561–564
2. McColl MA et al. (2000) Validity and community utility of Canadian Occupational Performance Measure. Can J Occup Ther 67:22–30
3. Rushton PW et al. (2002) Goal attainment scaling in the rehabilitation of patients with lower-extremity amputations: a pilot study. Arch Phys Med Rehabil 83(6):771–775
4. Wade DT (2005) Describing rehabilitation interventions. Clin Rehabil 19(8):811–818
5. Nair KP et al. (2003) Satisfaction of members of interdisciplinary rehabilitation teams with goal planning meetings. Arch Phys Med Rehabil 84(11):1710–1713
6. Wade DT (2004) Assessment, measurement and data collection tools. Clin Rehabil 18(3):233–237
7. Wade DT (2003) Community rehabilitation, or rehabilitation in the community? Disabil Rehabil 25(15):875–881
8. Wade DT (2002) Rehabilitation is a way of thinking, not a way of doing. Clin Rehabil 16(6):579–581

2 Physical Forces Used in Musculoskeletal Rehabilitation

Contents

2.1   Use of Radiation

2.1.1   Lasers

2.1.1.1   Meaning of the Word "LASER"
■ LASER = light amplification by stimulated emission of radiation (Fig. 2.1)

2.1.1.2   Historical Note
■ Concept of stimulated emission of radiation was first put forward by Albert Einstein
■ The first laser was built using the Ruby crystal in 1960
■ Followed by the later development of the HeNe gas laser, and semiconductor or diode lasers

2.1.1.3   Relevant Biophysics
■ Laser light features the following:
   – Minimal divergence despite travelling long distances (collimated)
   – Photons of same phase and direction (coherent)
   – Waves are of the same wavelength (monochromatic)

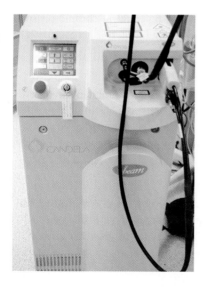

Fig. 2.1. A laser machine

2.1.1.4 Chief Components of a Laser Device
- Energy source
- Active medium (e.g. Ruby)
- Resonant chamber (houses the active medium)

2.1.1.5 Five Key Steps in Laser Generation
- Pumping (of the active medium)
- Population inversion
- Spontaneous emission
- Stimulated emission
- Amplification (via resonant chamber)

2.1.1.6 Lasers Used in Industry
- High power
- Can cause destruction of body cells (some lasers used in surgery), or materials (lasers used in industry)

2.1.1.7 Lasers Used in Rehabilitation
- Low level laser therapy = LLLT
- So named since lasers used in rehabilitation medicine are low energy, and may be conducive to processes like cell photobiomodulation (Schindl, 1999)
- Mester was the first to note the healing potential of chronic resistant ulcers with lasers with low levels of energy (Mester, Am J Surg 1971)

2.1.1.8 Mechanism of Action of LLLT
- Not fully known
- Believed to exercise a dose-dependent photobiomodulation effect on tissues (may trigger a stimulant effect, but possible inhibition effect at high doses)
- Thus, cell behaviour may be modified without significant heating, reason for the name "cold laser"

2.1.1.9 Absorption and Penetration
- Laser energy emitted gets mainly absorbed by the photosensitive molecules of the body called chromophores, an example is melanin
- The biologic action relies mainly on its monochromacity feature
- HeNe lasers cause effect at depths of 0.5–1 cm, not as deep as GaAlAs lasers

2.1.1.10 Clinical Use in Rehabilitation Medicine
▦ Promotes tissue healing via photobiomodulation
▦ Use of LLLT in pain management has also been described in the literature

2.1.1.11 Practical Examples
▦ Recalcitrant ulcers (Photodermatol Photoimmunol 2000)
▦ Osteoarthritis – experimental (Osteoarthr Cartil 2005)
▦ Trigger points (Lasers Surg Med 2003)
▦ DM neuropathic foot ulcer (Dermatology 1999)
▦ Hypertrophic scars (Ann Plast Surg 2005)

2.1.1.12 Administration
▦ Delivery is via probes, in either a contact or non-contact mode
▦ Grid technique has been described to ensure more even administration over the area of application
▦ Lasers of the proper wavelength should be selected, the area of application carefully defined, and the duration of administration determined, besides the energy and power density

2.1.1.13 Precautions/Contraindications
▦ Eye precautions and wearing protective devices is a must
▦ Tumours
▦ History of photosensitivity
▦ Infected area

2.1.2   Short Wave Diathermy

2.1.2.1 Meaning of Short Wave Diathermy
▦ Diathermy means "to heat up", a term first used in the early 1900s after the observation of tissue heating without muscle contraction can occur with high frequency electromagnetic currents
▦ Short wave refers to the later (more modern) invention of machines that has higher frequency thus shorter wavelength (as the speed of light is constant) to replace the traditional machines of longer wavelength

2.1.2.2 What Constitutes "Short Wave-Lengths" in "Short Wave"
▓ Commonly used devices have wavelengths 7 m, 11 m, 22 m
▓ Most devices in use have 11 m

2.1.2.3 Relevant Biophysics
▓ Short-wave diathermy (SWD) treatment is based on the principle of electromagnetic resonance. Thus, transfer of electromagnetic energy is maximal when resonance occurs between the tissue and the device oscillating at the same frequency

2.1.2.4 Clinical Use
▓ Continuous SWD mode: used for its heating (thermal) effect
▓ Pulsed SWD mode: used both for its thermal and athermal actions (such as possible effects on ATP and protein synthesis)

2.1.2.5 Practical Examples
▓ Chronic neck pain (Scand J Rehabil Med 1992)
▓ Back pain (Spine 1992)
▓ Osteoarthritis (Phys Ther 2006)
▓ Whiplash injury (Scand J Rehabil Med 1992)
▓ Pressure sores (Physiother Can 1996)
▓ Trigger points (J Orthop Sports Phys Ther 1984)
▓ Ligament sprains (Physiotherapy 1974)

2.1.2.6 Administration
▓ Modern devices can choose from continuous or pulsed administration
▓ During administration, ensure not to change electrode arrangement or position or electromagnetic resonance will be affected
▓ The proper pulse frequency, duration, mean and peak power outputs have to be set

2.1.2.7 Contraindications
▓ Inflamed/infected areas
▓ Over electronic equipment, e.g. pacemakers
▓ Tumours
▓ Avoid the foetal area in pregnancy
▓ Insensate skin
▓ Confused subject

2.2   Use of Magnetic Fields (Pulsed Electromagnetic Fields and Magnetopulse Therapy)

2.2.1   Pulsed Electromagnetic Fields

▥ These are devices that produce low energy (much lower than SWD) and time-varying magnetic fields, usually for the purpose of achieving bone healing effects and mainly act on bones (Clin Orthop Relat Res 1998)

2.2.1.1   Application

▥ These devices have been used mainly in treating non-unions and osteonecrosis
▥ They are applied daily for a few hours each session
▥ Degree of magnetic field strength produced: 1–2000 Gauss

2.2.1.2   Practical Examples

▥ Non-unions (Calcif Tissue Int 1991; Foot Ankle Int 2004; Clin Orthop Relat Res 2001)
▥ Osteonecrosis and Perthes (J Prosthet Orthot 1997)

2.2.2   Magnetopulse Therapy

▥ This is another recent type of pulsed electromagnetic therapy. Since it is a non-touch technique, can use the technique even in face of skin lesion. Possible mechanisms include tissue oxygenation effect, as well as possible enhanced healing and circulation
▥ Said to be useful for treatment of chronic tendinitis, pain and venous ulcers

2.2.3   Practical Examples

▥ Chronic tendinitis (Arch Phys Med Rehabil 1991)
▥ Chronic pain (Arch Phys Med Rehabil 1997)
▥ Venous ulcers (Br J Dermatol 1992)

2.3   Sound Waves (Acoustic Radiation)

2.3.1   Meaning of Ultrasound

▥ Normal range of sound audible to the human ear 20–18 000 Hz
▥ Ultrasound is therefore acoustic radiation with a frequency of >18 000 Hz

■ Ultrasound was found to be the most widely used appliance among physical therapists in many countries

2.3.2   Historical Note

■ The Piezoelectric phenomenon (natural crystals like quartz when subjected to stress, will have different charges on their opposite surfaces) was discovered in the late 18th century
■ The reverse Piezoelectric phenomenon (mechanical deformation occurs upon passage of alternating electricity to a piezoelectric material, being manifested as oscillations with cycles of contraction and expansion creating periodic cyclical pressure waves) was later discovered in the 19th century
■ Modern ultrasound machines work on the principle of the reverse piezoelectric phenomenon

2.3.3   Relevant Biophysics

■ By inducing a reverse piezoelectric phenomenon in the piezoelectric material in the transducer an ultrasound beam is formed
■ The ultrasound beam consists of a sinusoidal waveform featuring cycles of compression and rarefaction

2.3.4   Biological Effects

■ Thermal: as a result of induced molecular vibrations by the cycles of compression and rarefaction of the mechanical effects of the waveform produced. The thermal effect may increase metabolism and enhance soft tissue healing
■ Athermal:
   – Alteration of cell membrane activity via the actions of microstreaming and cavitation
   – Possible positive action on bone healing

2.3.5   Promotion of Osteogenesis

■ Mechanism: related to piezoelectric effect and low level of mechanical force to fracture area
■ Result: increased soft callus, vascularity, rate of endochondral ossification

2.3.6   Clinical Use
- Shoulder pain (Physiotherapy 1978)
- Phantom pain in amputees (Am J Phys Med 1953)
- Lateral epicondylitis elbow (Physiother Can 2001)
- LBP (Arch Phys Med Rehab 1983)
- Myofascial pain (Arch J Phys Med Rehab 2000)
- Venous ulcers (J Dermatol Treat 2004)

2.3.7   Special Use
- Phonophoresis has also been described (use of ultrasound energy to aid delivery of topical medications)

2.3.8   Application Techniques
- Use the proper coupling agent in the near field
- One should select the proper mode (continuous vs pulsed, the former causes more heating), frequency, application technique (direct, water immersion etc.), and note the beam non-uniformity ratio (BNR) of the device, ratio should be <8)

2.3.9   Contraindications
- Haematoma/bruised areas
- Tumours
- Local ischaemic areas
- Over electronic implants
- Over/near the foetus if pregnant
- Insensate areas

2.4   Shockwave

2.4.1   Definition
- A shockwave (Fig. 2.2) can be defined as an acoustic wave with the following features:
  - Acute rise in positive pressure build-up
  - Then, an exponential fall in pressure
  - Typical duration is only a few hundred nanoseconds

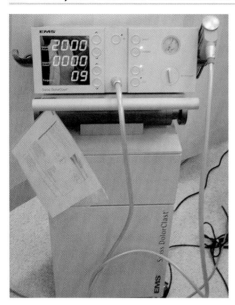

Fig. 2.2. Machine used in extra-corporeal shock-wave treatment described in this chapter

2.4.2   Potential Sources
▪ Electromagnetic source – commonly used. Works via passage of strong current through electromagnetic coil, thus inducing high magnetic field and current induction at an opposing metallic membrane. The latter produces shockwaves in the surrounding water
▪ Electrohydraulic source – an electric spark across submerged electrodes produces explosive vaporisation of H_2O and shockwave
▪ Piezoelectric source – via application of high voltage to piezoelectric crystals attached to a spherical surface

2.4.3   Characterisation of Shockwave Machines
▪ Peak positive pressure
▪ Peak negative pressure
▪ Rise time
▪ Duration
▪ Frequency spectrum
▪ Energy density
▪ Size of area of application

2.4.4   Study on Shockwave Safety
- Animal studies did not reveal signs of significant tendon damage with the usual energy density that is in clinical use
- Can induce compound motor action potential (CMAP) in peripheral nerves in animal studies; hence, one should not focus shockwave along the course of peripheral nerves when used clinically

2.4.5   Clinical Applications
- Plantar fasciitis (chronic)
- Elbow lateral epicondylitis
- Delayed union
- Shoulder calcific tendonitis and chronic Achilles tendinitis (Clin Orthop Relat Res 2006)

2.4.6   Contraindications
- Open wound
- Bleeding tendency
- Presence of local tumour
- Presence of sepsis
- Peripheral vascular disease
- Pregnancy
- Patient intolerance

2.4.7   Use in Plantar Fasciitis
- Mechanism of action not known for certain
- Possibly involving controlled internal fascial disruption that may initiate a healing response

2.4.7.1 Papers in Support of Use in Plantar Fasciitis
- Sems et al., J Am Acad Orthop Surg 2006
- Ogden et al., Clin Orthop Relat Res 2001
- Maier et al., J Rheumatol 2000

2.4.7.2 Current Recommendation
- Low-energy shockwave treatment preferred to high-energy treatments
- High-energy shockwave treatments may produce side effects in the form of periosteal detachments and even small fractures on the inner surface of the cortex

■ In 2000, the FDA approved the use of shockwave in the treatment of heel pain

2.4.8   Use in Delayed Unions
■ Although there are occasional positive results in some but not all studies, including animal studies, comparison is not easy due to differences in types of machines and details of administration, and the timing of wave application, frequency of follow-up, and paucity of prospective studies in the past
■ Overall quoted rate of success was around 50% according to authorities like Heller (1998)
■ It is the author's opinion that true pseudoarthrosis is best excised, as opposed to ordinary cases of delayed union

2.4.8.1   Papers in Support of Use in Delayed Unions
■ Senge and Schleberger, 1992
■ Michailov and Valchanou, 1991

2.4.9   Use in Elbow Lateral Epicondylitis
■ Recent prospective (controlled) trials suggest almost 50% good results in the treatment group compared with 6% among controls
■ Most experts suggest the use of low-energy density shockwave protocols, and reservation for resistant cases only
■ Exact mechanism for improvement not yet certain

2.4.9.1   Methods for the Localization of the Correct Site of Application
■ Fluoroscopic method[1]
■ Ultrasonic method

2.4.9.2   Papers in Support of Its Use in Lateral Epicondylitis
■ Prospective controlled trial by Niethard and Heller, 1998
■ Brunner et al., 1997
■ Lohrer et al., 1998

---

[1] This method sometimes results in focusing shockwave directly on the periosteum and may cause discomfort

2.4.10 Use in Calcific Tendinitis of the Shoulder

■ Possible mechanism: focused administration of shockwave may cause fragmentation and cavitation effects upon the deposits of calcification

■ Pearl for getting a good result: use adequate energy fluxes to ensure complex deposit disintegration

■ So far, studies have not mentioned cuff tear as a complication

■ Non-responsive, resistant cases may need open or arthroscopic surgery

2.4.10.1 Papers Supportive of Its Use in Calcific Tendinitis of the Shoulder

■ Sems et al., J Am Acad Orthop Surg 2006

■ Loew et al., 1995

■ Spindler, 1998

■ Rompe et al., 2001

2.5   Fluidotherapy Treatment

2.5.1   Historical Note

■ This technique is relatively new, starting in the early 1970s (Fig. 2.3)

■ Works on the concept of improved heat transfer with fluidisation of particles, proposed by a chemical engineer

2.5.2   Relevant Biophysics

■ The principle of fluidotherapy is based on forced convection as the chief mode of heat transfer to the body's tissues. This was made possible by making finely divided particles acquire the characteristics of a fluid in a closed chamber

2.5.3   Biological Effects

■ Said to possibly have the following effects:
   – Promotion of soft tissue healing (via heat transfer)
   – Prevent limb oedema
   – Helps in cases where skin desensitisation is needed
   – Some patients also feel elated or notice a "light" feeling

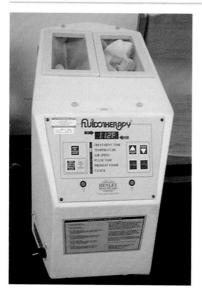

Fig. 2.3. A "fluidotherapy" machine for delivery of dry heat

2.5.4   Clinical Use

▓ Some painful joint conditions
▓ Among podiatrists to improve the local circulation (J Am Podiatr Assoc 1979; Phys Ther 1981)

2.5.5   Advantage Over Other Common Forms of Heat Treatment

▓ A form of dry heat, less messy
▓ Limb is elevated while treated, which helps prevent oedema
▓ Presence of a wound is not regarded as a contraindication (but obviously need to provide a dressing over the wound)

2.5.6   Contraindications/Cautions

▓ Some patients love the experience of fluidotherapy, but excess duration of treatment should be avoided
▓ Insensate skin
▓ Infection
▓ Ischaemia
▓ Tumours

2.6   Other Forms of Heat Treatment

2.6.1   Introduction
- Included under this category are hot packs, paraffin wax, infrared lamp
- These are sometimes referred to as "superficial thermotherapy" agents, but studies reported that deeper tissues may sometimes be heated

2.6.2   Mechanism of Action
- Works by reflex vasodilatation via release of acetylcholine by sympathetic fibres
- May stimulate tissue metabolism, but have to attain the correct temperature range of between 40 and 45 °C (too low is not effective, too high causes tissue/cell damage)
- In general, a temperature > 45 °C will cause tissue damage. Notice also a temperature of between 42 and 45 °C may produce temporary neural blockade

2.6.3   Clinical Use
- Relieve of joint stiffness
- Pain relief

2.6.4   Hot Packs
- Very frequently used in physiotherapy departments
- There are also microwavable packs on the market
- Application of hot pads – dry or moist towels need to be used; avoid having the patient putting pressure on the pads

2.6.5   Paraffin Wax
- Since the melting temperature of paraffin wax is 54 °C and is beyond the therapeutic range, mineral oil is added to adjust the temperature to within the correct range
- Can administer by dip immersion with or without wrapping. Does not require coupling medium

2.6.6   Clinical Use of "Superficial Thermotherapy"
- Neck and shoulder pain (Arch Phys Med Rehabil 1959)
- LBP (Phys Ther 1967)
- Trigger point (J Orthop Sports Phys Ther 1984)
- Burn contracture (J Burn Care Rehabil 2001)

2.6.7   Contraindications/Cautions

- Do not exceed the therapeutic range of heating (40–45 °C)
- Ensure wax bath sterilised before use in burns patient
- Avoid application near foetus in pregnancy
- Tumours
- Infected bed
- Confused patient

2.7   Cryotherapy

2.7.1   Historical Note

- Cryotherapy was popularised in physiotherapy medicine in the 1960s after influential works like Grant (Arch Phys Med Rehabil 1964)
- Many forms available on the market including ice packs, gel packs, vapour coolant preparations etc.

2.7.2   Relevant Biophysics

- Vapour coolants work by evaporation
- Most other cooling agents cools the surface by conduction (energy exchange through temperature gradient)
- Besides the cooling action, believed to help lessen secondary tissue hypoxia, thus limiting injury extent after trauma, by decreasing the metabolic rate in the area near the injury zone. If used for this purpose, should be applied within 5 min, as seen in ice treatment of professional athletes by team physicians (Knight)
- Ice also helps reduce oedema after acute injury and has a positive effect on rehabilitation effort (Curl, J Bone Joint Surg 2002)

2.7.3   Clinical Use

- Muscle spasm (J Am Podiatr Assoc 1976)
- Spasticity (Spinal Cord 2002; Int J Rehabil Res 2001)
- Sprained ankle and other soft tissue sprains (J Orthop Sports Phys Ther 1994)
- Postoperative anterior cruciate ligament (ACL) reconstruction, after shoulder surgery (J Knee Surg 2005)
- Knee arthritis (Rheumatol Rehabil 1974)

2.7.4   Administration
▦ There are different methods of delivering cryotherapy:
  – Cryostatic: static application (20–25 min)
  – Cryomassage: dynamic with added massage to the treated area
  – Cryokinetic: application alternating with bouts of voluntary exercise
  – Cryostretch: three sessions of cold applications each followed by passive stretches and isometrics (Knight). Others propose only a few 2–3 s duration of ice strokes following in succession, then passive stretching will be performed

2.7.5   Contraindication/Cautions
▦ Cold urticaria
▦ In lower limb with peripheral vascular disease (PVD)
▦ Caution in elderly with myocardial ischaemia and/or vasomotor instability

2.8   Use of Electric Currents

2.8.1   Radiofrequency

2.8.1.1 Historical Note
▦ Radiofrequency is a form of surgery used with fluoroscopy to attain a highly localised burning or lesioning of tissues; as such it is used by an interventional physiatrist or radiologist, instead of a physiotherapist (Fig. 2.4)
▦ It replaces the use of old DC electricity generators since the DC generators produced irregular, poorly controlled unpredictable heating of tissues

2.8.1.2 Biophysics
▦ Radiofrequency lesioning is effected by ionic means
▦ This is unlike traditional DC generators, which cause lesioning by a dielectric mechanism
▦ The lesion produced is usually like an inverted cone, and the radius is maximal furthest away from the electrode tip (Neurosurgery 1987)
▦ Controlling the lesion only to the size desired important; a temperature $> 45\,°C$ can cause irreversible tissue damage

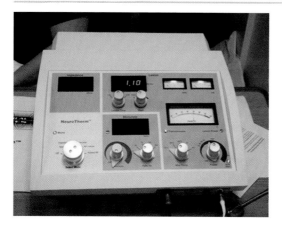

Fig. 2.4. A "radio-frequency" machine at work

2.8.1.3 Biological Effects

▨ The heat generated by the active electrode depends on the current density: the amount of current per unit area

▨ Refer to the ensuing discussion on how to control the lesion position and size

▨ Most procedures in practice are aimed at denervation. The histology of lesions produced corresponds to that of a local tissue burn. After lesioning the neural structure, Wallerian degeneration occurs. Theoretically, since the perineurium is usually destroyed, neuroma formation is possible. There is no concrete evidence that the device can selectively destroy only the pain sensory fibres

2.8.1.4 Examples of Clinical Uses

▨ Lumbar facet denervation (Clin J Pain 2005)

▨ Dorsal root ganglionotomy (Spine 2005)

▨ Cervical facet denervation (Spine J 2003)

2.8.1.5 Administration

▨ Active electrode that will deliver the current

▨ Radiofrequency generator equipped with temperature control

▨ Passive electrode (of large surface area)

2.8.1.6   Pitfalls

▓ Important to control the size and position of the lesion by:
- Using an electrode of the correct size, too big may cause more unwanted tissue damage including unwanted neural damage
- Use an active electrode with a low thermal coefficient, thereby attaining quicker thermal equilibrium
- Use fluoroscopy in most cases (e.g. lumbar facet denervation), similarly electrical stimulation can help locate the correct neural structure
- Use devices with automatic temperature control to prevent overheating
- Preferable to measure the tissue impedance as this has a bearing on the size of the lesion

2.8.1.7   Cautions

▓ Refer to the pitfalls just discussed
▓ If impedance that is too low is detected, this may indicate a short circuit
▓ If impedance is too high, may indicate a disconnection somewhere in the circuitry
▓ Be sure the patient's condition indicates the procedure

2.8.2   Transcutaneous Electrical Nerve Stimulation

2.8.2.1   Historical Note

▓ Concept of transcutaneous electrical nerve stimulation (TENS) initially came about after the inception of the "Gate theory" proposed by Melzack in the 1960s.
▓ Investigators used stimulation of the dorsal column of the cord in an attempt to relieve pain
▓ The TENS is a device that delivers a pulsed electric current through the skin via the electrodes

2.8.2.2   Relevant Biophysics

▓ Believed to work by selective depolarization of either sensory nerve, sensory-motor nerve, or sensory-motor-nociceptive nerve fibres
▓ The type of nerve depolarisation depends on the mode of administration (see later)
▓ Chief goal is to decrease pain

2.8.2.3   How to Achieve "Selective Fibre Activation"

- Depolarisation of sensory-only fibres more likely with short pulse duration, low amplitude current
- Depolarisation of both sensory and motor and/or nociception fibre more likely with long pulse duration and high amplitude

2.8.2.4   How Does Depolarisation of Nerve Fibres Decrease Pain?

- Done through two mechanisms – based on the gate theory, which was discussed in the section on pain management:
  - Pain relief by a mechanism at spinal level: selective depolarisation of large diameter A-beta (sensory) fibres > those fibres of the pain pathway (A-delta and unmyelinated C fibres)
  - Pain relief by a mechanism from the supraspinal level (via the opiate system): somehow the negative feedback of pain relaying cells at spinal level to higher centres (T cells) are inhibited by secretion of opiate substances

2.8.2.5   Evidence that Opiate System is Sometimes Responsible

- By experimentation with opiate antagonist: the existence of this mechanism was surmised after the observation that sometimes pain relief by TENS can be promptly counteracted by the action of naloxone
- This pathway is believed to be more likely at work using TENS device in certain modes, e.g. acupuncture modes, or as brief bursts of stimulation (see later)

2.8.2.6   Clinical Use

- Neck pain (Clin Rehabil 2005)
- LBP (Spine 2005)
- Whiplash injuries (Pain 2004)
- Osteoarthritis (Aust J Physiother 1992)
- Reflex sympathetic dystrophy (Stereotact Funct Neurosurg 1989)
- Phantom pain (J Bone Joint Surg Br 1988)
- Post-herpetic neuralgia (BMJ 1974)

2.8.2.7   Administration: Common Modes

- Basic: most often used, high-frequency – short-duration pulses
- Acupuncture: of low frequency – long duration
- Burst: administer as bursts not as pulse, of low frequency

- Brief intense: high frequency – long duration
- Modulation: random modulation of amplitude and frequency

2.8.2.8 Administration Details
- The type of nerve fibre depolarisation must be decided upon, or in other words the pain modulation desired
- Set the relevant amplitude, frequency and pulse duration
- No apparent muscle contraction is expected and the patient only perceives electrically evoked sensation in sensory-only depolarisation mode
- Sensory-motor depolarisation is expected if muscle contraction is also detected
- Depolarisation of sensory-motor + nociceptors likely if besides muscular contraction, evoked sensation had reached the point just below the pain threshold
- Since duration of TENS on the patient is often lengthy, one needs to ensure balanced waveform to prevent net accumulation of charges under the electrodes

2.8.2.9 Contraindication/Caution
- Cardiac pacemakers – caution if asynchronous type, contraindicated if synchronous type
- Other electrical implanted devices
- Pregnancy requires caution
- Insensate skin
- Tumours
- Confusion

2.8.3 Interferential Therapy

2.8.3.1 Relevant Biophysics
- The aim of the treatment is to provide pain relief by depolarization of peripheral sensory and motor nerves
- Involves the interference or interaction of 2–3 medium frequency, one of which is the carrier of a frequency of a few thousand Hz, the other had a lower frequency range

2.8.3.2 Administration Modes

▦ Bipolar: the interference between the two medium-frequency currents occurs inside the machine and is premodulated

▦ Quadripolar: two frequencies each from two different circuits, a total of four electrodes and interference occurred outside the machine

▦ Quadripolar with vector scan: like the above, but current amplitude in one circuit allowed to vary, and a more circular field of results. The field here is also dynamic, not static

▦ 3D stereodynamic format: this needs to be custom-made and a 3D field results from three medium currents and six electrodes

2.8.3.3 Clinical Use

▦ Pain relief in osteoarthritis (Rheumatol Int 2006)

▦ Pain relief in other musculoskeletal conditions (Aust J Physiother 1981)

▦ Pelvic Floor Rehabil (Clin Rehabil 1997)

2.8.3.4 Contraindication/Caution

▦ Tumours

▦ Over electronic built-in devices

▦ DVT

▦ Pregnancy

2.8.4 High-Voltage Pulsed Current Therapy

2.8.4.1 Historical Note

▦ High voltage pulsed current therapy came into the clinical arena in early 1990s although first reported two decades prior

2.8.4.2 Relevant Biophysics

▦ By high voltage, we mean a voltage in excess of 150 V

▦ The device generates twin peak monophasic short pulses of current; the time between the peaks can be adjusted

▦ Owing to the short pulse duration, voltage needs to be high in order to effect attempted neural depolarisation

▦ Can be used to stimulate muscle or nerve

2.8.4.3   Biological Effects

- Can be adjusted to depolarise nerve or muscle
- Claimed to have tissue healing functions, including healing of wounds allegedly increase the voltage of weak endogenous skin batteries in attempted healing by local tissues (see section on microcurrents in Chap. 4)
- May decrease limb oedema by induced muscular contractions, or microvascular exchanges (Phys Ther 1983)
- Relief of muscle spasticity and relief of pain from prolonged muscle spasm by inducing fatigue

2.8.4.4   Clinical Use

- Improve circulation in DM foot ulcers (Arch Phys Med Rehabil 2001)
- Decubitus ulcers (Phys Ther 1988)
- LBP (Physiother Can 1984)
- Spastic levator ani (Phys Ther 1987) – via anal probes

2.8.4.5   Administration

- Needs coupling media like electro-conduction gels
- One has to select pulse frequency, voltage, duration of treatment. Continuous mode sometimes for pain relief as opposed to pulsed mode say in oedema control

2.8.4.6   Contraindications/Cautions

- Pregnancy
- Presence of bruising or bleeding
- Bleeding tendency
- Over in-built electronic devices
- Tumours

2.8.5   High Intensity Electrical Stimulation and Russian Currents

2.8.5.1   Historical Note

- The late 1970s saw reports from Russia that a so-called "Russian current" as it has come to be know can:
    - Create significantly (33%) more forceful muscle contraction than maximum voluntary contraction
    - That so-doing is painless

   – That any resultant gain in muscle strength can be long lasting in
     healthy athletes

2.8.5.2 Word of Caution

■ It is not in theory impossible to create more forceful contraction than
  maximum voluntary contraction. This is because even in normal individuals, we found asynchronous firing of motor units – with the slow
  twitch type I fibres followed by fast twitch type II fibres. With this
  technique, synchronous firing in addition with frequently reverse firing sequence type II followed by type I can theoretically result in
  more forceful contraction
■ That such a forceful contraction is painless is doubtful and debatable.
  Pain is a subjective experience, and different people having different
  thresholds. Tetanic contraction of this nature is expected to give rise
  to pain, unless the degree of contraction is such that it just depo-
  larises all nociceptors (besides motor and sensory fibres) thereby lessening pain
■ Lasting resultant gains has not been recorded in experiments in patients, but seem to be possible in healthy athletes

2.8.5.3 Relevant Biophysics

■ Creation of tetanic muscular contractions via a sine-wave burst-modu-
  lated current of 10-ms fixed period and with inter-burst intervals of
  10 ms. The neuromuscular structure recognize these bursts as if it
  was a pulse
■ The current is believed to depolarize both motor and sensory fibres

2.8.5.4 Potential Clinical Use

■ Strengthen quadriceps post knee surgery have been reported (Phys
  Ther 1986; J Orthop Sports Phys Ther 1986)

2.8.5.5 Administration Pitfall

■ It is uncertain that whatever machine on market claiming can produce
  Russian current is exactly of the same performance and quality as the
  originator

2.8.5.6 Contraindication/Caution
■ Pain is possible with tetanic contractions, although the originator claims painless
■ Pregnancy
■ Tumours
■ Bleeding tendency
■ Built-in electronic devices
■ Avoid use along the courses of major nerve or nerve trunks
■ Confusion

2.8.6   Microcurrent Therapy

2.8.6.1 Historical Note
■ Subsequent to initial observations of regeneration of amphibian stumps may be driven by skin batteries in the 1970s
■ It was surmised in the 1980s by investigators that such a current of injury in the microampere range may be present in humans after trauma, as in finger amputation stumps of children. It was further theorised that different cell types possess their own endogenous current of injury that is instrumental in the healing process (Fig. 2.5)

2.8.6.2 Relevant Biophysics
■ Involves the use of direct current in the microampere range or microcurrent (< 1 mA) electrical stimulation

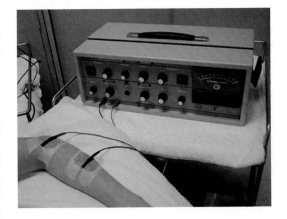

Fig. 2.5. A machine delivering microcurrent

2.8.6.3 Biological Effects

▦ Attempts to promote wound and tissue healing, subsequent to the finding of the presence of skin batteries in healing human tissue cells. These skin batteries are less well developed in humans as opposed to amphibians which have great regeneration potentials

2.8.6.4 Clinical Uses

▦ Venous ulcers (Am J Surg 1968)
▦ DM ulcers (Diabetes Care 1997)
▦ Ischaemic ulcers (Phys Ther 1976)

2.8.6.5 Administration

▦ Either used as constant or pulsed manner
▦ Lower pulsed frequencies is usually used in wound therapy

2.8.6.6 Contraindications/Cautions

▦ Tumours
▦ Infected bed
▦ Over electronic implants

2.9   Hydromechanics and Hydrotherapy

2.9.1   Introduction and Common Myths

▦ Even in this day and age, the use of hydrotherapy is being deferred until rather late in the treatment of various common orthopaedic conditions such as osteoarthritis and back pain (Figs. 2.6, 2.7)
▦ In addition, it is not yet widely used in other clinical conditions such as rehabilitation of cruciate ligament injuries

2.9.2   Clarification of Myths

▦ In fact, hydrotherapy can and should be introduced early on in the rehabilitation of patients with painful arthritic conditions as well as many LBP patients, provided there is no contraindication (see Sect. 2.9.8 below), rather than being used as a last resort
▦ The use of hydrotherapy in the rehabilitation of common patients with sports injuries (such as ACL injury) has been found to be fruitful in Scandinavian countries and is widely practiced

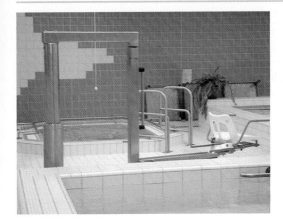

Fig. 2.6. Many hydrotherapy units are equipped with instrumentation for controlled lowering of patients with poor mobility to the pool

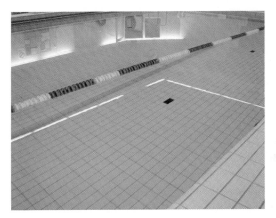

Fig. 2.7. Hydrotherapy should preferably be performed in standard sized pools like the one illustrated (in Orton) where therapists can also teach patients in groups

2.9.3 Physiology of Water Immersion
■ Fluid redistribution due to the effect of hydrostatic pressure
■ Increased cardiac venous return and stroke volume

2.9.4 Main Difference of Motion in Water with Respect to Motion in Land
■ For motions in land, one find that more resistance will be encountered with longer lever arm

■ In water, a longer lever arm, e.g. more arm abduction creates more assistance so that exercise is made easier. (But resistive exercises same as in dry land)

2.9.5   Hydromechanics of Immersed Bodies in Water

■ Hydrostatic pressure
■ Buoyancy
■ Drag force

2.9.5.1   Hydrostatic Pressure

■ Hydrostatic pressure is applied in all directions of submerged objects (Pascal's Law)
■ The deeper the depth of submersion the greater the force. Thus, magnitude of this pressure can be adjusted by depth of immersion
■ On common beneficial effect on LL with submersion is to decrease oedema.
■ Normal pressures used to decrease LL oedema in inflatable boots vary from 40–70 mm Hg, and the hydrostatic pressure on the feet with in hydrotherapy usually also falls within this range

2.9.5.2   Buoyancy Force

■ Submerged objects in water also experiences an upward force (anti-gravity force) according to the Principle of Archimedes
■ The upward force = weight of fluid volume displaced by the object

2.9.5.2.1 Relation of the Buoyancy Force and Rotational Torque

■ A rotational torque is often experienced by the submerged object since this buoyancy force acts on the "centre of buoyancy" and not the "centre of gravity"
■ These two centres do not coincide in humans, and the result being existence of a rotational torque until the two centres become vertically aligned

2.9.5.2.2 Practical Uses of the Buoyancy Force

■ Depending on the instructions of the therapist, the buoyancy force can be made use of as either an assistive force or a resistive force for the training of the patient during hydrotherapy
■ To some extent, one can put this buoyancy force to good use by adjusting the position of the patient in water

2.9.5.3 Total Drag Force

▓ These act as resistive forces to movement of the objects in water
▓ The total drag force consist of a surface drag (due to friction), a profile drag (providing the major resistance, and magnitude increase with size of limb), and a wave drag (due to waves created, and can be minimised by effecting body's movement at deeper water level

2.9.6   Administration

▓ Hydrotherapy may be given in different modes:
  – Tank/bath immersion therapy
  – Spa therapy
  – Pool therapy
    (Mostly we use water temperatures in the range of 32–36 °C, but occasionally one uses a slightly higher temperature (for arthritis), and in selected cases of lower temperature)

2.9.7   Common Uses of Hydrotherapy

▓ Painful arthritic conditions (Orthop Clin North Am 2004; Clin J Pain 2004)
▓ Back pain (Clin J Pain 2002)
▓ Patients on protected or non weight bearing as in after some fractures (extent of weight bearing can be fine tuned using different pool depths)
▓ Patients that need improvement in balance and support
▓ Can cater for patients requiring a variety of resistive or assistive training
▓ Sometimes of use in disabled and cerebral palsy patients, e.g. use of rotation with the help of water buoyancy to initiate motion in disabled persons
▓ Oedema control

2.9.8   Contraindications

▓ Open wounds, especially with bleeding or discharge
▓ Presence of macerated tissue
▓ Severe cardiopulmonary diseases
▓ Insensate limbs
▓ Incontinence of urine or faeces

2.9.9   Precautions

- The pool must be of the correct temperature, ideally from 34–35.5 °C, but 32–36 °C is the quoted maximum variation
- Excess temperature will create tachycardia which will be dangerous to patients of limited cardiopulmonary reserve
- Proper warm up especially in cool weather
- Have a drink before entering the pool is advisable as prolonged submersion tend to have a diuretic effect
- Precautions should be exercised in prescribing hydrotherapy for burn patients, since these patients are prone to infection if the wounds have bacterial colonisation

General Bibliography

Cameron MH (2003) Physical agents in rehabilitation, 2nd Edition, Saunders, Missouri, USA

Greenman PE (2003) Principles of manual medicine, 3rd Edition, Lippincott Williams & Wilkins, Philadelphia, USA

Rompe Jan-Dirk (2002) Shock wave applications in musculoskeletal disorders. Thieme, Stuttgart

Selected Bibliography of Journal Articles

1. Schindl A, Schindl M et al. (1999) Diabetic neuropathic foot ulcer: successful treatment by low-intensity laser therapy. Dermatology 198:314–316
2. Mester E, Spiry T et al. (1971) Effect of laser rays on wound healing. Am J Surg 122:532–535
3. Docker M, Bazin S et al. (1992) Guidelines for the safe use of continuous shock-wave therapy equipment. Physiotherapy 78:755–757
4. Foley-Nolan D, Moore K et al. (1992) Low energy high frequency pulsed electromagnetic therapy for acute whiplash injuries. Scand J Rehabil Med 24:51–59
5. Esenyel M, Caglar N et al. (2000) Treatment of myofascial pain. Am J Phys Med Rehabil 79(1):48–52
6. Rompe JD (2005) Shock wave therapy for plantar fasciitis. J Bone Joint Surg 87(3):681–682
7. Rompe JD, Theis C et al. (2005) Shock wave treatment for tennis elbow. Orthopade 34(6):567–570
8. Rompe JD (2006) Shock wave for chronic Achilles tendon pain: a randomized placebo controlled trial. Clin Orthop Relat Res 445:276–277

9. Sems A, Dimeff R et al. (2006) Extracorporeal shock wave therapy in the treatment of chronic tendinopathies. J Am Acad Orthop Surg 14(4):195–204
10. Ogden JA, Alvarez R et al. (2001) Shock wave therapy for chronic proximal plantar fasciitis. Clin Orthop Relat Res 387:47–59
11. Schleberger R, Senge T (1992) Non invasive treatment of long bone pseudoarthrosis by shock waves. Arch Orthop Trauma Surg 111(4):224–247
12. Clinkingbeard KA (1981) Heat from fluidotherapy. Phys Ther 61(3):391
13. Wong RA (1986) High voltage versus low voltage electrical stimulation. Force of induced muscle contraction and perceived discomfort in healthy subjects. Phys Ther 66(8):1209–1212
14. Strauss-Blasche G, Ekmekcioglu C et al. (2002) Contribution of individual spa therapies in the treatment of chronic pain. Clin J Pain 18(5):302–309
15. Stener-Victorin E, Kruse-Smidje C et al. (2004) Comparison between electro-acupuncture and hydrotherapy both in combination with patient education and patient education alone on the symptomatic treatment of osteoarthritis of the hip. Clin J Pain 20(3):179–185

3 Basic Science on Injury and Repair of Skeletal Muscle, Ligaments and Tendons

Contents

3.1   Muscle Basic Science

3.1.1   Basic Functional Anatomy

3.1.1.1 Basic Structural Hierarchy

▧ Starting from the sarcomere → myofibril → muscle fibre → fascicle → muscle
▧ The "skeleton" of each muscle fibre consists of endomysium – the sarcoplasmic reticulum rather like endoplasmic reticulum, which is Ca-rich; T-tube penetration helps spread the action potential
▧ The exoskeleton consists of perimysium surrounding each fascicle, and epimysium around each bundle of muscle

3.1.1.2   The Musculotendinous Junction

▧ The weak link between muscle and tendon
▧ Usually injured during eccentric exercise
▧ Although sometimes it is either the muscle proper that is partially or completely torn or sometimes the tendon itself (tendon has stronger tensile strength than muscle)
(P.S. tendon more likely to be injured with greater muscle force (eccentric) and also depend on any weakness of the tendon itself and ratio of cross-section of muscle vs tendon)

3.1.1.3   Contraction Coupling

▧ Z-lines are locations of actin
▧ "Zone of actin"=I band
▧ "Zone of myosin"=A band
▧ Normal resting state: portion of myosin prevented from binding to actin by troponin – tropomyosin binding. But release of Ca causes uncovering of strategic sites and binding occurs. Then, Ca pumped back into the sarcoplasmic reticulum

3.1.1.4   Two Main Muscle Fibre Types

▧ Type 1 – slow acting, red in colour since aerobic with much mitochondria – involved in endurance activities
▧ Type 2 consists of A and B types
These are explosive, fast acting, anaerobic metabolism – white in colour since less myoglobin – involved in resistance training like weight lifting

3.1.1.5 Neural Innervation
- Motor unit – number of muscle cells innervated by a single motor neuron between 10 and 2000
    - All or none phenomenon
    - In large (e.g. bi-articular) muscles, ratio is high
    - In fine coordination (e.g. eye) muscles, ratio is small
- Motor end plate – can waste away after denervation going on too long (around 2 years)
- Neuromuscular junction – release of Ach across synapse on arrival of impulse
    - Negative inhibition effect can be either competitive, e.g. curare, which binds Ach receptors, or non-competitive, e.g. depolarising agent like suxamethonium
- Reversal agents include neostigmine, which prevents Ach break-down and reverses non-depolarising agents

3.1.1.6 Normal Motor Unit Recruitment
- At the time of ordinary voluntary muscle contraction, there is asynchronous recruitment of motor units: usually fires from slower Type 1 motor units to fast-twitch Type 2 motor units (J Neurophysiol 1965)

3.1.1.7 Changes with Aging
- With aging, there is a preferential loss of Type 2 muscle fibres
- It is possible that loss of Type 2 fast-twitch fibres in the elderly may potentially affect the body's adaptive movement or reactions to falling; we will discuss these points in the last two chapters

3.1.1.8 Is There Any Situation with Reversed Pattern of Recruitment?
- Yes
- Synchronous firing of motor units or firing in reverse order (Type 2 first, then Type 1) can occur in some special form of electrically induced muscular contractions such as the "Russian Current" (Delitto et al., Phys Ther 1990)
- Caution: *not* each and every individual can achieve this type of motor unit activation, as will be discussed shortly

3.1.1.9 Evidence from the Study of the "Twitch Interpolation Technique"

▨ Originally published in J Physiol 1954 by Merton, and supported by subsequent studies of other workers like Behm et al., J Appl Physiol 1996

▨ Physiological testing supports the concept that not every individual can attain really complete motor unit activation despite maximum stimulation

3.1.1.10 Clinical Implications

▨ Those patients in whom synchronous firing of motor units can be achieved, theoretically have the potential to effect not only restoration of weakened muscle power, but might achieve muscular strength not easily achievable with conventional methods

▨ Another obvious implication is the theoretical potential use in older postoperative patients (say, after hip fractures) where muscle re-training, even to pre-injury levels, is not always achievable

▨ More research is needed to access the effects on training in older individuals as opposed to young adult volunteers or athletes

3.1.1.11 Newer Studies

▨ Two newer studies seem to support the role of neuromuscular stimulation in the elderly:
  - Pfeifer et al. showed favourable outcome with neuromuscular electrical stimulation compared with volitional isometric contractions in adults over 65 years (Physiother Can 1997)
  - Positive role of Type 2 fibre firing and recruitment shown by neuromuscular stimulation in patients with chronic disease and the elderly which as we know predominantly affects Type 2 muscle fibres (Delitto et al., Phys Ther 1990)

▨ Previous reports of special techniques like "Russian Current" may bring about strength gains that can be long-lasting in around 40–50% of subjects after a period of stimulation of 30 sessions (Kubiak et al., J Orthop Sports Phys Ther 1987; Soo et al., Phys Ther 1988)

▨ Research is needed to ascertain if the above can benefit our older patients who frequently need this extra strength to ambulate, such as after surgery

3.1.2   Prevention of Muscle Injury

3.1.2.1 The Intrinsic Reflexes

■ Skeletal muscle stretch reflex involves two types of receptors:
  - Golgi organs – sensitive to tension
  - Muscle spindles – sensitive to length changes, and rate of length changes
■ Muscle stretch → increased firing of muscle spindles → message relay to SC → increased motor nerve impulse and increased resistance of muscle to stretch
■ But if increase in tension → Golgi organ fires → inhibit motor impulse and muscle relaxes

3.1.2.2 Optimising Muscle Length During Warm-Ups

■ The functional unit of muscle = sarcomere
■ Optimising length/tension relation is necessary for optimal muscle performance
■ Excess overlap of muscle contractile units – contraction compromised
■ Inadequate overlap of muscle contractile units – contraction also compromised
■ Thus, rather narrow optimal window should be exercised

3.1.2.3 Rationale for Warm-Up

■ If start out slightly stretched, enhances muscle's ability to generate force
■ Warming up also helps to increase core temperature and prepare muscles for more physical activity
■ The capacity of Golgi tendon organs to effect its inhibitory reflex is increased upon increased core temperature on warming up

3.1.2.4 Practical Example

■ In normal gait, many of our muscles tend to lengthen prior to contracting, this is to attempt to maximise the amount of force generation
■ Example: in human gait, the gastrocnemius-soleus unit undergoes eccentric contraction during the second rocker, but then gives back significant energy during the end of the stance phase or third rocker when it undergoes concentric contraction

3.1.3   Muscle Injury and Healing

3.1.3.1 Basic Terminology: "Concentric", "Isometric", "Eccentric" Contractions

▨ Under a given load, the tension generated across the tendon depends on the type of muscle contraction:
  - Concentric → the musculotendinous unit (MTU) shortens in length resulting in positive work
  - Isometric → the MTU length remains constant while resisting force and no work generated
  - Eccentric → the MTU lengthens in response to load resulting in negative work

3.1.3.2 Muscle Response to Injury

▨ Notice that muscle has rather limited regenerating potential except in newborn
▨ In adults, although injured skeletal muscle may repair itself to a certain extent via spontaneous regeneration (if there is an intact basal lamina as a scaffold, myofibrils can sometimes regenerate); however, the overproduction of extracellular matrix and excessive collagen deposition lead to fibrosis
▨ One key cytokine producing fibrosis is believed to be transforming growth factor-beta 1; we will come back to this point later

3.1.3.3 Broad Types of Muscle Injury

▨ Muscle sprain
▨ Delayed onset muscle soreness – can occur after unaccustomed exercise (especially eccentric variety)
▨ Partial muscle rupture – especially more in two jointed muscles, especially MT junction – wait until healing is complete before returning to sport. Prevent further injuries by warm-up exercises and stretching
▨ After healing, contraction only 60% as forceful, but has full ability to shorten
▨ Complete muscle rupture – heals by scarring mostly, contracts only 50% as forcefully as before, and 80% ability to shorten

3.1.3.4 Classification by Mechanism

▨ Direct injury (e.g. laceration, direct blow)
▨ Indirect:
  – Three types of muscle sprains (see below)
  – Delayed onset muscle soreness

3.1.3.5 Indirect Injuries

▨ Most indirect injuries of muscles result from eccentric contraction
▨ This is more likely to occur in muscles that span two joints, e.g. hamstrings
▨ Clinical example: hamstring injuries in runners. Injury commonly occurs either during the action of decelerating the extended knee during a forward swing or during take-off. Injury came about by a sudden change in function (of the hamstring) from stabilising a flexed knee joint to that of assistance in paradoxical extension of the knee
▨ Note: avulsion injuries of bi-articular muscles such as hamstring can also occur, this is usually due to a forceful contraction with one of its ends relatively fixed. In the case of the hamstring, this less common avulsion injury can result from, say, sudden severe knee flexion with the knee in a fully extended posture (Sally et al., Am J Sports Med 1996)

3.1.3.6 Word of Caution Concerning MTJ Being a Common Rupture Site

▨ Some muscles have their MTJ spanning fairly long distances, and an apparent "mid-substance" tear may still represent an MTJ injury
▨ Example: the MTJ complex covers as much as 60% of the length of the biceps femoris muscle! (Garrett et al., Med Sci Sport Exerc 1989)

3.1.3.7 Further Classification of Types of Muscle Sprains

▨ Type 1: mild, <5% disruption of MTJ integrity
▨ Type 2: moderate, incomplete rupture of MTJ
▨ Type 3: severe, complete (avulsion injuries also fall into this category; Zarins, Clin Sports Med 1983)

3.1.3.8 Key Issues to Note in Healing Response of Muscle After Injury

▨ Quantity and quality of fibrous scar formation. The amount of scarring boils down to the relative contribution of this process of scar formation vs muscle regeneration (if any) at the phase of remodelling after muscle injury

■ Given an intact basal lamina as a scaffold, myofibrils can sometimes regenerate, although a properly aligned extracellular matrix is necessary to obtain proper myofibril orientation

3.1.3.9 Key Rehabilitation Principle (According to Stauber)

■ The above-mentioned points form the basis of the repair model suggested by Stauber and Leadbetter: that of advocating early range of motion of strained muscles to prevent disorganised scar formation and re-injury

3.1.3.10 New Drug: Relaxin

■ A recent observation is that administration of relaxin may significantly improve skeletal muscle healing
■ Clinical relevance: these findings may facilitate the development of techniques to eliminate fibrosis or perhaps lessen scarring, enhance muscle regeneration, and improve functional recovery after muscle injuries (Am J Sports Med 2005)

3.1.3.11 New Drug: Suramin

■ Another drug with possible positive effect in producing less scarring with a similar mechanism of action was also described (Am J Sports Med 2005)

3.1.4   Principles of Rehabilitation After Muscle Injury

3.1.4.1   Introduction

■ There are six main areas essential for proper rehabilitation after muscle injury such as those sustained in sports
■ We will repeatedly refer back to this concept with more elaboration in many chapters of this book. In this chapter on basic science, we will only elaborate on the importance of bi-articular muscles during rehabilitation of the kinetic chain

3.1.4.2   Cornerstones of Restoration of Proper Musculoskeletal Function

■ Proper limb alignment and biomechanics
■ Proper joint kinematics, stability and proprioception
■ Proper neuromuscular control including sequence of firing (among individual muscles and between different functional groups, concept of muscle synergism)

- Proper length–tension relationships
- Proper force couple relationships
- Proper pain management

3.1.4.3   Role of Bi-Articular Muscles in Coordination Between Muscles of the Kinetic Chain

- The importance of bi-articular muscles has only been recognised and highlighted in recent years. One of their key functions is for proper energy transfer between and linking different segments in the kinetic chain
- Rehabilitation and restoration of function of the kinetic chain after injury should always involve proper retraining of the bi-articular muscles

3.1.4.4   Function of Bi-Articular Muscles

- Help in energy transfer: this needs precise timing and intensity of firing. Example: this action of bi-articular muscles helps lower the energy consumption of normal gait in humans (see Chap. 8)
- Enables rapid, coordinated and linked motions of the joints spanned by them

3.2   Ligaments Basic Science

3.2.1   General Functions

- Neurosensory role
- Stabilising joints
  (mechanical behaviour is like other viscoelastic soft tissues, but with adaptations that allow joints to be flexible, yet stable)

3.2.2   Important Feature

- Different ligaments heal differently
- ACL in particular, often fails to show any healing response
- Medial collateral ligament (MCL) seems to have much better healing potential – perhaps because of its environment, nutrition sources and other intrinsic advantages

3.2.3   Anatomy
- Types 1 and/or 3 collagen
- Non-linear portion represents unwinding of the collagen
- Two main types of ligament–bone attachments:
  - Like femoral attachment of MCL – attaches via fibrocartilage, then bone
  - Like MCL tibial attachment (indirect variety) – attaches to periosteum/bone through Sharpley's fibres

3.2.4   Anatomy
- Water 60–70% total weight
- Collagen 80% dry weight (90% Type 1, others mainly Type 3)
- Proteoglycans 1% – but their hydrophilic nature plays an integral part in viscoelasticity
- Elastin – resists tension by reverting from globular to coiled form under stress
  (other content: minor amount of actin and fibronectin)

3.2.5   Gross and Microscopic Structure
- Gross: white, shiny, band-like
- Hypocellular, a few fibroblastic cells, interspersed within the tissue matrix
- Under polarised light, the fibrils have a sinusoidal wave pattern or crimp – which is thought to have significance in the non-linear functional properties

3.2.6   Biomechanics
- Viscoelastic behaviour
- Stress–strain behaviour is time-rate dependent
- During the cycle of loading and unloading between two limits of elongation, the loading and unloading curves of a ligament follows *different paths* – the area enclosed by the two curves is called the area of hysteresis, which represents the energy loss
- Other viscoelastic behaviour:
  - Stress relaxation – decrease in stress when subjected to constant elongation
  - Creep – a time-dependent elongation when subjected to a constant load

3.2.7   Viscoelasticity – (Using ACL Reconstruction as Illustration)

- The phenomenon of stress–relaxation predicts that the initial tension applied to the graft in ACL reconstruction can decrease 30–60% over the course of surgery; however, it has been shown that cyclic stretching of patella tendon grafts prior to graft tensioning reduced the amount of stress relaxation. Hence, preconditioning a graft will lessen the loss of tension after its fixation
- Although stress relaxation is reduced via pre-conditioning, the replacement graft continues to demonstrate cyclic stress relaxation, e.g. a large number of cyclic loads like running reduces stress in the graft with each elongation cycle; fortunately, this behaviour is recoverable
- Also, cyclic stress relaxation contributes to prevention of graft failure, the viscoelastic behaviour also illustrates the importance of warm-up exercises before physical testing to decrease maximum stresses in the ligament

3.2.8   Shape of the Stress–Strain Curve

- Non-linear toe area
- Linear area
- Ultimate tensile strength
- Area under curve is energy absorbed

3.2.9   Effect of Strain Rate

- Savio Woo's group seemed to think that strain rate plays a relatively minor role with regard to mechanical properties
- Other workers, however, believed that strain–rate sensitivity is important, the ligaments becoming slightly stronger and stiffer at higher loading rates

3.2.10   Site of Ligament Rupture and Age

- Young age – ligament–bone junction (e.g. rabbit MCL model, all tears before skeletal maturity at tibial insertion area)
- After growth ceased and physis closed – the ligament–bone junction is no longer the weakest link
- Older age – mid-substance tear is commoner; there is also overall decrease in tensile strength of the ligament

3.2.11   Healing of the Injured Ligament
■ Inflammation
■ Matrix and cell proliferation
■ Remodelling
■ Maturation

3.2.12   Factors Affecting Healing
■ Systemic factors
■ Local factors – especially immobilisation, vs early motion
■ Prolonged immobilisation can cause joint stiffness and damage healthy ligament by synovial adhesions
(Cooper, J Bone Joint Surg 1971: immobilisation of a joint can lead to sharp decline in ligament–bone junction strength, especially in the collateral ligament that inserts via the periosteum)

3.2.13   Effect of Immobilisation and Exercise
■ Rabbit model, structural properties of MCL decrease dramatically at 9-week immobilisation, the elastic modulus and ultimate tensile strength of MCL are also reduced; histologic evaluation shows marked disruption of the deeper fibres that attach the MCL to the tibia by osteoclastic absorption in the subperiosteum. Resorption was prominent, especially in the femoral and tibial insertions – the structural properties are slow to recover
■ Ligament substance recovers more quickly from immobilisation than the insertion areas. Takes months of rehabilitation for full recovery

3.2.13.1 Example 1: Isolated MCL Injury
■ Operative vs conservative results comparable, but both are inferior to the natural ligament (although adequate for most knee functions)
■ MCL was shown to heal spontaneously and yielded good knee function – though tensile strength reached only 60% at 1 year
■ No major difference in orthopaedic treatment/conservative group at 6 out of 52. The healed MCL adequate for knee function due to the larger cross-section area of the healed ligament
■ Gap vs in-contact healing in laboratory experiments: in-contact healing yielded slightly better results

3.2.13.2 Example 2: MCL + ACL Injury

- Still debated whether need to repair MCL *after* ACL been reconstructed
- Currently, some laboratory experiments are being carried out in support of comparable results with conservative vs operative treatment
- Checking the overall limb alignment and for any associated other ligamentous injury is very important
- In cases of ACL tear with Grade 3 MCL injury, it may be wise to treat the MCL conservatively for a period (most heal with conservative treatment) before proceeding to definitive reconstruction of the ACL

3.2.13.3 Example 3: ACL Reconstruction

- Pre-conditioning is advisable for the graft
- At 6 out of 52 laboratory experiments in Savio Woo's lab – Bone-patellar tendon-bone incorporation good, not for semi-tendinosus graft
- Recommend go slower if soft tissue (hamstring) graft was used since it incorporates more slowly, also future use of growth factors possible to speed healing
- Recent robotic experiment in laboratory – strain was maximal postoperatively in knee extension; hence, some suggest avoid full knee extension in postoperative rehabilitation after ACL reconstruction

3.3   Tendon Basic Science

3.3.1   Tendon Structure

- Cells 20%
- Water 70%
- Collagen type 1
- Small amount of proteoglycan/glycoprotein as "cement" function + small amount of elastin
- Collagen arrangement absolutely parallel – can withstand high tensile stress
- Weak area is MTJ
- Rupture risk depends on → muscles force generation, cross-section ratio between muscle and tendon, eccentric muscle force, and any weakness in the tendon proper

3.3.2   General Features
■ Low blood supply
■ Low metabolic rate and demand (tendon is predominantly an extra-cellular tissue)
■ Therefore, it can stand high tensile loads, since low metabolic demands
■ But the drawback is that healing is slow

3.3.3   Function
■ Anchors muscle to bone
■ Withstands large amounts of tensile stress
(adaptations can occur with age, exercise, and disuse)

3.3.4   Anatomy
■ Follows the blue-print of connective tissue: "Mesenchymal cells in a supporting matrix", with cells making the matrix
  – Tenocytes (longitudinally aligned)
  – Matrix contain proteins – collagen Type 1 + elastin; ground substance has water and glycoproteins

3.3.5   Structural Hierarchy
Collagen secreted as tropocollagen → microfibrils (after x-linked), molecules overlap as quarter-stagger/striations → fibril → fascicle (with crimp structure) → tendon (covered with paratenon)

3.3.6   The Junctional Zones
■ MTJ: how the tension generated by muscle fibres transmits from intracellular contractile proteins to extracellular connective tissue: "The collagen fibrils insert into *recesses* formed between the finger-like processes of the muscle cells" – this folding increases the contact area = less force/area. But the weakest link is still in the muscle–tendon–bone unit (e.g. after eccentric loads in young sportsmen)
■ Osteotendinous junction (OTJ) with four zones viz.:
  – Tendon
  – Fibrocartilage
  – Mineralised fibrocartilage
  – Bone
    (border distinct between b and c called "cement line" or tide mark = place where avulsion fractures occur)

3.3.7   Structure vs Function Correlation

■ Elastin contributes to tendon flexibility
■ Ground substance gives structural support and diffusion of nutrients and gases – the proteoglycans regulate matrix hydration and contain glycosaminoglycans
■ Collagen aligned in the direction of stress, orderly and parallel. But at rest, fibres are wavy with crimped appearance
■ Low metabolic rate withstands high tensile stresses
■ Tenocytes squeezed in between collagen
  (low metabolic rate enables it to remain under tension for long periods without risk of ischaemia and necrosis)

3.3.8   Blood Supply

■ Perimysial at MTJ
■ Periosteal at OTJ
■ Paratenon – major supply
  – Paratenon vessels enter the tendon substance and, passing longitudinally within the endotenon sheath, form a capillary loop network
  – Tendons enclosed in synovial sheaths are supplied by vinculae
  – Vascularity compromised at junctional zones and areas of friction/torsion/compression – no capillary anastomosis – (e.g. supraspinatus near its insertion, and tibialis anterior where the combined tendon of gastrosoleus undergo a twist that raises stresses across this site)

3.3.9   Nerve Supply

■ Nerve endings mostly at MTJ
■ Four types of nerve-endings:
  – Free – pain reception
  – Golgi – mechano-reception
  – Paccinian – pressure sensors
  – Ruffini

3.3.10   Biomechanics

■ Tendon = strongest component in the muscle–tendon–bone unit
■ Tensile strength = half stainless steel (e.g. 1 cm^2 cross-section area can bear weight of 500–1000 kg)

3.3.11 Force Elongation Curve

■ Less useful than the stress–strain curve because unlike the stress–strain curve it not only depends on the mechanical behaviour of the tissue, the shape of the curve also depends on the length and cross-section area (the larger the cross-section area, the larger the loads that can be applied; the longer the tissue fibres, the greater the elongation before failure)

3.3.12 Stress–Strain Curve

■ Four regions:
   – Toe region
   – Linear region
   – Micro-failure
   – Macro-failure
■ Toe – disappears at 2% strain as the crimpled fibres straighten. Non-linear in shape
■ Linear portion – tendon deforms in linear fashion due to the inter-molecular sliding of collagen triple helices. This portion is elastic/reversible and the tendon will return to original length when unloaded, if strain <4%. Slope = elastic modulus
■ Micro-failure: collagen fibres slide past one another, intermolecular cross-links fail, and tendon undergoes irreversible plastic deformation
■ Macroscopic failure: occurs when tendon stretched >10% its original length. Complete failure follows rapidly once the load-supporting ability of the tendon is lost, and the fibres recoil into a tangled ruptured end

3.3.13 Viscoelasticity

■ The stress–strain behaviour of the tendon is time-rate dependent
■ The sensitivity to different strain rates means that the tendon is viscoelastic
■ Hence exhibits associated properties of "stress relaxation" (decreased stress with time under constant deformation) and creep (increased deformation with time under constant load)
■ At higher rates of loading, the tendon becomes more brittle – exhibits a much more linear stress–strain relation prior to failure (under these circumstances, the ultimate strength is greater, energy absorbed [toughness] lesser, and more effective in moving heavy loads. At slow

loading rates, the tendon is more ductile, undergoing plastic deformation and absorbing more energy before failure)

3.3.14 Storage of Energy

■ During movement, part of the kinetic energy created by muscle transiently stored as "strain energy" within the tendon. This gives the tendon the capability to passively transfer the muscle force to bone, as well as control the delivery of the force. A stronger, stiffer tendon exhibits a higher energy storing capacity – but if pre-stretched, its energy absorbing capacity is reduced, and risk of rupture is higher should added loading occur

3.3.15 Tendon Injury

■ MTJ – the weakest link
■ Especially during eccentric contractions → since maximum tension created in such contractions (>isometric/concentric types by 3-fold) and especially if speedy – hence increasing the speed of eccentric contraction will increase the force developed
■ If the loading rate is slow, bone breaks and avulsion fraction likely occurs. If loading is fast, more likely to cause tendon failure (especially if degenerated to start with)

3.3.16 Other Terms Concerning Injury Mechanics

■ Direct: penetrating, blunt, (thermal-chemical)
■ Indirect: acute tensile overload (macro-traumatic partial/complete tear), chronic repeated insult (micro-traumatic subthreshold damage – cause can be exogenous, e.g. acromial spurs, and endogenous)
  – Acute tensile failure when strain beyond 10%
  – But less strain can cause the same if pre-existing degeneration (chronic repeated overload occurs when there is failure to adapt to repeated exposure to low magnitude forces <4–8% strain)

3.3.17 Four Types of Micro-Traumatic Tendon Injury

■ "Tendinitis" – tendon strain or tear
■ "Tendinosis" – intra-tendinous degeneration
■ "Paratenonitis" – inflamed paratenon only
■ "Paratenonitis with tendinosis"

3.3.18 Three Phases of Tendon Healing

▧ Inflammation – fibrin links collagen, chemotactic to acute inflammatory cells – leukocytes, monocytes, and macrophages; clear damaged tissue

▧ Repair – macrophage as co-ordinator of migration and proliferation of fibroblasts, tenocytes and/or endothelium. These cells secret matrix and form new capillaries, replace clot with granulation tissue. Type 3 collagen produced, Type 1 later around second week

▧ Remodelling – started in third week, scar maturing, collagen more densely packed and orientated. The scar never has same properties – final tensile strength 30% less; biochemical and mechanical deficiencies will persist

3.3.19 Rehabilitation

▧ Knowledge of the *phased* healing response → allows the proper time frame within which to introduce our rehabilitation programme

▧ From first few days to end of week 2 – inflammatory response, significant decrease in tendon tensile strength, Type 3 collagen deposition. Our programme should avoid excess motion, as excess stress at this time *disrupts* healing instead of promoting it

▧ As from second to third week – this is the repair phase. Gradual introduction of motion, and prevention of excess muscle and joint atrophy

▧ In the rehabilitation phase – there is remodelling, progressive stress can be applied, but note that the tendon can require 10–12 months to reach the normal strength levels

3.3.20 The Scar

▧ Much collagen Type 3 persists in the scar – with thinner, weaker fibrils and fewer x-links

▧ Collagen – deficient in content, quality, and orientation

3.3.21 Effects of Use, Disuse and Immobilisation

▧ Use: will slowly hypertrophy – more action of tenoblast, accelerated collagen synthesis, more collagen thickness and cross-links, improved stress orientation of fibres, larger diameter and total weight

▧ Disuse: opposite changes

▧ Immobilisation: tendon atrophies, seen only after a few weeks and these adaptations more rapid than changes after exercise

General Bibliography

Ip D (2005) Orthopaedic Principles – A Resident's Guide. Springer, Heidelberg Berlin New York

Bulkwalter J, Einhorn T, Simon S (2000) Orthopedic Basic Science, 2nd Ed. American Academy of Orthopedic Surgeons Press

Selected Bibliography of Journal Articles

1. Delitto A, Snyder-Mackler L (1990) Muscle stimulators. Arch Phys Med Rehabil 71(9):711–712
2. Behm-DG, St-Pierre DM et al. (1996) Muscle in-activation – assessment of interpolated twitch technique. J Appl Physiol 81(5):2267–2273
3. Soo CL, Currier DP et al. (1988) Augmenting voluntary torque of healthy muscle by optimization of electrical stimulation – a review. Phys Ther 68(3):333–337
4. Sallay PI, Friedman RL et al. (1996) Hamstring muscle injuries among water skiers – functional outcome and prevention. Am J Sports Med 24(2):130–136
5. Zarins B, Ciullo JV (1983) Acute muscle and tendon injuries in athletes. Clin Sports Med 2(1):167–182
6. Negishi S, Li Y et al. (2005) The effect of relaxin treatment in skeletal muscle injuries. Am J Sports Med 33(12):1816–1824
7. Laros GS, Cooper RR et al. (1971) Influence of physical activity on ligament insertions in the knees of dogs. J Bone Joint Surg Am 53:275–286

Contents

4.1   Introduction

■ This chapter reveals the key and common physical therapy techniques used in orthopaedic rehabilitation
■ They are presented in the order of the time sequence of administration in most rehabilitation protocols
■ The important technique of proprioceptive neuromuscular facilitation (PNF) is discussed in Chap. 11, while Sects. 4.11.2 and 4.11.3 touch on chiropractics and osteopathic medicine respectively

4.1.1   Cornerstones of Restoration of Proper Musculoskeletal Function

■ Proper limb alignment and biomechanics
■ Proper joint kinematics, stability and proprioception
■ Proper neuromuscular control including sequence of firing (among individual muscles and between different functional groups)
■ Proper length–tension relationships
■ Proper force couples
■ Proper pain management

4.1.2   General Time Sequence of Rehabilitation

■ Regain range of motion (ROM) and flexibility, pain and oedema control
■ Training of muscle strength
■ Proprioception and neuromuscular control training
■ Endurance training added (and circuit training)
■ Co-ordination and motor re-learning
■ Sports- (or job-) specific training, plyometrics

4.2   Regaining Range of Motion and Flexibility

4.2.1   Definition of ROM

■ Range of motion refers to movement of a body part through a particular joint's complete, unrestricted, normal motion (according to Heyward)

4.2.2   Definition of Flexibility

▧ Flexibility refers to the musculotendinous unit's ability to elongate with the application of a stretching force (according to Heyward)

4.2.3   Essential Difference Between ROM and Flexibility

▧ It can be seen that ROM mainly refers to movement of a joint, while "flexibility" is based on concepts of muscle stretching

4.2.4   Common Causes of Joint Stiffness

▧ Stiffness of joints may originate from different structures, including the articulating bone surfaces, joint capsule, ligament, muscle, tendon, subcutaneous tissue and even skin
▧ The following classification is preferred for clarity

4.2.5   Categories of Joint Stiffness

▧ Intra-articular
▧ Extra-articular
▧ Both

4.2.5.1 Intra-Articular Causes

▧ Congenital, e.g. bony dysplasia
▧ Acquired, e.g. previous fracture
   (In this chapter, we will only concentrate on discussion on regaining "flexibility" from muscle tightness rather than discussing intra-articular causes of joint stiffness. The use of machines like the continuous passive motion (CPM) will be discussed in Chap. 14)

4.2.5.2 Extra-Articular Causes

▧ Skin – e.g. hypertrophic burn scarring (Chap. 13)
▧ Soft tissue – e.g. ectopic calcification, burns and rarer causes like fibrodysplasia ossificans progressiva (with heterotopic ossification)
▧ Muscle – e.g. "functional" like reactive muscle spasm due to local painful condition, muscle imbalance from poor training, and other, rather less common, causes like myositis ossificans

4.2.5.3 Both

▧ In fact, any long-standing joint stiffness can influence extra-articular structures that create further stiffness, e.g. (adhesions between myo-

fascial planes) and the initially unaffected joint structures like ligaments and capsules can lose elasticity or in fact shorten by relative immobility
▨ Conversely, any long-standing extra-articular causes of joint stiffness can have a significant influence on the joint itself or its kinematics (e.g. kinetic chain dysfunction), see Chap. 9

4.2.5.4   Muscular Causes of Joint Stiffness
▨ Common: causes like poor posture, poor training techniques in athletes causing neuromuscular imbalance and muscle tightness, and joint stiffness
▨ Rarer causes:
  – Myositis ossificans

4.2.5.5   Options to Tackle Commonly Encountered Muscle Tightness
▨ Muscle stretching exercises
  – Static stretches
  – Ballistic stretches
▨ Muscle energy techniques[1]

4.2.5.6   Techniques to Improve Flexibility

4.2.5.6.1 Muscle Stretching Techniques: General Rationale
▨ Stretching to effect muscle lengthening is based on the principle of:
  – Muscle autogenic inhibition
  – With prolonged stretching, viscoelastic and/or plastic change can occur in the connective tissue elements that have elastin and collagen
▨ The contractile actin-myosin elements respond more to high-velocity deforming forces, while the connective tissue non-contractile portion responds mainly to the degree of stretch

---

[1] The technique of PNF is based on somewhat similar principles, but since this technique is best suited to patients with neuromuscular disorders (after Knott and Voss) it will be discussed under the section on cardiopulmonary (CP) rehabilitation instead

4.2.5.6.2 Pre-Requisite Before Stretching

▦ Adequate warm-up is needed to increase core temperature, easing the deformability of the connective tissue elements

▦ Most recommend warming up to 103°F

4.2.5.6.3 Static Stretches

▦ Involve stretching the muscle in question in a position that allows for maximum stretching and hold there for 15–30 s

▦ Advantage: less chance of injury than ballistic stretching, and does not usually cause delayed onset muscle soreness

▦ Disadvantage: in stretching the upper limb, can need an assistant or instrument to perform

4.2.5.6.4 Ballistic Technique

▦ This usually involves jerking and bouncing movements, usually of the lower limb

▦ Disadvantage: may cause injury if not adequately warmed up or preceded by static stretch; the timing may not be adequate for the Golgi tendon to fire its inhibitory reflex

4.2.5.6.5 Combined Use of Cryotherapy and Stretching

▦ This was discussed under the section on cryotherapy in Chap. 2

▦ Cold stretching can sometimes be effective in managing delayed onset muscle soreness

4.2.5.6.6 Others

▦ See "muscle energy" techniques in the following discussion

▦ As mentioned, PNF techniques are best described for rehabilitation of patients with neuromuscular disorders, and will be described separately

4.2.5.6.7 General Precautions for Stretching

▦ Patient must be relaxed and preferably seated

▦ Do not attempt ballistic stretches without adequate warm-up and static stretches, do not commence these exercise if there is recent injury to the musculotendinous unit

▦ Avoid overdoing the muscle stretches to the point of pain

4.2.5.7 "Muscle Energy" Techniques

4.2.5.7.1 Definition

▦ Muscle energy techniques is a type of manual muscular stretching technique based on sound neurophysiology and involves ways of relaxing and stretching overly active muscles

▦ This technique can be useful in tackling complex dysfunction of the kinetic chain

4.2.5.7.2 Rationale of Using Muscle Energy Techniques

▦ Many a times when a group of muscles becomes tight or overactive (produced by, e.g. poor posture, abnormal nearby joint kinematics, or improper training techniques in athletes) it may cause an abnormal length–tension relationship of the kinetic chain, and also produce concomitant weakness of antagonist by reciprocal inhibition, and abnormal compensatory firing of associated synergistic musculature

▦ Muscle energy techniques attempt to relax overactive muscles, stretch over-tight muscles or shortened muscles, and prevent the complications of altered neuromuscular control and firing of the muscles of the kinetic chain; also prevents unwanted inhibition of the antagonist of the overactive musculature

4.2.5.7.3 Main Underlying Neurophysiological Principles

▦ Principle 1: post-contraction inhibition

▦ Principle 2: reciprocal inhibition

Principle 1: Post-Contraction Inhibition

▦ This makes use of the observation in neurophysiology that after a muscle contracts, it will be rendered in a more or less relaxed status for a brief period of around half a minute, which provides a "window of opportunity" for the therapist or the surgeon to stretch it

Principle 2: Reciprocal Inhibition

▦ The principle of "reciprocal inhibition" states that upon contraction of a muscle, its antagonist will be reciprocally inhibited

▦ This is a normal physiological phenomenon that helps to allow proper and smooth functioning of the kinetic chain

▦ This can be put to good use to help relax the overactive agonist

4.2.5.7.4 Common Indications for Muscle Energy Techniques

- Dysfunction of the kinetic chain, the main underlying cause of which is not mainly due to alignment problems, bony deformity, or joint instability
- Useful in managing many problems of the kinetic chain in both amateur and professional athletes, e.g. involved in jumping sports like basketball or in running

4.2.5.7.5 Tricks for Proper Performance of Muscle Energy Techniques

- Identify the point in the ROM at which resistance is first encountered
- Effect agonist contraction at 25% strength while the therapist resists the isometric contraction for about 10 s
- During the window of opportunity that follows as aforementioned, the agonist is stretched
- Patient uses the antagonist to effect further inhibition of the agonist to achieve further improvement in the ROM

4.2.5.7.5 Clinical Examples: Tight Gastrocnemius

- Tight gastrocnemius is rather common; causes include:
  - Pathology in the tendon proper, e.g. Achilles tendinitis
  - High heeled shoes in women
  - Painful heels, e.g. plantar fasciitis
  - Gait anomalies
  - Flexed posture of the hip or knee
  - Painful ankle, etc.

4.2.5.7.6 Effect of Tight Gastrocnemius

- Can affect nearby subtalar joint, or Chopart's joint
- Gait anomalies (affect first and second rockers)
- Altered shock absorption, and increased force transmission up the ipsilateral kinetic chain (ankle, knee, hip)
- Sometimes predispose to back and sacroiliac joint (SIJ) discomfort

4.2.5.7.7 Application of Muscle Energy Techniques

- Put your relaxed patient supine on the couch
- Ensure ipsilateral subtalar joint is neutral
- Ankle dorsiflexion (thus stretching the Achilles tendon) up to first point of passive resistance

- Patient asked to actively perform ankle plantar flexion at 25% of maximum strength (i.e. agonist firing)
- Continue agonist firing for 10 s
- Then ask patient to actively perform ankle dorsiflexion (i.e. firing of antagonist) until a new improved ROM is achieved

4.2.5.7.8 Precautions
- Patient education: patient taught to continue stretching exercises at home; both warm-up and warm-down are needed
- Concomitant training of the patient in techniques of proper core exercises and neuromuscular stabilisation training

4.3   Muscle Strength Training

- General principle of muscle strength training (according to Geffen)
  - Overload principle
  - Specificity principle
  - Individual differences principle
  - Reversibility principle

4.3.1   Overload Principle
- Overloading a muscle can be effected by an increase in frequency of training or its intensity or duration
- The overload principle involves exercise that is carried out at a level greater than that to which an individual has been accustomed, in order to achieve gains in physiological function

4.3.2   Principle of Specificity
- Another name of this principle is specific adaptation to imposed demand (SAID)
- During the later stage of rehabilitation of athletes for example, the individual needs to simulate the task required of the sport (sport-specific) in order to optimise the neural firing pattern and timing of the required task

4.3.3   Individual Differences Principle

▨ This essentially highlights the fact that rehabilitation of patients should not be in a stereotyped or cook-book fashion; with due consideration paid to individual differences in, say, preoperative fitness, time lapse between surgery and the start of rehabilitation, and gender differences, etc.

4.3.4   Reversibility Principle

▨ Even strong athletes can suffer from the phenomenon of "detraining" since gains from exercise can be rapidly lost within a few months of exercise cessation (Jeffreys, 2002), sometimes even earlier

4.3.5   Types of Muscle Strength Training

▨ Isometric
▨ Isotonic
▨ Isokinetic

4.3.5.1   Isometric Training

▨ Method of muscle strengthening where despite the fact that the muscle is contracting, there is no change in length or joint angle (Komi 1992)
▨ Commonly employed mode of rehabilitation in early phase of rehabilitation
▨ Another advantage is no need for expensive equipment

4.3.5.1.1 Why Strength Can Improve with Isometrics Without Motion

▨ Due to the $20°$ physiologic overflow that accompanies this type of training

4.3.5.1.2 Key Concept

▨ Isometric exercises are joint angle-specific; thus, gains in strength only occur within a small range of motion corresponding to the joint angle at which the contraction is undertaken

4.3.5.1.3 Disadvantage/Caution

▨ Avoid doing the Valsalva during isometric training, or BP may increase
▨ This type of training needs to be done under supervision since patient may overload the healing structures

4.3.5.2   Isotonic Training
■ A typical example is the use of free weights where the load is constant, but the speed of motion varies
■ Isotonic muscle activity can be subdivided into concentric and eccentric movements

4.3.5.2.1 Disadvantage of Isotonics
■ Muscle is maximally loaded at its weakest point in the range of motion; thus, not safe to perform this kind of exercise in the early postoperative period
■ But for the rest of the ROM the muscle can be under-loaded
■ May induce unnecessary pain
■ Injury can result from falling weights or by weights that exceeded the limits of the muscle

4.3.5.3   Isokinetic Training
■ Isokinetic contraction is featured by contraction at a pre-defined rate and usually performed using special machines like a dynamometer (Figs. 4.1, 4.2)

4.3.5.3.1 Key Concept
■ It works by the principle of "accommodative resistance"
■ The patient connected to the isokinetic machine encounters a resistance no greater than the amount of force applied to the muscle, per-

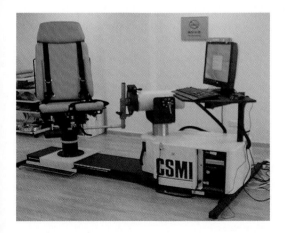

Fig. 4.1. Machine for isokinetic training

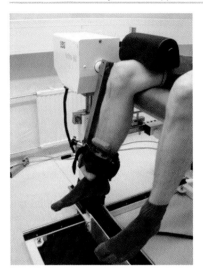

Fig. 4.2. Close-up of another isokinetic machine preparing to initiate training for this patient after anterior cruciate ligament reconstruction

mitting the muscle to exert its own maximum force and strength throughout an ROM

- The machine keeps the angular velocity of the moving limb constant by changing the force generated by the isokinetic machine to resist the intended movement

4.3.5.3.2 Main Advantages
- Can be applied relatively early on in the rehabilitation of many sports injuries
- Forces generated are usually well tolerated by the soft tissues and the joint
- Thus, less chance of re-injury
- Provides an objective measurement of dynamic strength for better documentation and comparison between different methods
- Allows the muscle to exert its maximum strength throughout the ROM
- Isokinetic testing can help identify the cause of the patient's (especially an athlete's) problem, e.g. by use of torque analysis
- Data collected serially (and on both sides for comparison) are useful for imparting decisions on the progress of rehabilitation

■ In short, on the one hand avoidance of undue stresses on the joint, and yet can avoid excessive maximum dynamic loads

4.3.5.3.3 Details of Isokinetic Training

■ It is best to test the type of motion the patient performs in daily life, and (in the case of the athlete) reproduce the plane of motion pertaining to his sports
■ The machine needs calibration before use and monthly thereafter
■ Minimise motion above and below the joint in question
■ Adequate warm-up
■ Give rest interval between each test of about 2 min
■ Test speed depends on the joint in question – in general higher for knees and shoulders and low for ankles and wrist, etc.
■ Each training session consists of around ten exercise repetitions

4.3.5.3.4 Recording of Data

■ Traditional method: the details of reporting are outside the scope of this book, but we are mainly interested in looking at parameters like average power, peak torque and total work
■ New isomapping method: essentially a method that involves graphical representation plus qualitative analysis of neuromuscular performance. Like the traditional method, it can help identify, say, in which muscle group or contraction mode or in which part of the ROM the problem lies (Med Sci Sports Exerc 2000)

4.4   Closed Chain and Open Chain Exercises

4.4.1   Introduction

■ Closed kinetic chain rehabilitation protocol is commonly used and started early in many rehabilitation protocols
■ Most applications in the past have been used for LL rehabilitation (e.g. with the feet on the ground), although it is now increasingly used in UL rehabilitation as well

4.4.2   Differences Between Open and Closed Kinetic Chain Exercises

■ Open-chain: refers to those exercises in which the distal end or terminal of the chain is freely mobile and not loaded, e.g. back extension exercises against gravity
■ Closed-chain: here, the distal end or terminal is immobile or loaded

4.4.3   Definition of "Closed-Chain" Exercises

■ Those in which the distal (terminal) end of the lower or upper limb is kept immobile or being loaded with considerable resistance

4.4.3.1   Advantages of Closed Kinetic Chain Exercises

■ Simulate more normal biomechanical and physiologic function
■ Little shear stress across the injured joint or peri-articular soft tissue
■ Provision of proprioceptive stimuli

4.4.3.2   Key Principle

■ The force and transmission of closed kinetic chain exercise works on the principle of summation of speed
■ According to Putnam (J Biomech 1993), the total energy of force in the closed kinetic chain is a summation of the contributions of the individual segments of the kinetic chain

4.4.3.3   Practical Application

■ Keys to success besides ensuring the distal end of the kinetic chain is loaded or stationary:
  – Small joint movements
  – Decreased joint shear
  – Proprioceptive stimulation
  – Dynamic joint stabilisation through muscle co-contraction
  – Translation of instantaneous centre of motion should occur in a predictable manner based on the local biomechanical forces at work

4.4.3.4   Pitfall or Contraindication

■ May not work if there is an altered sequence of firing of the muscles in the kinetic chain

4.4.3.5 Key Concept

■ Importance of rehabilitating the whole kinetic chain in sports injury cannot be over-emphasised, see the section on rehabilitation in sports injury in Chap. 9

4.5 Training of Proprioception and Neuromuscular Control

4.5.1 Definition of Proprioception

■ Proprioception involves aspects of joint position sense, sensing of motion, vibration and pressure via mechanoreceptors located in joints, ligaments and musculotendinous units

■ It is sometimes also referred to as the "somatosensory system" and is made up of muscle spindles, Golgi tendon organs and joint/skin receptors (Hogblum, 2001)

4.5.2 Importance of Proprioceptive Training

■ There is an increasing trend toward emphasising proprioceptive training in rehabilitation of the kinetic chain (Fig. 4.3). Moreover, training should start as early as possible after commencement of weight-bearing (Kinch, 2001)

■ This is because diminished afferent proprioceptive input can deactivate coordinated neuromuscular activation

■ If severe, the functional effects can be comparable to actual anatomic disruption of the ligament or tendon (Laskowski, 1997)

4.5.3 Proper Sequence of Proprioceptive and Co-ordination/Agility Training

■ It is essential to note that re-training of proprioception and balance should precede coordination training

■ Agility training can only start *after* training of proprioception and later coordination

4.5.4 Proprioception Exercises

■ Should proceed from simple to complex

■ Slowly progressing in degree of difficulty, e.g. from one-leg stands, to wobble board, to mini-trampoline, etc.

■ Further discussion of this topic will be found in Chaps. 9 and 19

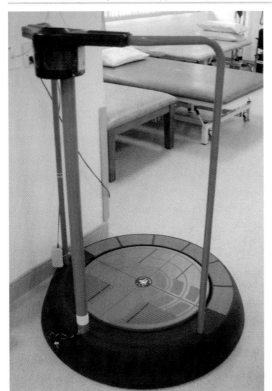

Fig. 4.3. Machine for proprioceptive training

4.6   Biofeedback

4.6.1   Introduction
■ Neuromuscular control will be discussed in Chap. 9
■ But we will take this opportunity to describe yet another technique, i.e. biofeedback

4.6.2   Definition of Biofeedback
■ The technique of using electronic equipment to reveal to humans their internal physiologic events, usually in the form of visual or auditory signals

- With an aim to teaching them the way to manipulate these otherwise involuntary events by the manipulation of displayed signals (Basmajian et al., Arch Phys Med Rehabil 1975)

4.6.3   Reports on the Clinical Use of Bio-Feedbacks

- Field of orthopaedics
  - SCI patients and posture training in scoliosis
  - Retraining hand function after tendon transfer
  - Retraining the proper firing of muscle as in voluntary shoulder dislocators
  - Retraining the vastus medialis obliquus (VMO) of the knee
  - Pain control
- Other fields
  - Relaxation therapy
  - Stroke patient rehabilitation
  - Possible effect on heart rate and blood pressure

4.6.4   Most Popular Feedback: Myoelectric

- Here, the myoelectric signals from the muscle are translated into acoustic and visual signals, as in buzzing sounds and lights
- Usually displayed as spikes on a cathode ray oscilloscope or as popping noises on a loudspeaker

4.6.5   Other Clinical Uses of These Myoelectric Signals

- These signals can also be put to good use in other clinical areas such as the control of myoelectric prostheses
- Myoelectric prostheses are discussed in Chap. 10

4.6.6   Principle of Use

- One of the great advantages of biofeedback = enables small changes in the correct direction to be detected and rewarded as success so that with time these build up into larger changes
- Patients may ultimately be able to learn to perceive these changes in the absence of the instruments and practice themselves

4.6.7   Another Possible Mechanism

■ Occasionally, the extreme plasticity of the nervous system may allow the individual to learn to use alternative pathways that bypass the faulty tissue (JAMA 1985)

4.6.8   Advantages of Biofeedback

■ Acts as a form of encouragement and motivation
■ Engenders a coping response and helps alleviate stress
■ Many patients feel the technique improves his or her own recognition of the clinical problem at hand
■ Increased confidence

4.6.8.1   Use in Pain Relief

■ Tracts were discovered in the brain, which, when stimulated in unanaesthetised animals, can effectively relieve pain
■ The stimulation of these tracts is believed to produce opiate-like substances and have in the past had variable success in the relief of some patients with chronic excruciating and intractable pain. Whether occasional reports of pain relief with biofeedback uses these pathways needs further research

4.6.8.2   Use in VMO Training and in Voluntary Shoulder Dislocators

■ Here, the patient will relearn to:
  – Contract the correct muscle or muscle groups
  – Or to strengthen the weakened or atrophied muscle, in this case the VMO

4.6.8.3   Use of Biofeedback in SCI

■ Chronic SCI with little neuromuscular activity are probably not good candidates
■ Refer to discussion in Chap. 12 on SCI
■ Requires extra motivation from patient, very labour-intensive

4.6.8.4   Posture Training in Scoliosis

■ New training devices can be worn under the clothes without movement restraints (Wong et al., Prosthet Orthot Int 2001). When the patient is not in a good posture for, say, 20–30 s, an audible sound will be made, but this ceases upon restoration of a better posture:

- The general move towards the miniaturisation of electronic devices provides the potential to provide the patient with training in the friendly home environment
- Newer training devices can readily be worn by the patient and readily incorporated in daily life

4.6.8.5 Incorporation of Endurance and Cardiovascular Training

4.6.8.5.1 Endurance vs Strength Training

- Alongside the rehabilitation programme, a fitness schedule is required to allow the patient to maintain cardiovascular fitness and muscular endurance
- To promote cardiorespiratory adaptations, use of dynamic exercises involving contractions of large muscle groups need be performed over an adequate period with sufficient oxygen or aerobic exercise and under guidelines as set out by the American College of Sports Medicine (ACSM 1990). A detailed comparison of endurance vs strength training is given in Chap. 9.

4.6.8.5.2 Circuit Training

- Newer regimens like "circuit resistance training" (where the individual goes through a number of stations training both strength and endurance) that de-emphasise the traditional, very brief intervals of heavy muscle strengthening in standard resistance training protocols are gaining in popularity
- This is because this form of training provides a more general conditioning, with demonstrated improvements in body composition, muscle endurance and strength, as well as cardiovascular fitness (Haennel, Med Sci Sports Exerc 1989)
- In addition, circuit resistance training also provides supplementary off-season conditioning even for sportsmen and women who demand high levels of strength and power. There will be more discussion in Chaps. 9 and 19

4.6.8.5.3 Timing of Cardiovascular Conditioning

- Total body aerobic conditioning should be initiated as early as possible after injury or surgery if this does not aggravate pain or impair healing

▦ This minimises effects of disuse and also has a positive psychological impact on our patients

▦ Timing and administration of endurance training and the way to incorporate with strength training if your patient is a professional athlete will be discussed in Chap. 9

4.7   Plyometrics and Sports Training

4.7.1   Introduction
▦ Plyometrics is only one of the different methods of preparing the athlete to return to sports or even competition

▦ Other adjuncts include fast-velocity isokinetic and isotonic training, sports-specific muscle conditioning and strength training, and agility exercises

4.7.2   History of "Plyometrics"
▦ The term literally means "to increase", translated from Greek

▦ This technique of training is well known to have been applied to the jumping sports, but now the term usually encompasses any type of exercise utilising the stretch reflex to increase the power output of the contracting muscle

4.7.3   Definition
▦ Essentially a form of training, usually in athletes, consisting of combined strength and speed training

▦ This may also form part of the *late* rehabilitation of injured athletes in preparation for their return to the field or athletic arena

4.7.4   Mechanism Behind the Use of Plyometrics
▦ Normal movement patterns of the musculoskeletal system work by stretch-shortening cycles of muscle

▦ The technique of plyometrics works by pre-stretching the muscle and activating the stretch-shortening cycle, causing a more powerful subsequent concentric contraction

▦ Energy stored in the pre-stretch will be released as kinetic energy in an opposite direction, and if applied correctly will result in an explosive movement

4.7.5   Normal Functioning of the Muscle Spindles
- Muscle spindles are parallel to the muscle fibres; they fire in response to stretch and the impulse goes to the brain, which ultimately results in muscle contraction
- The firing is increased with more rapid muscular stretch

4.7.6   Normal Functioning of the Golgi Tendon Organs
- The Golgi tendon organs are in series and embedded in the tendon; they fire when there is increased tension in the tendon and induces an inhibitory reflex to prevent tension build-up – with inhibitory signals sent to the muscle, which contracts, and its synergists

4.7.7   Determinants of the Efficiency of Plyometrics
- Increased effectiveness with decreased interval between lengthening and shortening
- Rate of stretch
- Degree of stretch – which depends on magnitude of stretch force, the extent of firing of muscle spindles, and the strength of individual fibres
- It is believed that prolonged training can raise the firing threshold of the Golgi tendon organs, allowing enhanced force generation

4.7.8   Metabolic Pathway Involved
- Plyometrics mainly involves anaerobic pathways
- Adequate rest between sessions is warranted

4.7.9   Main Mechanisms Causing Power Increase
- Shortening the time interval between the eccentric contraction and the subsequent concentric contraction (Acta Physiol Scand 1979)
- Usually, fast-twitch muscle fibres are involved

4.7.10   Importance of Speed
- This has just been discussed
- Speed improvements may be partly due to improved and additional recruitment of motor units

4.7.11 Importance of Adequate Strength

▧ Plyometrics training will not succeed in the absence of adequate strength

▧ Also, increased muscle strength and cross-sectional area allows greater storage of energy not only in the contractile unit, but also in the elastic connective tissue elements

4.7.12 Prerequisite Before Commencing Plyometrics Training

▧ Adequate flexibility and warm-up

▧ Adequate strength and muscle cross-sectional area

▧ Stable base and proper alignment and stability of the kinetic chain (including static and dynamic stability)

4.7.13 Precautions Necessary for Plyometric Training

▧ Adequate rest

▧ Periodisation among strength training, plyometric training, general conditioning (while off season), in addition to sports-specific training

▧ Beware of over-training, adequate nutrition and fluid replenishment, prevent boredom by introducing variability of training manoeuvres

4.8   Concept of "Core Stability"

4.8.1   What Constitutes the "Core"

▧ The "core" is composed of the lumbar vertebrae, the pelvis, and hip joints, together with the active and passive structures that either produce or restrict movements of these motion segments

4.8.2   What Is "Core Stability"

▧ "Core stability" refers to the ability of the lumbopelvic hip complex to prevent buckling and to return to equilibrium without perturbation. This is mainly dependent on the active structures consisting of contractions or co-contractions of the muscles, since the stiffness of the lumbopelvic hip complex has been shown in the past to be mainly dependent on the active stabilisers for its stiffness as opposed to passive stabilisers

▧ Core stability is also dynamic; hence, the local anatomy must be able to continually adapt to changing postures and loading conditions in order to maintain the integrity of the vertebral column thus providing a stable base for the extremities

4.8.3 Importance of Core Stability

■ Contraction of the muscular elements of the core can increase the stiffness of the hip and trunk. To achieve stability, not only is the ability of co-contraction of the antagonistic trunk muscles required (in response to anticipated spinal loading), but the contraction of the hip and trunk muscles must also be coordinated, as prolonged co-contraction is also detrimental and may lead to excess compressive loading to the system

■ Another important factor underscoring the importance of core stability is that although normal trunk muscle reflexes are automatic and may stiffen the spine for loading, this system tends to have an innate neuromuscular delay and may offer inadequate protection in the face of a sudden spinal load, thus underscoring the importance of training of core stability

4.8.4 Three Main Mechanisms of Provision of Stability

■ Increased intra-abdominal pressure can be effected by simultaneous contraction of the diaphragm and the pelvic floor muscles, or by abdominal muscles, particularly the transversus abdominis

■ Increased axial load can be effected by muscle co-contractions of the trunk extensor and flexor muscle groups

■ The large, superficial muscles of the hip and trunk are architecturally best suited to producing movement and increasing hip and trunk stiffness to counteract destabilising forces during functional activities

4.8.5 Example of the Concept of Core Stability in Patient Rehabilitation

■ Example: back injury in a game of golf, due to poor technique, over-swing, improper warm-up or improper equipment

■ The golf swing has four components: take-away, acceleration, impact and follow-through

■ During the swing, trunk rotation and high shear forces can cause injury to the thoraco-lumbar spine, thus causing back pain

4.8.6   Important Element
in Rehabilitating Golf-Related Back Injuries

■ Pain relief
■ Training in flexibility
■ Training in core stability
■ Proper coaching and warm-up
■ Proper technique and equipment

4.8.7   Anatomical Note

■ Anatomically, the chief muscles that function in the sagittal plane include the rectus abdominis, transversus abdominis, erector spinae, multifidus and hamstrings. The rectus abdominis and multifidus, together with tonic contraction of the transversus, can produce increases in intra-abdominal pressure. The gluteus maximus is important to help transfer lower extremity forces to the trunk. Chief lateral muscles of the hip and trunk that function in the frontal plane include gluteus medius, gluteus minimus and quadratus lumborum. These glutei help maintain a level pelvis in closed chain motion. Co-contraction of bilateral quadratus lumborum help stiffens the spine. Chief medial muscles acting in the frontal plane include adductor magnus, adductor longus and brevis, and pectineus. Their role in core stability is smaller than that of the aforementioned muscles. Trunk rotation is provided for by internal and external oblique muscles, the iliocostalis lumborum and the multifidus. Bilateral activation of these muscles also aids core stability by increasing intra-abdominal pressure

4.9   Acupuncture Therapy

4.9.1   Introduction

■ As acupuncture therapy (Fig. 4.4) is increasingly used by physiotherapists and other health professionals (either alone or as part of a treatment programme) in the US and abroad, it will not be included under Sect. 4.11 on alternative medicine

■ It is interesting that despite being based on theories very different from western medicine, acupuncture has now received wide clinical acceptance because it has been proven to be efficacious in both clinical and basic science research

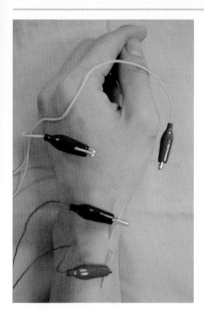

Fig. 4.4. Electro-acupuncture therapy at work

▓ In fact Melzack, the originator of the gate theory of pain, found a 70% correlation between acupuncture points and trigger points used in the treatment of myofascial pain (Melzack et al., Pain 1977)

4.9.2 Historical Note
▓ First practised in China >2 millennia ago, with published works in writing around 100 BC
▓ Owing to significant differences from western medicine theories, it was not popularised in US until the 1970s
▓ Currently has a well-accepted place in US after the NIH consensus development conference on acupuncture with well-proven efficacy in postoperative pain, postoperative dental pain and chemotherapy-induced vomiting (J Am Med Assoc 1998)

4.9.3 Popularity
▓ All along has been popular in Asian countries, and increasingly popular in USA and other western nations
▓ Practised by both physiotherapists, acupuncturists, and some traditional Chinese medicine practitioners

▨ Owing to increasing acceptance in US, some insurance companies are willing to cover costs incurred in acupuncture treatment

4.9.4   Training in Acupuncture
▨ Most USA states use the National Commission for Certification of Acupuncturists (NCCA) standards during certification
▨ Most licensed acupuncturists need to go though 3 years of training
▨ It is interesting to note that virtual reality was reportedly being used to help teach acupuncture in some centres (IEEE Trans Inf Technol Biomed 2006)

4.9.5   Basic Philosophy of Chinese Medicine
▨ Basic thinking includes:
  – Concept on yin vs yang: these two opposing forces need to be balanced. A good balance of yin–yang is needed to promote the flow of "chi" which is essentially visualised as a form of energy. Illness will result if there is an abnormal flow of "chi" through the body's meridians
  – Concept of five elements including fire, earth, metal, water and wood. Their correct dynamic interaction is needed for health

4.9.6   Basic Philosophy of Acupuncture
▨ The flow of "chi" can be potentially restored by needle insertion at some of the acupuncture points (a total of 365 in the body)
▨ One needs to select the correct point combinations, have the correct technique, correct positioning, and correct depth in order for the treatment to work
▨ Several treatment sessions or even longer periods are needed depending on the condition treated

4.9.7   Acupuncture Needles
▨ Traditionally used needles in the distant past in the times of the emperors were made of gold
▨ The fine needles used nowadays are made of stainless steel, most are reusable upon proper sterilisation to prevent disease transmission

4.9.8   Stimulation Method

■ Traditional needles are in involved various methods, e.g. twisting, twirling, lift-and-thrust techniques, etc.

■ Some centres use both low (2 Hz) and high frequency (100 Hz) electrical stimulation to accompany the needling procedure – "electrical acupuncture"

4.9.9   Scope of Clinical Use

■ Acute pain, e.g. postoperative dental pain, and after abdominal surgery (Pain 2002)

■ Chronic pain and reflex sympathetic dystrophy (RSD; see Chap. 15)

■ LBP (Furlan et al., Spine 2005)

■ SCI (see Chap. 12)

■ Cerebrovascular accident (Sze et al., Stroke 2002)

■ Nausea and vomiting (Vickers, JR Soc Med 1996)

■ Psychological disturbance, e.g. depression (Psychol Sci 1998), and sleep disturbances

■ Neck disorders (Trinh et al., Cochrane Review 2006, CD004870)

4.9.10   Support from Basic Science Studies

■ On pain relief: three possible mechanisms:
  – By the gate theory (see Chap. 15)
  – By endogenous opioid peptides (Acta Physiol Scand 1977) and reversal by naloxone (Brain Res 1977)
  – By descending pain inhibitory pathways (Pain 1987)

■ On possible effects on higher centres besides spinal cord, e.g. higher brain centres that can be stimulated include:
  – Limbic system by functional MRI studies (Human Brain Mapping 2000)
  – Pituitary–hypothalamus area and midbrain (according to Pomeranz 1987)

4.9.11   Common Side Effects

■ Pain especially if needle inserted in incorrect position

■ Bruising

■ Infection

■ Tiredness

4.9.12 Rare Side Effects
- Pneumothorax
- Aggravating the presenting systems
- Systemic feeling of being unwell
- Syncope and even more serious effects (White et al., BMJ 2001)

4.9.13 Precautions or Contraindications
- If using reusable needles, need proper sterilisation
- A small number of patients develop significant systemic sickness after the start of acupuncture; they should preferably avoid the use of this therapy
- Therapist with newly acquired acupuncture skills should ideally be supervised by colleagues experienced in this technique

4.10   Massage Therapy

4.10.1 Introduction
- Since many physiotherapists use massage therapy, myofascial and trigger point techniques in their daily practice, this form of therapy is arbitrarily not grouped under "alternative medicine" in this book
- The number of professional massage therapists in the USA is increasing and estimated to be 200 000, according to the American Massage Therapy Association

4.10.2 Brief History
- The roots of massage therapy lie in the oldest of civilisations, e.g. Chinese, Greek, Egyptians centuries ago
- The more widely used modern Swedish techniques originated from the works of Per Henrik Ling in the early 18th century based on ideas of proper motion and massage to benefit the lymphatic and circulatory systems

4.10.3 Place in the Field of Rehabilitation
- Massage therapy is widely practiced by many health professionals e.g.:
  - Professional massage therapist
  - Physiotherapist
  - Physiotherapist assistants

- Some orthopaedic nurses
- Some osteopathic practitioners
- Some chiropractors

4.10.4 Licensing and Setting of Standards

- Only 30 out of 50 US states require formal licensing
- Abundant massage training courses in USA and other countries
- Some US states offer professional degree courses in bodywork and massage therapy

4.10.5 Scope of Massage Therapy

- Majority of patients going to seek massage therapists are suffering from musculoskeletal disorders or desire feelings of wellness or relaxation
- As discussed, massage therapy techniques are used by many different fields of different health care professionals

4.10.6 Basic Philosophy

- This varies somewhat from that of the country of origin
- Most are based on:
  - Movement re-education to obtain a more normal kinesiology
  - Superficial and deep massage techniques to effect relaxation, pain relief, improve circulation among other effects
  - Accompanied by exercise, energy techniques and stresses the adequacy of fluid intake
  - Beliefs in the philosophy of aiding the body to heal itself
  - Finally, deep massage therapy is aimed at tackling restricted motion, pain relief and myofascial trigger point release
    (Discussion of trigger points and myofascial pain syndrome closely follows this discussion)
  - There are some claims regarding positive effects on digestive, immune and hormonal systems

4.10.7 Types of Massage Therapy

- The majority of massage therapy techniques practiced in the USA tend to follow the Swedish techniques
- Other countries have other techniques based on different underlying ideas or philosophies

4.10.8   Techniques Used in the Swedish Methods
- Petrissage – including kneading and lifting
- Effleurage – gliding movements
- Friction – involves "moving the layers under the skin"
- Percussion
- Vibration

4.10.9   Massage Therapy Principles in Other Countries
- India: stresses the combined use of oil and hand to restore the flow of energy
- China: stress on treating imbalance of body's energy or "chi". Techniques include acupressure, tuina, etc.
- Japan: popularised a type of finger pressure called "shiatsu", essentially a variety of acupressure

4.10.10 Papers in Support of Massage Therapy
- In a recent Cochrane Collaboration review of nine previous publications (Spine 2002) the effectiveness of massage therapy for LBP was assessed
- In many studies in the Cochrane review, massage therapy was found to be superior to relaxation therapy, acupuncture and education, but seemed less efficacious than TENS and spinal manipulation

4.10.11 Common Precautions
- Infected field
- Tumour
- Bleeding tendency
- Extreme osteoporosis
- Insensate skin
- Instability or fracture of local musculoskeletal structures

4.11   Brief Outline of "Alternative Medicine"

4.11.1   Overview
- As orthopaedic surgeons, we frequently encounter patients having sought treatment by chiropractors or osteopathic practitioners prior to their clinic visit; it therefore pays to have a brief outline of the methods of treatment of the practitioners of these disciplines

4.11.2 Chiropractics

4.11.2.1 Brief History
- It was Daniel David Palmer who performed the first chiropractic manipulation in 1895
- Despite initial conflicts with traditional mainstream medicine including lawsuits, the two professions finally came to a consensus in the 1970s, and subsequently the National Center for Complementary and Alternative Medicine was set up in the USA

4.11.2.2 Popularity
- There was a resurgence of popularity in alternative medicine in the USA and in many other countries, and relaxation therapy and chiropractics ranked among the most used forms of alternative medicine
- In the USA, the number of chiropractors rose from 13 000 to 50 000 between 1970 and 1995, owing to the increase in patients seeking alternative medicine

4.11.2.3 Licensing and Setting of Standards
- There are 14 accredited chiropractic colleges in the USA
- Candidates need to pass college examinations before practice; the same occurs in Canada and the UK
- The scope of their practice is governed by state law in the USA

4.11.2.4 Scope of Chiropractics
- In practice, most patients seek chiropractors for treatment of musculoskeletal system problems
- The most common diagnoses are LBP and neck pain

4.11.2.5 Basic Philosophy
- The traditional thinking of this trade involves the idea of "subluxation" or "misalignment" of the spine, causing abnormal pressure and interfering with nerve function
- These concepts are altered in modern chiropractors who learned about basic science, biomechanics and theories on the neurophysiology of pain

4.11.2.6 "Mobilisation" vs "Manipulation"

▓ These two terms are often confused
▓ "Mobilisation", if passive, means giving an external force to move the joint within its physiological range of motion
▓ "Manipulation" implies and involves movements induced at the end of the normal ROM and may well lie slightly beyond the usual range, but less than that which creates breaches in spinal integrity

4.11.2.7 Goal of Modern Chiropractics (Using LBP as an Example)

▓ Pain relief
▓ Muscle relaxation
▓ Improved joint ROM
▓ Some modern chiropractors also give vitamins, nutritional advice, pain killers, order adjunct rehabilitation techniques like ultrasound, cryotherapy, etc.

4.11.2.8 Spinal Manipulative Therapy

▓ The details of the spinal manipulative therapy (SMT) trade cannot be discussed here, but some techniques used include:
  – Long lever arm technique (e.g. enlist the help of the limbs and/or special tables)
  – Short lever arm techniques (most commonly used)
  – Recoil techniques

4.11.2.9 Papers in Support of SMT in Back Pain Treatment

▓ A more recent trial by Cherkin (N Engl J Med 1998) compared three groups: chiropractic manipulation, McKenzie exercise and education leaflet. He did not find any difference among the three groups with regard to pain recurrence or days off work. The chiropractic group performed significantly better than the minimal intervention group at 4 weeks, but not at 3 months and the 1 year mark
▓ Triano et al. published a report in Spine 1995 comparing SMT vs education programme. He noted greater improvement in pain and activity tolerance in the SMT group
▓ Other support comes mainly from journals on manipulative therapy, e.g. a prospective randomised trial in J Manipulative Physiol Ther 1992 compared TENS, SMT and massage or use of corset. The SMT group showed the greatest improvement at 3 weeks with regard to pain score, patient confidence, and improvement in lumbar flexion

4.11.2.10 Possible Mechanism of SMT (Author's View)

- The exact mechanism is unknown as written in most textbooks
- However, if the underlying neurophysiological principles (such as autogenic inhibition of skeletal muscles by the induction of Golgi tendon organ firing) work for strategies like PNF and muscle energy techniques (discussed in Sect. 4.2.5.7), there is no reason why proper stretching of paraspinal muscles with a knowledge of local muscular anatomy and fibre direction need not work for skeletal muscles of the spine, at least in theory

4.11.2.11 Limitations and Contraindications

- Infected field
- Haematoma/bleeding tendency
- Tumours
- Spinal instability and fractures
- Extreme osteoporosis
- Congenital insensitivity to pain
- Caution if congenital ligamentous laxity
- Pre-existing neurology
- Whenever unsure, perform investigations to rule out significant pathology first

4.11.2.12 The Future

- More research is needed to investigate the efficacy and mechanism of chiropractics
- In the author's own personal view, special caution is needed in performing SMT for the normally very mobile cervical spine to prevent damage to the underlying neural structures

4.11.3   Osteopathic Medicine

4.11.3.1   Brief History

- Originated by Andrew Taylor Still who was a physician, and the American School of Osteopathy was founded in 1892
- The word "*osteo*" means bone, "*pathos*" means suffer

4.11.3.2 Popularity

▦ In the USA, osteopathic medicine has generally received wide acceptance since the 1970s. Currently, osteopathic medicine is a recognised profession in all states of the USA

▦ There are 50,000 osteopathic physicians in the USA, with >20 colleges of osteopathic medicine

4.11.3.3 Licensing and Setting of Standards

▦ There are board examinations in the USA set by the National Board of Osteopathic Medical Examiners that have to be passed before licensing. The curriculum includes osteopathic manipulation therapy (OMT) and neuro-musculoskeletal medicine plus a stress on basic science, anatomy and physiology. A final but key element in the curriculum is the use of palpatory diagnosis (e.g. including teaching of trigger points)

4.11.3.4 Scope of Osteopathic Medicine

▦ As there is a stress on the fascia as the "origin" of dysfunction, many patients with diffuse pain and suspected myofascial pain syndrome are referred or volunteer to go to osteopathic practitioners themselves

▦ The reader can refer to the section on myofascial pain syndrome in Chap. 16

4.11.3.5 Basic Philosophy of Osteopathic Practice

▦ It is regarded as both a science and an art by osteopathic practitioners

▦ It is a science because throughout the past and present history since its inception, there is a great deal of research on the subject, including that by scientists and physiologists

▦ It is an art because it is based on very "natural" concepts such as its emphasis on the interplay between human structure and function, and the appreciation that the body has the ability to heal itself, that disease occurs when there is a disruption of the anatomy

4.11.3.6 Basic Philosophy of Osteopathic Manipulation

▦ Although the name osteopathy has the word "bone" in it, many manipulative strategies are based on the search for fascia as the cause of disease and the place to commence therapy. The aim of manipulation was to "release soft tissue and bone barriers affecting the circulation or neural function and the homeostatic mechanics of the body will do the rest"

- In short, mainly based on provision of adequate nutrition, and stressing the ideas of drainage and neural innervation, plus the importance of a normal anatomical and structural relationship

4.11.3.7 Goal of Modern Osteopathic Medicine (Using Musculoskeletal Pain as an Example)

- Stress on palpatory diagnosis and management, especially arising from the fascia
- Based on principles already mentioned
- Managing segmental dysfunction
- Promoting the natural healing potential of the body

4.11.3.8 Papers in Support of Osteopathic Manipulation Therapy

- There is support for some of the concepts put forward in osteopathy, e.g. the goal of neural facilitation (e.g. facilitation of spinal cord segments) and its associated physiological changes were confirmed by experiments and reported in J Neurophysiol and Am J Physiol

4.11.3.9 Limitations

- Some of the manipulation strategies are difficult in practice to understand for non-osteopathic physicians, since the selection is not based on a disease (such as what orthopaedists do when referring a patient to a physiotherapist), but by continuous feedback between the patient and the osteopathic practitioner to tackle the personalised somatic dysfunction, and assess the local and systemic response
- There is a relative lack of more clinical outcome-orientated research so far, which is needed to grant the profession further support

4.11.3.10 The Future

- Although there has been some scientific support for techniques like neural facilitation, there is a need for more clinically-orientated outcome studies
- Further research is eagerly awaited

General Bibliography

Garrett WE Jr (2000) Principles and Practice of Orthopaedic Sports Medicine. Lippincott Williams & Wilkins, Philadelphia

Atkinson K (2005) Physiotherapy in Orthopaedics, 2nd edn. Elsevier/Churchill Livingstone, UK

Selected Bibliography of Journal Articles

1. Putnam CA (1993) Sequential motions of body segments in striking and throwing skills: descriptions and explanations. J Biomechan 26 (Suppl 1):125–135
2. Sheth P, Laskowski ER et al. (1997) Ankle disk training influences reaction times of selected muscles in a simulated ankle sprain. Am J Sports Med 25(4):538–543
3. Baker M, Basmajian JV et al. (1977) Developing strategies for biofeedback – applications in neurologically handicapped patients. Phys Ther 57(4):402–408
4. Petersen SR, Haennel RG et al. (1989) The influence of high velocity circuit resistance training on VO2 max and cardiac output. Can J Sports Sci 14(3):158–163
5. Tesch PA, Dudley GA et al. (1990) Force and EMG signal patterns during repeated bouts of concentric and eccentric muscle actions. Acta Physiol Scand 138(3):263–271
6. Heng PA, Wong TT et al. (2006) Intelligent inferencing and haptic stimulation for Chinese acupuncture learning and training. IEEE Trans Inf Technol Biomed 10(1):28–41
7. Deal DN, Curl WW (2002) Ice reduces edema. A study of microvascular permeability in rats. J Bone Joint Surg Am 84A(9):1573–1578
8. Chiu TT, Hui-Chan CW et al. (2005) A randomized clinical trial of TENS and exercise for patients with chronic neck pain. Clin Rehab 19(8): 850–860

5 Principles of Assessment: A Holistic and Case-Based Approach

5.1   Introduction and Key Basic Principles

5.1.1   Introduction and Concept of a "Holistic Approach"

- Although there are dozens of books on physical assessment in orthopaedics, very few in fact tell the reader about the real "train of thought" that must go through the mind of the clinician when the patient comes for rehabilitation. Traditional books concentrate mainly on a cook-book type of regional approach to our skeletal system that has been taught for generations
- But we all know that our body does not work this way!
- Two of the chief functions of our musculoskeletal system are maintenance of posture and mobility. The body is not going to achieve this by seeing itself divided into isolated small regions as depicted in textbooks
- Our musculoskeletal system is controlled by a central nervous system (CNS) that controls not only muscle tone and sequence of firing, but also patterns of muscle firing
- The traditional way of teaching a regional approach works for medical students sitting for an examination. But it is less useful in real life. I prefer the "holistic approach" to physical assessment, which is much more appropriate
- In this chapter, we will first talk about principles, then three very common case scenarios for illustration follow. The answers to the cases are not given in point form, but in essay format to highlight the "train of thought". The author hopes the reader will excuse him for doing this

5.1.2   Key Principle 1

- Being an orthopaedic rehabilitation specialist, or physiatrist, or therapist, we need to think several steps ahead and not just examine the part that is injured
- We also need to concentrate on structures and areas that are of relevance to our present and future rehabilitation of the patient. To this end, a good knowledge of functioning anatomy and physiology is important

5.1.3   Key Principle 2

- When we assess injuries to the upper or lower limbs that are often seen in sports for example, it is essential for the whole kinetic chain to be assessed
- This is contrary to traditional texts on physical examination, when you were told how to examine each region. Our limb simply does not work in this fashion, our limbs work as a kinetic chain and each and every portion of the chain must be assessed
- To illustrate the importance of assessment and rehabilitation of the kinetic chain, there is a worked example in Case Number 3 in the Sect. 5.3, "Case-Based Approach"

5.1.4   Key Principle 3

- When a limb muscle is injured for instance, in addition to the whole kinetic chain, we need to know the status of the antagonist, e.g. is it injured, is it in spasm, etc.
- This has a strong bearing on the rehabilitation of the patient. Proper stretching of the injured muscle to regain flexibility cannot occur in the presence of an antagonist that is in spasm or not adequately relaxed

5.1.5   Key Principle 4

- We should never underestimate the effect of pain on the process of rehabilitation
- Although there is a whole chapter on pain management in this book (Chap. 15), it is very important to highlight that pain should not only be controlled, but controlled very early in the course of rehabilitation. This point has not been stressed enough in many texts
- The reasons are manifold. First, pain in the injured musculotendinous unit will cause muscle shutdown. The common example is a patient with a sprained knee with mild effusion and pain causing quadriceps shutdown. Wasting can occur promptly if pain is not properly dealt with
- Secondly, pain in one part of the kinetic chain will affect and hinder the rehabilitation of the whole kinetic chain
- Thirdly, persistent pain may cause our CNS to alter the pattern or sequence of firing of muscles, thus affecting our subsequent effort to retrain the synergists in order for the patient to regain adaptive movements to possible future injury. Recent literature support can be found

in an article entitled "Muscular activation patterns of healthy persons and low back pain patients performing a functional capacity evaluation test" (Fabian et al., Pathophysiology 2005)

5.1.6   Key Principle 5

■ The concept of muscular synergism was discussed in the last chapter of this book. Our body tends to adopt different kinds of strategies like "ankle" strategy or "hip" strategy, etc. in order to avoid perturbations to our gait and our posture. These adaptive strategies are even more important if our patient will resume contact sports in future

■ These different adaptive strategies that the body adopts to avoid injury (such as a fall when being struck by a tackle from behind in sports) depends on a pre-programmed pattern of firing of synergistic muscles that allows a particular strategy to be performed. Hence, to avoid re-injury to a sporty patient or the elderly, re-training of *all* the components of synergistic muscle groups is important

■ Examples of this concept will be given in Chap. 19 when we talk about preventing injuries and falls in the elderly

5.2   History Taking and Physical Examination

5.2.1   Principle 1: A Proper History Guides Us with What to Look for in Examination

■ Example 1: accurate description of the injury mechanism of, say, the knee can not only suggest what was injured (e.g. heard a pop during the incident suggesting ACL injury), but also the type of possible concomitant injury of either the knee or other parts of the kinetic chain (since the ACL can have different types of tear, as found in recent studies as opposed to old textbook descriptions, which state that there is only one or two mechanisms)

■ Example 2: in patients with more severe trauma, analysing the direction of the injurious force and the position of the body of the patient help predict the direction in which the energy dissipates, i.e. the direction and type of possible concomitant fractures or soft tissue injury. (In the case of fractures, knowing the detailed mechanism may allow one to predict concomitant injuries elsewhere at body parts not shown by the X-ray film showing the primary fracture lines)

5.2.2 The Two Faces of a Physical Sign (Principle of Careful Inspection)

▦ Example: just as the author pointed out in the companion volume of this book *Orthopaedic Traumatology, A Resident's Guide*, concerning two faces of a fracture, or a fracture reduction; to identify more subtle physical signs warrants more careful inspection from different planes or directions

5.2.2.1 Illustration of the Principle: Description of a Brand New Physical Sign

▦ The author coined this as "on-profile test" in carpal tunnel syndrome (CTS)
▦ Description is hereby made of a new physical sign which is itself an illustration of the point we just made
▦ To the author's knowledge, this physical sign has not been recorded or described before and the new name is now coined as above (Fig. 5.1, 5.2)

5.2.2.2 The On-Profile Test in Carpal Tunnel Syndrome

▦ The sign helps us to detect early muscle wasting in the setting of CTS
▦ In undergraduate days we were taught about the Tinel and Phalen test for the diagnosis of CTS

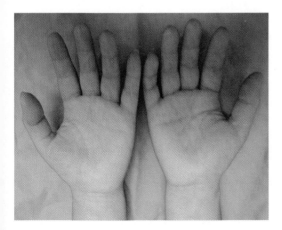

Fig. 5.1. When viewed in the antero-posterior direction, the small muscles of both hands appear rather unremarkable

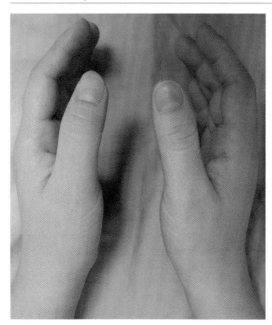

Fig. 5.2. The loss of the smooth contour of the thenar eminence of the left hand is obvious when both hands are re-positioned. When the author showed this to the patient, she immediately jumped up from her chair asking how it is possible that she did not notice the wasting for the past 2 years

- But I notice many a clinician misses the early muscle wasting that can be seen by positioning both hands of the patient in about 70–90° pronation (see Figs. 5.1, 5.2)
- It should be stressed that while late and severe muscle wasting is easy to see on inspection of the patient's hands in an AP direction, it is the detection of early muscle wasting that is most important in order for timely release of CTS to prevent extensive thenar wasting
- The on-profile test will aid the clinician in diagnosing early wasting, particularly of abductor pollicis brevis (APB) muscle – which if present, warrants surgical intervention rather than allowing the patient to adopt a "wait-and-see" approach. The author has also found more than 95% positive correlation between electro-physiological evidence of CTS and patients with hand numbness who have this physical sign (paper submitted for publication)

5.2.2.3 Importance of the New On-Profile Sign

■ A recent Canadian study showed a large amount of permanent pain and suffering, significant loss of work productivity, and considerable financial cost as a result of work-related CTS in an article entitled: "Carpal tunnel syndrome: cross-sectional and outcome study in Ontario workers" (Manktelow et al., J Hand Surg 2004)

■ Detection of early muscle wasting with the help of the new physical sign aids decision-making to persuade the patient to go for surgery instead of procrastination

5.2.3 Principle of "Feel and Move"

■ We have dealt with the importance of proper inspection or "look"

■ "Feel" or palpation is important in rehabilitation to distinguish between, say, dynamic vs static contractures; the degree of spasticity (e.g. grading and documenting R1 vs R2 in the Tardieu Scale in CP children); or pin-pointing the area of tenderness and location of trigger points, etc. One should always be gentle and take care not to hurt the patient

■ Documentation of joint ROM by goniometer is a necessity in rehabilitation. Muscle strength against gravity and with the effects of gravity negated can be tested during the documentation of ROM

5.2.4 The "Special Tests" in Orthopaedics

■ Bedside examinations in orthopaedics are full of many "special tests"

■ Their aims are mainly to reproduce the direction or orientation of the limb segment in order to reproduce the patient's symptoms

■ To fully understand these special tests, we need to:

  – Understand the sensitivity and specificity of each test in order to enhance the overall diagnostic accuracy of our bedside examination (see ensuing example on shoulder impingement as an illustration)

  – We need to use real-time investigations, be it, say, radiographic or arthroscopic, etc., to verify these traditional time-honoured special tests to check how good or accurate they are when diagnosing the condition. Example: use of functional MRI to verify the many different special tests in the physical examination of the shoulder

5.2.5   Example of the Combined Use of Signs for Diagnosing Impingement Syndrome (after McFarland)

■ The three main signs used by shoulder experts to diagnose shoulder impingement include Neer's sign, Hawkin's sign and "Painful Arc" sign

■ However, a knowledge of the level of sensitivity and specificity of each of these commonly used physical signs will improve our overall diagnostic accuracy at the bedside, viz.:

	Specificity	Sensitivity
Neer's sign	68%	69%
Hawkin's sign	71%	66%
Painful arc	73%	81%

5.2.6   Another Example – Diagnosis of Cuff Tears (after Murrell et al.)

■ Three most important signs:
  - Weakness on supraspinatus testing (empty can sign)
  - Weakness in external rotation
  - Positive impingement sign
■ All three positive: probability (p) of rotator cuff tear: 98%
■ Any two of the above + age >60: $p = 98\%$
■ Any two of the above + age <60: $p = 64\%$
■ Any one sign + age >70: $p = 76\%$
■ Any one sign + age 40–60: $p = 45\%$
■ Any one sign + age <40: $p = 12\%$

5.2.7   Importance of Serial Assessment

■ Assessment specific to a disorder have been described in the respective sections in this book
■ Gait analysis and applications as well as functional capacity assessment in worker's compensation cases will also be dealt with in separate chapters
■ Proper documentation and serial assessment by relevant tools pertinent to the disorder at hand are most important (e.g. physically the neurological deficit of SCI patients may change with time; and psychosocially, their goals may also change with it)

5.3   Case-Based Approach with Worked Examples

5.3.1   Introduction: Format of this Section

▪ In the following case-based approach, we will describe three different scenarios of sports injuries very frequently seen in your office

▪ The chief learning point of Case 1 is to stress the importance of a proper knowledge of sports mechanics besides a basic orthopaedic knowledge

▪ Case 2 serves to illustrate the concept you have just learned in Chap. 4 on the topic of core stability. This case was chosen since the concept of core stability may not be familiar to every orthopaedic surgeon

▪ Case 3 serves to illustrate an important point indicated in this chapter: namely, the importance of tackling the whole kinetic chain in sports injury of the extremity

▪ The proposed answer was written in an essay format instead of as a list of points, since it helps clarify the train of thought

5.3.2   Case 1: Shoulder Pain After Tennis

▪ Clinical scenario: a 40-year-old bank manager who is a keen amateur tennis player has been having increasing right shoulder pain in his dominant right upper limb. He has no neck pain. Describe your management of this patient, including the possible mechanisms and source(s) of his pain, assuming it was related to tennis

5.3.2.1 Proposed Answer

▪ We will start by analysing the functional anatomy and relevant biomechanics of the shoulder girdle, especially during abduction. The shoulder is a very mobile joint and thus prone to instability. Stability is offered by:

  – Static restraints mainly referring to the superior, middle and inferior glenohumeral ligaments. In addition, the coraco-acromial ligament also prevents superior subluxation of the humeral head

  – Presence of an intact labrum and the vacuum effect from negative pressure inside the capsule. Thus, a capsular tear or a breach of the rotator interval (between the supraspinatus and subscapularis muscles) for instance will make the shoulder unstable, the concept that dislocation always involves a Bankart lesion is obsolete as was pointed out in the most recent literature. The relative articular mismatch of the articulating surfaces is improved by the glenoid labrum. Thus, injury to the labrum as seen in superior labral anterior and posterior (SLAP) lesions in throwers by a peeling mechanism can also cause instability

- The dynamic restraints, which can be viewed functionally as consisting of two groups of muscles: the rotator cuff muscles (supraspinatus, infraspinatus, teres minor and subscapularis), and the scapula stabilisers (levator scapulae, rhomboids, serratus anterior, trapezius and pectoral muscles). Of the scapula stabilisers, the coordinated action of the trapezius, serratus anterior and levator are important in the necessary rotation needed to orientate the glenoid cavity for overhead sports

The act of shoulder abduction is usually initiated by the action of the supraspinatus, and then the main abduction force usually comes from the deltoid muscle. It is most important to note that proper abduction always involves rotation of the scapula; thus, there needs to be an intact rhythm of glenohumeral versus scapulothoracic movement and the ratio is usually 2:1. Without a stable base offered by the scapular stabilisers listed above, overhead activities will not be possible. This has been likened to a sea seal we see in television shows that tries to balance a ball on its nose. Another key point during abduction is the concerted effort of all four rotator cuff muscles plus the effect of the biceps long head, which acts as a humeral head depressor. It takes proper firing of all four rotator cuff muscles to centralise the humeral head inside the glenoid cavity, especially during the mid-abduction range. This is very important, as this so-called concavity-compression effect of the rotator cuff muscles will counteract the upward shear force of the deltoid. This is part of the key biomechanics involved in the act of abduction. Rotator cuff muscles act with force couples, and if one or more of the four muscles are not working, are torn, or weakened, the humeral head will not be exactly centralised in the glenoid cavity and impingement can occur in attempted overhead activity.

To understand impingement, which is essentially a clinical diagnosis, we must understand the local anatomy. Most people think that impingement is caused by one of the structures making up the supraspinatus outlet area namely: a hooked acromion, a thickened coraco-acromial ligament, osteoarthritis of the acromio-clavicular joint or even the distal clavicle. These cases do occur especially in the middle-aged patient (like ours) and can contribute to impingement pain and cuff tears and are referred to as "external impingement".

In the setting of overhead sports, a phenomenon called "internal impingement" can occur. The mechanism is due to repeated microtrauma and the hyper-angulation involved in overhead sports, causing rotator cuff weakness in particular and imbalance (e.g. repeated eccentric contraction of the supraspinatus, infraspinatus versus concomitant repeated concentric contraction of the subscapularis), with resultant element of shoulder instability and subluxation and causing internal posterosuperior glenoid impingement and even cuff tears despite the presence of a normal supraspinatus outlet (e.g. no hooked acromion, no osteoarthritis of the acromio-clavicular joint, etc.).

However, if one really wants to understand the pathogenesis of shoulder injury in tennis players, one needs to understand the biomechanics of the game of tennis itself, in addition knowing the basic biomechanics of the shoulder just discussed! One needs to know the following:

▓ The adaptations of professional and amateur tennis players are very different
▓ Difference between open stance versus square stance
▓ Analysis of body movement constituting the forehand serve, the proneness to injury with the high angular velocities of these serves, the increased chance of impingement during the overhead action and the potential for muscle imbalance and microtrauma between the eccentric firing of the supraspinatus and infraspinatus, versus the concentric firing of the subscapularis, especially in follow-through
▓ Analysis of the types of backhand serves, biomechanics involved and possible injuries
▓ Knowledge of techniques for both professional and amateur players to prevent injury to the shoulder viz.:
  – Physiological adaptations secondary to professional training and associated implications. A depression of the exercised shoulder is commonly found among highly trained professional athletes actively involved in overhead motions. This is caused by stretching of the shoulder elevating muscles, and generalised muscle hypertrophy of the racket-holding dominant upper extremity. There is reason to believe that this phenomenon further increases the chance of rotator cuff impingement, while the drooping of the

shoulder itself may predispose to thoracic outlet syndrome. This same phenomenon, however, is not seen in amateur tennis players. Other changes in the dominant upper limb include significantly greater range of motion of external rotation of the shoulder relative to the non-dominant arm, while there is frequently a deficit of internal rotation of the dominant arm. Prolonged microtrauma to the cuff frequently leaves the athlete with an overall deficit of the total range of motion; however, the overall demands of the game of tennis on the shoulder is such that it requires concentric work to stabilise the shoulder, with effective depression of the humeral head to prevent shoulder impingement. The added demands of forehand and back hand serves will now be discussed

- Open stance versus square stance technique: Comparisons have previously been made using a three-segment rigid body model in order to calculate the kinetics of the wrist, elbow and shoulder joints at the moment of impact. It was found that the open stance created lower resultant velocity of the racket at the moment of impact compared with the square stance, for professional tennis players and experienced amateurs. The largest component of the resultant joint torque was being generated by horizontal shoulder adductors, followed closely by varus torques on the elbow, and shoulder internal rotation torques. In addition, there was significantly greater peak shoulder internal rotation torques associated with the square stance than with the open stance. Overall, the peak upper extremity torques recorded were not dissimilar to those recorded for professional basketball pitchers and are of a magnitude that may well contribute to overuse injuries

- The tennis forehand and implications of high torque: it is common knowledge that the tennis forehand serve can produce enormously high angular velocity of the shoulder joint. Analysis using three-dimensional motion analysis revealed that these very high velocity tennis serves can be broken down and thought of as being made up of different segmental motions, including: trunk tilt, upper torso rotation, pelvis rotation, elbow extension, wrist flexion, and finally shoulder internal rotation during the final motion segment, which eventually involves sudden deceleration forces that can also harm the posterior structures of the shoulder. In addition, shoulder internal rotation torque was found to be greater in general for males, resulting in higher angular velocities attained relative to female professional athletes as expected

- The tennis backhand, and single versus double backhand: results of motion analysis of the single tennis backhand reveal the need for coordinated motion of the following body segments: hips, shoulder, upper arm, forearm, and hand/racket rotations. The same body segments are involved in the double backhand serve. Professional tennis players frequently produce comparable tennis racket horizontal velocities with either the double or single backhand techniques. The single backhand technique features a more rotated shoulder alignment than the double backhand technique upon completion of the backhand swing. During ball impact, the point of impact tends to be further in front, thus producing a slightly higher torque in the single backhand serve than the double backhand technique. The fact that the performance of professional players using the double backhand is comparable to the single backhand technique stems from the fact that players with the double backhand technique tend to delay the horizontal acceleration of the racket towards the ball, and thus are capable of comparable hitting motion at the time of ball impact

- Some coaching techniques for injury prevention: firstly, the motion analysis of professional athletes mentioned above can be recorded and played back to keen tennis players concerning the correct technique to adopt. However, other points worthy of note in injury prevention include: attention to the adequacy of knee bending since manoeuvres such as these are needed to exercise proper force transfer from the lower limbs through the arms during the tennis serve. If not performed properly, this will increase the demands on the shoulder to create the service speed needed and thus increase the chance of injury to the shoulder. Also, seemingly simple manoeuvres like ball tossing are in fact important, since if poorly done, this can result in excess spinal extension, encouraging shoulder impingement. Likewise, the likelihood of shoulder injury is increased if there is poor court positioning, which potentially can increase ground-stroke action and increase stress to the shoulder joint.

Analysis and differential diagnoses of pain in the shoulder in tennis players will now be discussed with regard to our patient present with pain. Owing to the complex anatomy of the shoulder complex that consists of four joints: sternoclavicular, acromio-clavicular, glenohumeral, and scapulothoracic articulations, analysis of pain arising from the shoulder girdle is not always straightforward. To complicate matters, we need to be mindful of the fact that pain can also be referred from the cervical spine, and other rarer causes like thoracic outlet syndrome, which was discussed previously. Previous literature analysis on shoulder pain in tennis players showed that in fact there are two most common causes that produce shoulder pain, namely the impingement syndrome and glenohumeral instability.

Tennis players with impingement syndrome typically present with pain during overhead strokes and serves. Bedside Neer's and Hawkin's test, we can consider that the use of the impingement test involving almost immediate pain relief on injection of anaesthetic to the subacromial area is often diagnostic if the diagnosis is unsure. Tennis players with instability present with pain and a sensation of the shoulder "slipping". Dislocation is rare. Most cases turn out to be in fact a form of internal impingement caused by fatigue of the rotator cuff muscles, particularly the supraspinatus and infraspinatus, thus causing difficulty in centralising the humeral head in position during overhead activity. An associated disruption of the normal ration of glenohumeral to scapulothoracic movement is not uncommon, causing further loss of sports performance, poor serve velocity, and easy fatigability.

Finally, some "external" factors that can contribute to the shoulder pain of our middle-aged patient who is involved in computer work potentially include:

- Technique and training errors: these have just been discussed above, including the methods of prevention of injury
- Improper equipment: notice that the game of tennis involves open kinetic chain activity of the upper limb. This, together with the high velocities encountered, can cause injury to the whole mobile kinetic chain, not just the shoulder. Thus, the use of improper equipment, like improper size of the racket, will increase the chance of injury to, say, the wrist and elbow as well. Other possible external factors that are sports-related include the playing surface, environment warm-up exercises, etc.
- An example of an external factor that is job related is that by the nature of his job as a computer worker, he frequently protracts his sca-

pula during work, and lack of exercise to the other scapular stabilisers that are essential for overhead sports can predispose to an abnormal glenohumeral to scapulothoracic rhythm

5.3.3   Case 2: Back Pain in a Golfer

▓ Your old friend, aged 48, who is a successful businessman, is a keen amateur golfer. He told you that his health has been good all along, and lately he has been playing many rounds of golf in preparation for next month's amateur golfing tournament. He complains to you of increasing back pain not radiating to the lower limbs that seems to get worse each time he finishes practicing his favourite sport. Discuss the management of this patient, assuming that his back pain is sports-related

5.3.3.1 Proposed Answer

Our patient is a middle-aged sedentary amateur golfer. He has been experiencing back pain hindering daily activities that may well be related to golfing, although other more serious causes of back pain must be ruled out. The following depicts the management of our patient.

Injury to the lumbar spine in fact ranks first among different possible injuries in amateur golfers, ranks second place in professional golfers and is of common occurrence. Other common injuries include rotator cuff injury of the shoulder, as well as elbow and wrist injuries.

There are a number of general mechanisms whereby golfing can cause musculoskeletal injuries including:

▓ Those caused by external forces such as hitting a stone
▓ Those due to overuse especially in the professional golfer
▓ Those due to poor swing techniques (which is commoner among amateur golfers than professional ones)
▓ The use of improper equipment, such as using clubs with an unsuitable grip or weight for the golfer

Obviously, predisposing back problems may well be triggered or exacerbated by the shear, rotatory and compressive forces to which the thoracic and lumbar spine is subjected during the golf swing. Previous studies found that the above-mentioned forces to the spine can be as great as eight times the individual body weight. In general therefore, the risk factors for injury in golf include age, improper equipment, poor swing mechanics, pre-existing pathologies before sports participation, inadequate warm-up, and low level of body fitness (with inadequate strength, flexibility, and endurance levels).

The golf swing can be divided into four stages: takeaway, acceleration, impact and follow-through. "Takeaway" involves movement of the club as a backswing; "acceleration" commences at the end of backswing when the club is brought down with increasing force and speed; "impact" occurs when the club hits the ball; while "follow-through" spans the period from the moment of impact to the completion of the golf swing.

One must understand the biomechanics of motion involved in the four stages before one can discuss aspects of prevention and treatment of injuries to the back. In the takeaway phase: there is rotation of the spine, hips and shoulders. During acceleration and impact: the forces and strains concentrate more on the elbows, wrist, and hand. Meanwhile, the arms and trunk continue to rotate back towards the ball with unlocking of the wrist. The follow-through phase involves spine and hip rotation, as well as some degree of hyper-extension of the cervical and lumbar spine.

Next we analyse the possible mechanisms of injury to the back during the golf swing. The motions just described during the golf swing result in forces that include lateral bending, shear, torsion and compressive forces. This is because the lumbar spine side-bends, rotates, compresses, flexes and hyper-extends during the swing. In addition, the shear forces are especially significant in amateur as opposed to professional golfers.

In contrast to professional golfers who have a smooth swing associated with coordinated muscle firing, amateur golfers tend to have a varied stance that leans away from the ball at impact and follow-through. This causes a "reverse C" posture of the lumbar spine at the end of the follow-through phase, which can result in increased torque on the vertebrae causing injury to the back.

As for the nature of injuries suffered by the back, commonly encountered conditions include:

- Lumbar disc herniations (herniated nucleus pulposus) with sciatica associated with radiating leg pain
- Lumbosacral back sprain, which is the most common type of possible back injury that can occur during activity with local soft tissue tenderness and relieved by rest, but without radiologic abnormalities
- Posterior facet joint degeneration characterised by pain being exacerbated by back extension and side-bending on the affected side

- In addition, owing to significant torque being produced during coiling and uncoiling of the lumbar spine, this may exacerbate and create symptoms in the presence of underlying spondylosis and/or spondylolisthesis. Severe cases may even cause fracture at the pars interarticularis, causing spondylolisthesis with the danger of nerve root impingement

- Compressive vertebral collapse in patients with pre-existing osteoporosis of the axial skeleton have also been described due to the increase in axial loading to the lumbar spine

- Lastly, improper techniques with significant rotatory forces as in over-swing can injure the thoracic spine as well, besides the lumbar spine

In summary, the anatomical structures that can be injured include muscle sprains, the osteoligamentous complex, the facet joints and injury to the intervertebral discs. The location of injury may involve either the lumbar or thoracic spine, or both.

Now that we have analysed the biomechanics of the swing and injury mechanics to the back; we can discuss practical aspects of management. Management of the patient at hand starts with a thorough history and physical examination. We have to look for any "red flag" signs that are suggestive of more serious underlying pathology to the lumbar spine, such as non-mechanical type of persistent back pain, the presence of associated neurological deficit, sphincter disturbances, etc. If red flag signs are absent, and especially if it is deemed likely that the pain is related to the game of golf, then the principle of management will be as follows.

Assessment of this patient starts with questions concerning how he performs his game of golf: i.e. whether a coach is available, the adequacy of warm-up exercises, any practice in the driving ranges, have a look at his equipment to see if properly selected, and most important of all is the step-by-step analysis of how he performs his golf swing. The patient should be asked about any changes in the frequency of golfing and use of new or novel techniques. This is because poor swing mechanics is the most frequent cause of back pain in amateur golfers. To this end, the patient can be shown pictures of serial manoeuvres of a proper golf swing so that he can compare with his own technique. We can also ask him to demonstrate his typical swing if there is enough space and a golf club is available in the clinic. One commonly seen form of poor swing mechanics is the so called "over-swing", whereby the spine is subjected to too much rotatory force.

After this initial analysis, it will be obvious that in order to prevent and treat back injuries related to a game of golf, the basic guiding principles include the training of flexibility, strength, and general fitness. Flexibility is essential since as mentioned, the swing involves flexion, rotatory, and extension moments of the lumbar spine; training of fitness can be effected by endurance exercise and cardiovascular conditioning exercises. Warm-up exercises that can include stretching, and driving range drills performed at around half the swing speed are useful to prevent injuries to the back. Strength training is of utmost importance and at this juncture, we would like to introduce the concept of "core stability" training.

Core stability is of paramount importance in both the prevention and treatment of back and lower limb injuries in a game of golf. The "core" is composed of the lumbar vertebrae, the pelvis and hip joints, together with the active and passive structures that either produce or restrict movements of these motion segments. "Core stability" refers to the ability of the lumbopelvic hip complex to prevent buckling and to return to equilibrium without perturbation. This is mainly dependent on the active structures consisting of contractions or co-contractions of the muscles, since the stiffness of the lumbopelvic hip complex has been shown in the past to be mainly dependent on the active stabilisers for its stiffness as opposed to passive stabilisers. Core stability is also dynamic, hence the local anatomy must be able to continually adapt to changing postures and loading conditions in order to maintain the integrity of the vertebral column, thus providing a stable base for the extremities.

Contraction of the muscular elements of the core can increase the stiffness of the hip and trunk. To achieve stability, not only is the ability of co-contraction of antagonistic trunk muscles required (in response to anticipated spinal loading), but also, the contraction of the hip and trunk muscles must be coordinated as prolonged co-contraction is also detrimental and may lead to excess compressive loading to the system. Another important factor underscoring the importance of core stability is that although normal trunk muscle reflexes are automatic and may stiffen the spine to loading, this system tends to have an innate neuromuscular delay and may offer inadequate protection in the face of a sudden spinal load, thus underscoring the importance of training in core stability.

It is important to realise that the muscular elements of the core contribute to stability by means of three mechanisms: intra-abdominal pressure, spinal axial compressive force, as well as hip and trunk muscle stiffness.

- Increased intra-abdominal pressure can be effected by simultaneous contraction of the diaphragm and the pelvic floor muscles, or by abdominal muscles, particularly the transversus abdominus muscle
- Increased axial load can be effected by muscle co-contractions of the trunk extensor and flexor muscle groups
- The large, superficial muscles of the hip and trunk are architecturally best suited to produce movement and increase hip and trunk stiffness to counteract destabilising forces during functional activities. Anatomically, the chief muscles that function in the sagittal plane include the rectus abdominis, transversus abdominis, erector spinae, multifidus, and hamstrings

The rectus abdominus, and multifidus together with tonic contraction of the transversus can produce increases in intra-abdominal pressure. The gluteus maximus is important to help transfer lower extremity forces to the trunk. Chief lateral muscles of the hip and trunk that function in the frontal plane include gluteus medius, gluteus minimus and quadratus lumborum. These glutei help maintain a level pelvis in closed chain motion. Co-contraction of bilateral quadratus lumborum help stiffens the spine. Chief medial muscles acting in the frontal plane include adductor magnus, adductor longus and brevis, and pectineus. Their role in core stability is lesser than that of the aforementioned muscles. Trunk rotation is provided for by internal and external oblique muscles, the iliocostalis lumborum and the multifidus. Bilateral activation of these muscles also aids core stability by increase in intra-abdominal pressure.

Besides the training of core stability, other methods of injury prevention include ensuring correct techniques and swing mechanism. The golf swing can be analysed by a professional golf instructor. The coach or instructor can correct the deficiencies in techniques to prevent undue stresses on specific anatomic regions (in this case the spine), and also prevent overuse injuries. In addition, equipment selection is essential; the patient's golf club should be of proper length and weight to enhance swing mechanics. Either excessive velocity and improper weight of the golf club can create high forces that can cause injury to the back and the shoulder.

In summary, golf is a demanding activity that requires both flexibility and strength to swing the club correctly and consistently. The mainstay of management of our patient therefore should include stretching exercises for the back, the lower and upper extremities, and flexibility exercises for both the thoracic and lumbar regions to prevent the effects of rotational stresses on the spine. The importance of core stability and strengthening of the muscles essential for core stability cannot be over-emphasised. Strength training of the hips and lower extremities is also an essential component in addition to core training since they provide much power to the swing. Adequacy and maintenance of the level of endurance fitness and cardiovascular conditioning is important, and a programme of jogging or cycling can prepare the patient for an 18-hole game. Finally, the use of proper warm-up exercises such as walking, practice swings on the driving range as well as the procurement and use of proper equipment will go a long way to making this game enjoyable yet safe for our patient.

5.3.4   Case 3: Knee Pain after Jogging

■ A young 29-year-old nurse working at a local hospital comes to your orthopaedic clinic complaining of increasing knee pain after jogging. She has been keen to keep fit since high school and likes to work out in the gym. For the past year, she has been jogging regularly, but the frequency has increased significantly lately as she wants to lose weight. She complains having increasing anterior knee pain over the past 3 months, made worse by negotiating stairs

■ Outline your management of this patient, assuming it is sports-related, with emphasis on the physical assessment

5.3.4.1 Proposed Answer

Our patient is a young lady who has recently been involved in excessive running several times a week to which she is probably unaccustomed. The fact that her anterior knee pain gets worse on getting up and down stairs is typical of pain of patellofemoral origin. A proper understanding of the underlying biomechanics is essential before proper treatment can be administered.

Relevant biomechanics of the tibiofemoral joint: during the last few degrees of knee extension, there is a "screw-home" mechanism. This represents an obligatory lateral rotation of the tibia that accompanies final knee joint extension, which is neither voluntary nor produced by muscle forces. This is a coupled motion, and involves rotation around the longitudinal axis of the tibia and provides more stability to the knee. What happens is that at the final 30° of extension, the shorter lateral tibial plateau/femoral condyle pair completes the rolling–gliding motion before the longer medial side articular surfaces. As extension continues, the longer medial plateau continues its roll and glide motion anteriorly. The outcome is lateral rotation of the tibia on the femur. Part of this motion in the final 5° of extension is due to the increased tension of the knee ligaments, bringing the knee into the locked position. To initiate knee flexion from the locked position, the knee must be unlocked. Thus, the laterally rotated tibia cannot simply flex, but must medially rotate concomitantly as knee flexion is initiated. This automatic rotation occurs in both the weight-bearing and non-weight-bearing knee. During weight-bearing, the freely moving femur medially rotates upon the fixed tibia.

Relevant biomechanics of the patellofemoral joint: the patella is the largest sesamoid bone in the body. It has several functions, but the most important lies in increasing the moment arm of the quadriceps tendon particularly at knee flexion angles of around 45–60°. This not only increases the efficiency of the quadriceps pull, but also helps to diminish the rapidly rising patellofemoral joint forces during knee flexion. This type of knee flexion angle (and thus the high patellofemoral forces) is usually seen on ascending and descending stairs as opposed to casual walking; thus, most patients with patellofemoral pain have aggravation of their pain on negotiating stairs, like our patient. The high patellofemoral joint forces on knee flexion when climbing stairs can reach as high as several times that of the body weight of the patient. There are several adaptations to accommodate these high stresses in the normal knee. It should be remembered that during full knee extension, there is only a minimal contact area of the patella with the articular trochlea. Luckily, as the knee flexes from 0–90°; the patella contact area also increases. This increase in contact area, together with increased compressive forces, acts to minimise patellofemoral joint stresses until about 90° of knee flexion, as the contact area diminishes again beyond 90° of knee flexion.

It should also be noted that the patellofemoral joint is not a very congruent joint. In the normal patellofemoral joint, the medial facet bears the brunt of the compressive force. Mechanisms exist to minimise the patellofemoral joint stresses on the patella in general, and upon the medial facet specifically. During full knee extension, there is minimal compressive force on the patella and no compensatory mechanism is needed. As the knee joint flexes, the area of contact gradually increases to spread out the stresses. As the knee flexes to between 30 and 70° of flexion, the magnitude of the contact force is highest at the thick cartilage of the medial facet of the patella under-surface near the central ridge. This articular cartilage is among the thickest hyaline cartilage in the human body, and can better tolerate the high local joint stresses. Also, within this range of knee flexion; the patella exerts its greatest effect as a pulley, maximising the moment arm of the quadriceps. Beyond 90°, the patella is no longer the only structure contacting the femoral condyle, since at this angle the quadriceps tendon contacts the femoral condyles and assists in dissipating the compressive forces on the patella.

Effect of hip, foot and vastus medialis: several common reasons or causes that may predispose to increased patella compression forces include a tight iliotibial band, large Q angle (as in females, patients with genu valgum, or patients with femoral anteversion with lateral tibial torsion), and relative vastus medialis weakness. In addition, foot hyperpronation is frequently associated with patellofemoral pain, particularly in adolescents. Each factor will now be discussed:

- Any alteration in the alignment that increases the Q angle is widely thought to increase the lateral force on the patella and may predispose or worsen anterior knee pain. This can be harmful because an increase in this lateral force may increase the compression of the lateral patella on the lateral lip of the femoral sulcus. In the presence of a large enough lateral force, the patella may in fact subluxate or even dislocate. Common causes of an increased Q angle have just been mentioned

- The presence of a tight iliotibial band can limit the mobility of the patella and limit its ability to shift medially during knee flexion, contributing to increased stress under the lateral patella facet. When the iliotibial band moves posteriorly with knee flexion, it exerts an even greater pull on the patella, which results in a progressive lateral tilting as the knee flexion increases, which causes further loading to the lateral patella facet

- Identification of excessive foot pronation is also important because pronation at the subtalar joint is associated with internal tibial rotation; this increases the Q angle as well as laterally tracking the patella. McConnell found that in adolescents and young adults, subtalar pronation rather than the Q angle was the single most important factor associated with patellofemoral pain. If hyper-pronation is diagnosed (sometimes a clue can be seen from the patient's footwear), supination exercises are prescribed to increase the awareness of the foot position. Orthotics to improve foot posture is also useful, especially in runners. However, just resorting to supination exercises and corrective footwear is not enough; we need to find any underlying forces. An example will be for instance: we need to correct a tight gastrocnemius muscle because this tightness may limit ankle dorsiflexion. The movement will be translated to the subtalar joint, increasing foot pronation

- Vastus medialis obliquus (VMO) is an important portion of the quadriceps musculature as it counteracts dynamically the lateral force or pull of the patella created by the Q angle, although the importance of the static medial restraints like the medial patellofemoral ligament should not be forgotten. In the past, there have been many attempts to selectively strengthen this muscle (VMO) by therapists to tackle patients with anterior knee pain who have a weakness of the VMO, or delayed firing of the VMO. However, it should be remembered that both portions of the VMO, like other components of the quadriceps, are innervated by the femoral nerve, making preferential recruitment of the VMO in fact difficult. More realistic training to strengthen the VMO will probably involve biofeedbacks. In addition, taping of the patella is employed to reduce pain and enhance VMO activity. Patella subluxation if not severe, can be corrected by firm taping from the lateral aspect of the patella medially. The addition of extra tape can also help tackle any tilting, However, some studies seem to indicate that the improvement in the patellofemoral after taping may be due more to the quadriceps strengthening rather than the act of taping itself and the high success rate of taping reported by McConnell is not always reproducible in other physiotherapy centres

After obtaining a careful history from our patient, we will pay particular attention to the following during physical examination: we start off with an assessment of the lower limb alignment, look for any genu valgum, check the Q angle, and look for evidence of squinting of the patellae –

the presence of which necessitates ruling out any torsional anomalies like excessive femoral anteversion, tibial torsion, or feet hyper-pronation. The foot-wear of the patient is inspected. Excess wear of the medial heels is suggestive of excess feet pronation (unless she is wearing a new pair of shoes). A quick assessment to check for any generalised ligamentous laxity will be performed. Local examination includes checking for any quadriceps wasting with particular attention being paid to the bulk of the VMO. Other local examinations include checking for the integrity of the extensor mechanism of the knee, the site of any local tenderness, say, at the retinaculum or the patella under-surface. The patella glide and tilt test should be performed. Gently bring the knee to flexion from full extension and look for the patella tracking.

Of relevance to our therapist includes: looking for tightness of the rectus femoris, iliotibial band, hamstrings, and gastrocnemius. The reason for the identification of tight gastrocnemius and iliotibial band was mentioned. Tight hamstrings increase midstance knee flexion during running and create extra loading to the knee extensor mechanism. Also, increased flexion of the knee requires increased dorsiflexion of the ankle to produce a plantigrade foot. If these cannot be accommodated at the ankle joint, the movement may be transferred to the subtalar joint, resulting in increased foot pronation with its consequences.

Main treatment principles for our patient include:

- Symptomatic control with relative rest
- Avoiding painful activities
- Conditioning the other parts of the kinetic chain, the opposite lower limb and upper body
- Identification of the cause of the anterior knee pain
- If any of the above named muscles (iliotibial band, rectus femoris, gastrocnemius, hamstrings) are tight, one may proceed to stretching exercises. Stretching should also be done to the tight lateral peripatellar structures
- McCornell taping is frequently tried, and may even correct cases with an element of patella subluxation or tilting on physical examination or radiographic examination (using the Merchant's and Laurin's views)
- Strengthening the quadriceps in general is important, but training specific to strengthening the VMO, such as the use of biofeedback, is useful. Also, since most of the fibres of the VMO originate from the

tendon of the adductor magnus, contraction of the adductors during knee extension facilitates VMO activity. Also, pain during exercise should be avoided because pain has an inhibitory effect on muscle contraction and can result in muscle atrophy. Besides the adductors, strengthening the gluteus medius is important because it causes a concurrent reduction in the activity of the iliotibial band. It should be mentioned in passing that stresses across the patellofemoral joint can be reduced with closed kinetic chain exercises that utilise co-contraction of the quadriceps, hamstrings and gastrocnemius muscle

- Later on, a graduated running programme can be initiated, sometimes preceded by water sports and water walking
- A proper maintenance programme should be adhered to

Lastly, it should also be emphasised that activity reduction is of utmost importance; but this does not mean that our sporty patient needs to give up her training all together. However, most patients with anterior knee pain who reduce their activity tend to have a higher success rate than those patients who did not

General Bibliography

Insall J, Scott N (2001) Surgery of the Knee, 3rd edn. Churchill Livingstone, Edinburgh

Ip D (2006) Orthopaedic Traumatology – A Resident's Guide. Springer, Berlin Heidelberg New York

Fu FH, Stone DA (2001) Sports Injuries, 2nd edn. Lippincott Williams and Wilkins, Philadelphia

Roberts PJ (2001) Clinical Examination for FRCS. The Institute of Orthopaedics (Oswestry) Publishing Group, UK

Selected Bibliography of Journal Articles

1. Sonnery-Cottet B, Edwards TB et al. (2002) Results of arthroscopic treatment of posterosuperior glenoid impingement in tennis players. Am J Sports Med 30:2, p 227–232
2. Priest JD (1988) The shoulder of the tennis player. Clin Sports Med 7(2):387–402
3. Schmidt-Wiethoff R, Rapp W et al. (2004) Shoulder rotation characteristics in professional tennis players. Int J Sports Med 25(2):154–158
4. Bahamonde RE, Knudson D (2003) Kinetics of the upper extremity in the open and square stance tennis forehand. J Sci Med Sport 6(1):88–101
5. Fleisig G, Nicholls R et al. (2003) Kinetics used by world class tennis players to produce high-velocity serves. Sports Biomech 2(1):51–64
6. Reid M, Elliott B (2002) The one- and two-handed backhands in tennis. Sports Biomech 1(1):47–68

7. McCarrol JR, Rettig AC, Shelbourne KD (1990) Injuries in the amateur golfer. Phys Sport Med 18(3):122–126
8. Metz JP (1999) Managing golf injuries. Phys Sports Med 27(7)
9. McCornell J (1996) Management of patellofemoral problems. Manual therapy 1:60–66
10. Grelsamer RP, McCornell J (1998) Conservative management of patellofemoral problems. Aspen, Maryland, p 119–136
11. Hungerford DS, Barry M (1979) Biomechanics of the patellofemoral joint. Clin Orthop 144:9–15
12. Murrell GA, Walton JR (2001) Diagnosis of rotator cuff tears. Lancet 357, 9258:769–770

6 Assistive Technology

Contents

6.1   Introduction

6.1.1   Definition of Assistive Technology

▧ Assistive technology (AT) includes any item, piece of equipment, or product system, be it commercially acquired or off the shelf, modified or customised, that is used to increase, maintain, or improve the functional capabilities of individuals with disabilities
("Technology-Related Assistance for Individuals with Disabilities Act", USA)

6.1.2   Author's Viewpoint

▧ The last sentence might well be modified to read thus: "assistive technology includes functional capabilities of individuals with impairments so as to minimise their disability (if any) in the community

▧ The reason for the proposed amendment should be very obvious to the reader after reading Chap. 1 of this book

▧ To recapitulate a little, our job as a team of health-care workers is to minimise the effect of the impairment of our patient, so that he or she is no longer being "disabled" by the impairment. This is done via the combined care of the physician; use of AT devices; environmental modifications like lift, housing or vehicle designs although aspects of housing design will depend on the local government. A point we should never miss is the accessibility and ease of referral to the AT centre itself

6.1.3   Question of Accessibility

▧ This is an important issue

  – No matter how good the AT team or how advanced our technology, if patients with impairment who require our help do not know about the service or the service is unavailable to patients who do not live in the city but in less accessible areas, this will defeat our purpose

  – Hence the importance of continuous quality evaluation projects to ensure easy booking, referral and ready accessibility of our AT service. One such continuous quality improvement project is under way in the US in Massachusetts, other AT centres should follow this good example in the author's view

6.1.4   Model on Which AT Works

■ Most AT teams work on the model proposed by Cook et al. (1995) called the Human Assistive Technology Model (HAAT), which explains the interaction between humans (our patient) and the environment

6.1.5   Elements of HAAT

■ The human–technology interface: e.g. use of head control or breath-control switches by a high SCI patient
■ The processor: acting to relay information from the human–technology interface. Transmission of information is commonly effected via:
  – Infrared radiation
  – Radiofrequency
  – Ultrasound waves
■ The activity output: a definite action performed, e.g. surfing web pages, switching on the lights, or television
■ The environmental interface or platform: has to have an adjustment and feedback role of the action or function so rendered

6.1.6   Scope of Patients Served by AT Centre

■ Very broad, if one refers back to the definition of AT. In practice, patients in need of only simple aids and walkers are infrequently referred to formal AT centres
■ Prosthesis and orthosis: will be discussed in other chapters
■ The related subject of "architectural accessibility" will be discussed in the appendix of the current chapter

6.2   Environmental Control and Modification Units

6.2.1   Environmental Control Units

■ Patients with impairments frequently make use of electronic aids to perform activities of daily living (ADL) and other daily functions like surfing the internet, this is done through the environmental control unit (ECU) established by the AT team with suitable controls tailor-made to the patient (frequently depending on what type of residual function he or she still possesses) and acting via interfaces as stipulated by the HAAT model just mentioned (Figs. 6.1, 6.2)

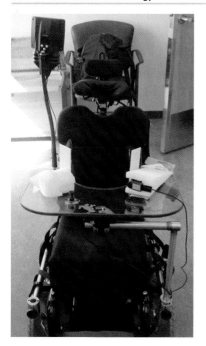

Fig. 6.1. Wheelchair tailor-made for a child with generalised muscle weakness. Note the small switches on the transparent table for the control of the environmental control unit

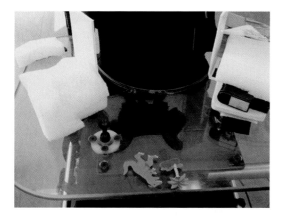

Fig. 6.2. Close-up of the switch for the environmental control unit

6.2.2   The Assistive Technology Team

- Team members include:
  - Patient
  - Family members
  - Care-taker
  - Occupational therapist
  - Physiotherapist
  - Rehabilitation engineer
  - Orthopaedist
  - Orthotists
  - Others, e.g. social workers, speech therapist, ENT surgeons, computing experts, AT provider's company's support staff, etc.
- Notice that:
  - The patient is the most important member of the team, since the team members all have him in mind during meetings, as the technology should be tailor-made to fit the patient and not the reverse
  - In the setting of the patient being a child, the patient + family will be viewed as a unit and become the most important, since if the family members do not exercise the team's recommendations, this will defeat the whole purpose

6.2.3   Overall Goal of the AT Team

- To provide necessary aids, equipment, or technology that may be needed to reduce the effect that the physical impairment has on the patient
- The patient always forms the centre of the team effort

6.2.4   Key Concept

- Every member of the AT team should remember that the technology should be adjusted to fit the patient (no matter how difficult or labour-intensive) and not manipulate the patient to adjust to the technology

6.2.5   Steps in Patient Assessment

- History:
  - Diagnosis and severity of the pathology
  - Whether the condition is going to be static or likely to progress is important, if unsure talk to the operating surgeon or clinician in charge of the patient
  - Expectations and goals of the patient

- Past medical health and previous functional status
- Examination with emphasis on:
  - Musculoskeletal examination
  - Neurological examination
  - Level of cognition and perception
  - Communicative skills of the patient
    (P.S. If the patient has very limited communicative skills available (e.g. locked-in syndrome), careful assessment needs to be made of the "kinds of access" that are available, e.g. even flicker of movement of the thumb, eye movements, etc.)
- Other aspects of physical examination:
  - Vision
  - Hearing
  - Cardiopulmonary status
- Deciding and setting up the use of controls and switches of the ECU
  - Deciding which movement is the most reproducible given our patient's impairment
  - If more than one method or reproducible movement is available, preference is usually given to the one preferred by the patient
  - Challenging scenarios: no reproducible UL or LL movement, triggers include, e.g. eyebrow motion, head-pointing device, chin controls, breath-controls, etc.
- Decide the rest of the components of the ECU: i.e. processor and type of signal relay, type of switches, etc.
- Practice the use of the ECU at the AT centre and make any necessary adjustments; if special equipment is needed, call in the company product technicians to help
- Home visit advisable by the team to assess modifications needed
- Try out the ECU at home by the patient
- Settle any concomitant problems that may exist, e.g. finance, WC application

6.2.6   Common Impairments that Require ECU
- Especially high dependency patients like:
  - High cervical cord C1–C4 lesions
  - Other SCI patients
  - Other neuromuscular disorder cases, e.g. multiple sclerosis, cerebral palsy, traumatic brain injury, etc.

6.2.7   Examples of Devices Provided by ECU

■ Communication devices (see Sect. 6.3 on alternative augmentative communication)

■ Assistive listening devices and hearing aids (see **Sect. 6.3**)

■ Electronic aids of daily living, e.g. text-to-screen readers, alternative keyboards and mice, head pointing devices, voice recognition software (see Fig. 6.3), screen magnification software

■ Impaired mobility will be discussed shortly, mainly concentrate on wheelchair technology

■ ADL aids for those less impaired

6.2.8   More Challenging Pathways of Access

Since physical impairments and severity do vary a lot among patients, the continuous search for access methods is an active on-going process

Examples of newer use of access pathways include MMG (mechanomyogram) – see Figs. 6.4, 6.5, eye-tracking, and push button sensors. Whenever possible visual/sensory feedback needs to be provided to make the patient improve the handling of the environmental control systems

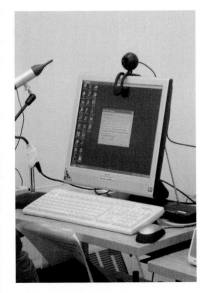

Fig. 6.3. Computer with built-in speech-to-text software

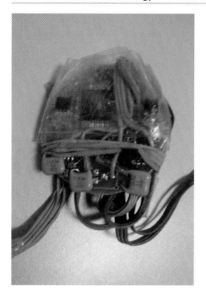

Fig. 6.4. Electronic equipment for mechanomyogram, being used here for a child with a forearm amputation

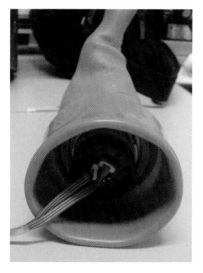

Fig. 6.5. The mechanical contraction of the residual stump muscles of the upper limb is transformed into EMG signals to operate the Otto-bock wrist unit, as shown here

6.2.9   Improving the Home Environment, ADL and IADL

6.2.9.1   ADL Performance by ECU

The most important function the ECU can serve in the author's viewpoint is calling for help via a switch triggered by, say, head control, text telephone, head-free, intercom, or other devices

This is especially important since even seemingly "stable" high SCI patients can suffer all of a sudden from autonomic disturbances

▪ Suitably placed processor and effectors can aid the patient in other ADL, e.g.:
  – Switching on the television
  – Flip over pages of a textbook (see Fig. 6.6)
  – Preparation of meals
  – Cleaning companies can be called via the Internet to perform more demanding tasks like cleaning and vacuuming
  – ADL aids for feeding, etc. will be discussed in Chap. 12 on SCI rehabilitation

6.2.9.2   IADL Performance by ECU

▪ The majority of instruments of daily living (IADL) can be replaced by the use of computers and surfing the internet
▪ Examples:
  – Purchasing goods and food

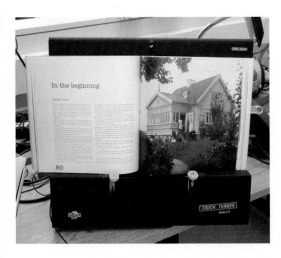

Fig. 6.6. Machine to help the patient to flip over the pages of a book

- Paying bills
- Internet banking
- Tele-conference with local and overseas colleagues
- Text phones for impaired hearing
- Placing orders for effecting repairs of the premises
- Even doing assignments and earning degrees by voice recognition software and distance learning

6.3   Alternative and Augmentative Communication Devices

6.3.1   What is AAC?
■ AAC = alternative augmentative communication
■ Communication systems can be non-electronic (e.g. papers, pen) or electronic
■ Electronic devices can be equipped with sound to arouse others' attention, but requires regular charging. Commonly used AAC therefore involves "voice output" AAC

6.3.2   Voice Output AAC
■ The "voice" can either be digitised or synthesised. The former resembles tape recorder function, stored in microchips. The latter are essentially microprocessor programs obeying set built-in rules of pronunciation, can be customised and versatile (can have different language settings)

6.3.3   Which Group(s) of Orthopaedic Patients Need AAC?
■ AAC are more commonly indicated with patients with medical disorders like cerebrovascular accident
■ Some patients with conditions like total body cerebral palsy with difficulties in communication may require AAC

6.4   Wheelchair Technology

6.4.1   Assessing the Patient
■ Type of musculoskeletal disorder
■ Emphasis on neurological and musculoskeletal systems assessment, besides cardiopulmonary screening

- Likelihood of disease to progress
- Does the patient need a manual WC or electric one or both?

6.4.2 Assessing the Environment
- Housing design
- Lift accessibility
- Does the furniture and bathroom need modification, etc., refer to the Sect. 6.8 on "architectural accessibility"

6.4.3 Assessing the Social Context
- Degree of support from family members
- Any financing difficulty
- If WC for temporary use, try to arrange for any available for loan

6.4.4 Other Aspects
- Patient's personal beliefs (some patients take quite some time to accept a WC as a form of mobility)

6.4.5 If WC for Temporary Use
- Cost will also be important

6.4.6 WC for Long-Term Use
- Durability issues become important
- Suitability for the individual also imperative, may need to be tailor-made

6.4.7 Key Concept 1
- There is not a type of WC that will suit every individual patient
- Long-term WC users should be provided with WC specially suited to the patient; this is particularly the case in those suffering from neuro-muscular conditions like cerebral palsy, and SCI (refer to the Sect. 6.5 on seating clinics)

6.4.8 Key Concept 2
- In patients with truncal and LL weakness or muscle imbalance, especially with associated scoliosis, the WC should be viewed as a "total body orthotic" device and not merely a machine to improve mobility

6.4.9   Elements of WC Design

- Components of design:
  - Position of axle
  - Wheel and tyre design
  - Seat support and design
  - Postural support
  - Posterior incline and support
  - Camber
  - Hand-rims

6.4.9.1   Rear Axle Position

- Pros and cons of more anterior placement: turning radius effectively decreases, as does resistance to rolling. But may lose balance and tip over backwards
- Pros and cons of more posterior placement: turning radius effectively increases, as does rolling resistance. But may have an edge in LL amputees (whose centre of gravity is displaced posteriorly) and patients with poor trunk control. A more posterior placement of the rear axle is necessary for WC equipped with a posterior recline option or tilt to ensure and maintain stability

6.4.9.2   Camber

- Pros and cons of increased camber: frequently seen in WC in "disabled" sports since not only protects the hand of the athlete (e.g. in a competitive game of basketball), but decreases effective turning radius and higher sideways stability. The disadvantage is increased tyre and wheel wear from eccentric loading
- The standard camber is around $7°$

6.4.9.3   Wheel Types

- Spoke wheels should be used with caution in those patients with finger deformity or loss of dexterity in case fingers get caught in-between the spokes, although this design is popular and also used in sports WC
- Plastic ones are safer for patients with associated hand pathology

6.4.9.4   Type of Tyres

- In home-bound patients, the solid rubber variety is adequate and durable, and will not go flat like pneumatic ones
- Pneumatic tyres are better on going outdoors as better shock absorption for slightly uneven ground, but there is a chance of them going flat

6.4.10 Use of Electric WC

- Main indication: poor cardiopulmonary reserve to drive WC (may add an outrigger to hold a small oxygen cylinder during outdoor use), high cervical cord lesions
- Pre-requisite: good cognition and have the required movement to use the control, be it hand control, chin, etc.
- Contraindication: poor motivation, perception, cannot reproduce the above said movement
- Caution: be sure the WC is of compatible size with lift and other access (the size may be different from the size of the manual WC that the patient may commonly also have)

6.4.11 Special Adaptations for High Cervical Cord Injury Patients

- This will be described in more detail in the section on SCI, the type of adaptation depends on the level, e.g.:
  - Sip and puff mouth sticks
  - Voice-triggered controls
  - Chin-triggered controls
  - Special hand controls

6.4.12 WC Design for Disabled Sports

- The design should suit the sporting event
- Prefer material of lighter weight if sporting event involves speed and manoeuvrability
- For sporting events requiring mobility over long distances, as in some para-Olympic athletes, the WC should be made to allow full use of the UL strength – hence better to be tailor-made to the sitting height as well as the UL length of the athlete in mind

6.4.13 One-Arm Drives

- Essentially referring to modified WC with both hand rims being on one side and excellent muscular strength is needed on that side since need to turn both the rims to move the WC. Only reserved for unilateral UL amputee with poor LL power or very occasionally for younger hemiplegics with good cognition, perception and coordination and good muscle strength on the good side

6.4.14 Special WC for Patients with Poor Standing Tolerance

■ Some WC equipped with rests for the UL can aid the patient to stand from a sitting position

■ This will help improve LL mobility, decrease chronic pressure on high pressure areas during sitting, may aid bladder and bowel habits in the elderly, and increase confidence in others

6.4.15 Advanced Technology WC that Helps to Manoeuvre Kerbs

■ Some technologically advanced WC are equipped with the special ability to overcome some obstacles like kerbs (see Fig. 6.7); developed by Independence Technology known as the iBOT mobility system

■ Although expensive, this new technology appears very promising

6.4.16 Pressure Relief and Postural Support

■ Pressure relief is particularly important for those with neuromuscular weakness and paralysis

■ Further illustrations of related technology will be found in the discussion in Sect. 6.7 on pressure sores

6.4.17 Types of Seat Cushions

■ Air filled compartments: frequently called by the brand name "ROHO", are ideal for those with pressure ulcers as the air-filled cells

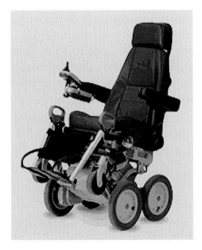

Fig. 6.7. An "intelligent" wheelchair that can negotiate kerbs or even ascend stairs

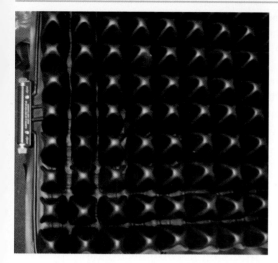

Fig. 6.8. An example of an air-cushion commercially produced and known by the name "ROHO"

give pressure relief. Because made of air sacs, they are light-weight and provide good heat dissipation. The disadvantage is cost (Fig. 6.8)

■ Gel cushion: frequently known by its brand name "Jay", ideal for patients with bony deformity, providing better fit and pressure equalisation and good heat dissipation. The disadvantage is their heaviness and cost. Notice that heaviness is not ideal for those patients with limited UL strength for WC propulsion

■ Foam cushion: although heat dissipation is poorer, they are cheaper and light weight. May work well in the absence of bony deformity, pressure ulcers, and the patient can do weight shifts by himself as in thoracic SCI patients (see discussion in Chap. 12)

6.4.18 Uses of WC Cushions

■ Equalise pressure
■ Increase height from floor
■ Improve sitting posture and balance
■ Comfort

6.4.19 Key Concept

■ No matter how well designed or advanced the technology of the cushion is, the need for weight shift should always be kept in mind

6.4.20   Truncal Support

▣ Those with cervical SCI or high thoracic complete SCI often have poor trunk support, as well as total body CP and other related neuro-muscular conditions, e.g. SMA

▣ In addition to truncal support, those with for instance CP or polio patients with significant structural scoliosis need to have moulding of the back support, and here the WC can be thought of as a total body orthotic

6.4.21   Need for Option of Reclining or Tilting

▣ Patients who lack ability to perform pressure shifts may need a reclining or tiltable WC for relief of pressure

▣ However, especially be aware that SCI patients can have spasms in the reclining position or BP fluctuations

6.4.22   Other Mobility Device for the Arthritic Patient

▣ Patients with generalised arthritis whose hands are also involved may have poor tolerance to WC manipulation (on their own) from the pain and stiffness of their hands

▣ If they have good trunk control, eye-hand co-ordination and no significant tremor, then scooters can be an option

▣ One precaution is to buy a scooter type that does not tip over easily

6.7   Setting up of Seating Clinics

6.5.1   Introduction

▣ The wheelchair is one of the most frequently prescribed mobility aid in the field of rehabilitation

▣ It is not usually stressed enough that WC have functions beyond mobility. For patients with significant motor and/or sensory disturbance, the WC is very much a "total body orthotic". It sometimes plays the role of pressure relief, correction of posture, accommodating deformity, etc. The importance of setting up of seating clinics cannot be over-emphasised (Coggrave et al., Spinal Cord 2003)

6.5.2 Team Members of Seating Clinic
- Orthopaedic surgeon
- Physiotherapist
- Occupational therapist
- Orthotist
- Rehabilitation engineer

6.5.3 Aim of Seating Clinics
- Provision of pressure relief
- Prevent development of pressure sores. A discussion on pressure sores will be found at the end of this chapter
- Postural controls and adaptations for accommodation of deformity or weakness
- Checking on the progress of the patient and assess need for adjustments

6.5.4 Example
- Figure 6.9 illustrates the use of a multi-axial head rest for the user of this WC with global weakness including weak neck control, notice the arms are well supported and a small switch for driving the power wheelchair, the other switch is for effecting environmental control

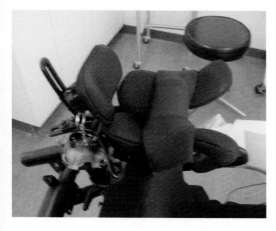

Fig. 6.9. Picture showing a multi-axial head rest for patients with muscle weakness and poor head and neck control

6.5.5   Cost Effectiveness of Seating Clinics

▪ The existence of seating clinics has caught the attention of medical administrators and many seating clinics are now under close scrutiny (Mulvany et al., Health Care Superv 1998)
▪ As usual, medical administrators like the use of "outcome measures" to see that its existence is justified. This will now be discussed. Further discussion on outcome measures is found in Chap. 18

6.5.6   Outcome Measures for Seating and WC Prescription and Usage

▪ There are few if any outcome measures tailor-made for assessing "seating clinics" usage and efficacy; one such measure is now being developed from the University of Pittsburgh

6.5.6.1 New Outcome Measure for WC Users (and Seating)

▪ A new outcome measure for wheelchair users was just developed by the University of Pittsburgh called "FEW" (functional evaluation in a wheelchair) that is potentially applicable to both manual and power WC users

6.5.6.2 Objectives of FEW

▪ Ascertain the level of functional change
▪ Provide documentation and justification of the efficacy of seating-mobility interventions
▪ Validate the cost effectiveness and functional value of seating-mobility technology

6.5.6.3 Ten Categories Reviewed by the FEW Measure

▪ Transfers
▪ Transportation accessibility
▪ Natural barriers
▪ Accessories
▪ Accessing task surfaces
▪ Transportation "securement"
▪ Human–machine interface
▪ Architectural barrier
▪ Transportation – portability
▪ Reach (Holm, Mills et al., University of Pittsburgh)

6.6   Conclusion and the Future

6.6.1   Conclusion

- In summary, AT that can be provided to our patients varies from simple to highly sophisticated technology
- Our technology must be made to suit the patient and not vice versa
- We need to select the best method in the light of the residual function of our patient. This does not, however, necessarily involve high technology in every instance
- There are still challenges facing the AT team when confronted with patients with limited motion. A few developing advanced technologies will now be discussed

6.6.2   The Future

6.6.2.1   What Lies in the Future?

- The challenges include:
  - Provision of AT for the extremely disabled, especially those that defy the best current technology available at the present moment. One type of research in this interesting field is the use of the patient's brain waves to effect computer controls (Birch et al., IEEE Trans Neural Syst Rehabil Eng 2006). Potentially, even patients with concomitant brain injury and locked-in syndrome will then communicate by brain waves to the outside word through a text-mediated interface or platform or via a virtual reality platform. Conversely, our patient will potentially be able to use brain waves to control the ECU (Wolpaw et al., Clin Neurophysiol 2002)

6.6.2.2   Virtual Reality

- Virtual environment uses computerised images and sounds to represent reality
- Besides its use in training future generations of surgeons, which has already started, the same kind of technology is of use in rehabilitation to teach, e.g. navigate in their environment, and as a tool to teach the activities of daily living (Fig. 6.10)
- The next step under active investigation is how to transfer techniques learned to real life. Research in this area is under way in the Toronto Rehab Institute, Toronto University, Canada. Similar tools of the virtual reality platform are developed in burns patients (Haik et al., J Burn Care Res 2006)

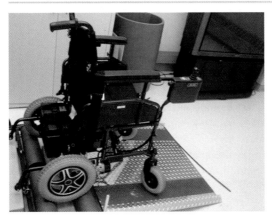

Fig. 6.10. A room devoted to "virtual reality" training of electric wheelchair users before they ambulate through the busy streets of the city

6.6.2.3 Communication with Severely Impaired Patients

■ We have talked about the possibility of the use of brain waves
■ Another technology to communicate with patients having marked impairment with difficulties in communication such as the locked-in syndrome is via the use of near-infrared imaging to detect changes in the haemodynamics of the brain's neural activity (PRISM Lab, Bloorview MacMillan Rehabilitation Center, Canada)

6.6.2.4 Increasing Role of Virtual Reality

■ The use of virtual reality has been mentioned throughout this book
■ Examples of some prior developments in this aspect include, e.g. virtual music as a form of therapy training, and entertainment of patients with limited hand function (developed in the PRISM Lab, Canada)
■ The above technology can in fact be modified to project the image in front of a specially made large arm-rest fitted to the WC. This, the author thinks, will even benefit patients who do not have the ability to raise their arm

6.6.2.5 Use of Holographic Screens and Virtual Keyboards

■ A technology that is deemed to be potentially complementary is the use of touch-sensitive holographic screens recently developed by a commercial company in Portugal (Fig. 6.11)
■ This cutting edge technology can be put to good use in the field of assistive technology for our patients in future

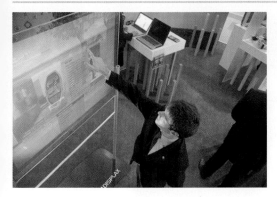

Fig. 6.11. The active touch-sensitive holographic screen equipped with the new Displax technology (courtesy of Edigma.-com)

■ If the patient has poor shoulder power, but reasonable finger dexterity, then the newly invented virtual keyboard (www.virtual-keyboard.-com) can be used, i.e. projection of the computer or related hardware keyboard to an arm support in front of the patient

6.6.2.6 The Coming of Age of Robotics

■ Since most of our patients with significant impairment will be home bound most of the time depending on computer controlled ECU; the coming of age of robotics (Fig. 6.12) will potentially allow the patient to use the computer to effect control of mobile robots or at least robotic arms to perform some fundamental housework, especially if he or she is lacking in carers

■ Robotic technology can also be of help in those rather less impaired patients. An example will be the newly invented "robotic arm" under study at MIT (USA) to benefit the re-training of UL strength (Fig. 6.13)

6.6.2.7 Legislation and Law

■ Legislation and laws in every country that will benefit patients with impairment, especially mandatory design of government and/or private owned housing estates to accommodate potential occupants with impairments, be it impaired mobility or otherwise, are important. Other areas as have already been mentioned include public lift access, design of washrooms, and of public vehicles plus provision of regional AT centres in areas that provide easy access to our patients with impairment

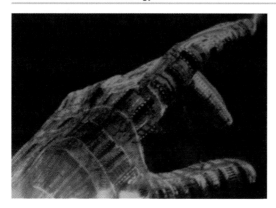

Fig. 6.12. Artist impression of a robotic hand pointing to the future in robotics

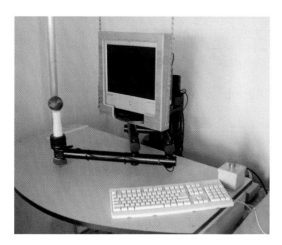

Fig. 6.13. Robotic arm developed at MIT in Boston, can potentially aid in the rehabilitation of patients with upper extremity disability

6.7   Appendix 1: Pathogenesis and Prevention of Pressure Sores

6.7.1   Classification of Pressure Ulcers

■ Most follow National Pressure Ulcer Advisory Panel guidelines:
  – Stage 1: intact epidermis with non-blanchable erythema
  – Stage 2: blisters or partial thickness skin loss present
  – Stage 3: full thickness involvement, with spared underlying fascia

– Stage 4: full thickness involvement with deep structures involved: muscle, bone, or tendon

6.7.2   Key Pathogenetic Factors for Sore Formation

■ Localised pressure concentration
■ Immobility
■ Shearing forces
   Others: advanced age, poor nutrition, sepsis, overweight, etc.
   P. S. All three most important pathogenetic factors can be improved by proper seating

6.7.2.1   Localised Pressure Concentration

■ Higher pressure concentrations are common over bony prominences, e.g. ischial tuberosities, trochanters, etc.
■ Posture is important – e.g. pelvic obliquity and spinal deformity will cause localised pressure elevation, underlying the importance of seating clinics
■ But even non-bony prominences cannot tolerate prolonged local pressure above the capillary (32 mmHg) from occlusion of tissue blood flow and oxygen deprivation

6.7.2.2   Tackling Immobility

■ Even in face of lower pressure level, if pressure is not relieved periodically and *sustained*, ulceration is common
■ The situation is aggravated in the presence of loss of sensation
■ Time-honoured study of the effect of time with different magnitudes of pressure by Reswick and Rogers should be noted
■ If the patient is intelligent, biofeedback can be taught with the help of pressure mapping
■ Carers should be taught the different methods of weight lifting (these will be discussed in Chap. 12)

6.7.2.3   Shearing Forces

■ Shear forces can cause deep tissue distortion and is a major contributing factor particularly for deep sores
■ On the other hand, surface sores are more often the result of repeated surface friction or abrasion
■ Surface friction tends to be higher with obesity

6.7.2.4 Other Adjunctive Measures

▦ Optimise nutrition

▦ Early detection and treatment of sepsis, treat anaemia, adequate vitamins, diabetes mellitus control, manage incontinence, keep perineum dry

▦ There are some factors that cannot be changed, such as the age, or take time to change, such as obesity

6.7.3   Scales for Assessment

▦ Some assessment scales were described in the past (e.g. Norton, Braden), but the modern tendency is to use more objective measures with technological advances

6.7.3.1 Assessing Skin Viability

▦ Screening: look for skin blanching

▦ Measurement of interface pressure (single site vs. mapping)

▦ Thermography

▦ Oxygenation of blood flow

▦ Other techniques: measurement of tissue deformation or stiffness reported by Brienza

6.7.3.2 Assessing Pressure

▦ Electropneumatic bladder

▦ Pneumatic bladder

▦ Fluid-filled bladder

6.7.3.2.1 Pros and Cons of Single Bladder Type Devices

▦ Single bladder type devices are:
  – More accurate and repeatable
  – More difficult to use
  – Provide limited information
  – Allow single or continuous measurements

6.7.3.2.2 Why Pressure Mapping is Preferred

▦ Provides posture and *relative* pressure (between individual cells) information, as well as distribution (Figs. 6.14, 6.15)

▦ Allows graphical displays; thus, can provide immediate feedback to therapist and patient about the pressure distribution with different postures

▦ Speedy response

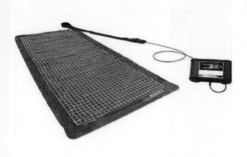

Fig. 6.14. Commercially available pressure mapping devices are indispensable in seating clinics

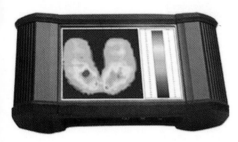

Fig. 6.15. Close-up of the pressure-mapping screen with differing pressure manifested as different colours. Device shown developed by the company that produces the 'ROHO'

▓ Allows either single or continuous measurements
▓ The only drawback is cost

6.7.4   Pressure Sore Management Principles

▓ Maximising the surface area will decrease the pressure concentration
▓ Redistribute body weight with proper support surface
▓ Proper moulding and proper selection of materials
▓ Minimise asymmetries to decrease unequal loading of pelvic structures and tissues, biofeedback sometimes helps, as mentioned
▓ Regular weight shift manoeuvres taught to patient and carers
▓ More details of weight shifts can be found in Chap. 12 on the topic of SCI
▓ Special "cut-outs" made of special softer foams may be needed for the ulcerated area (Fig. 6.16)
▓ Other measures:
  – Adjust arm and foot rests for optimal weight distribution
  – Use of recline vs tilt. Caution: use of recline can precipitate extensor spasms in a patient with high tone (e.g. total body CP), it may also slip the patient to the floor if we are not careful

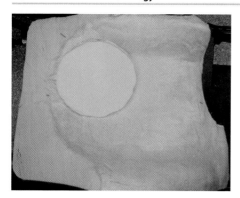

Fig. 6.16. Special cut-outs made of Liquid SunMate Foam for the ulcerated area of the patient (Dynamic System Inc)

6.7.5   Types of Support

- Generic contoured foam
- Air-filled, e.g. ROHO
- Water-filled
- Solid gel
- Others, e.g. viscoelastic, segmented foam
- The merits and demerits have been discussed already
- But the key properties to consider include:
  - Weight/volume ratio
  - Stiffness
  - Resilience – ability to recover shape
  - Dampening – load absorption
  - Envelopment – surface area covered
    (According to Sprigle)

6.7.6   Material for Moulded Seats

- The popular material used for moulding is liquid SunMate foam (Dynamic Systems)
- The active chemical here is diphenylmethane diisocyanate together with a catalyst
- Procedure:
  - Place the moulding bag on the WC
  - Mix the liquid SunMate foam
  - Pour to moulding bag, spread evenly
  - Position the patient still seated on the WC for 5 min
  - After 10 min, the foam is complete and ready to be trimmed for a snug fit

6.8 Appendix 2: Concept of Architectural Accessibility

6.8.1 What Constitutes Architectural Accessibility: Definition of "Architectural Accessibility"

■ In the present chapter, we mainly refer to housing and associated designs (such as lifts, doorways, etc.) that are compatible with and accessible to a person with impairment upon discharge from the rehabilitation centre to his home/work environment

■ In fact, the scope of AA goes far beyond the home of the patient, as the following discussion will show

6.8.2 Importance of Architectural Accessibility

■ In the absence of AA, the patient with impairment will be rendered house-bound and will encounter difficulty accessing the places he wants to go, thus creating and magnifying disability

6.8.3 With What Aspect of AA Can the AT Team Help the Patient?

■ If the main building design is satisfactory, a home visit by the occupational therapist may help to circumvent difficulties we envisage the patient encountering after discharge, e.g. providing a ramp to negotiate a few steps with his WC, enlarging some doorways for WC access

■ Liaise with relevant housing authority for compassionate re-housing if the housing design is not suitable for our patient

■ Liaise with his employer (if appropriate) concerning the problem of access upon his return to work

■ Although many employers are willing to accept the patient (now in a WC) back to work, it will also depend on the design of the building (and the passageways to the building in which he works, including the lifts) as to whether he can get unlimited access

■ Educating the patient about the local laws governing AA provision for patients with impairments

6.8.4 Relevant Laws Concerning AA in USA

■ In the USA, the Fair Housing Amendment Act makes AA a mandatory requirement for, say, WC users in the public and common areas in housing complexes. It provides the power for tenants to modify rental property at their own expense although the patient frequently needs to restore the amendments upon expiry of the rental agreement

■ That all public facilities should be made accessible to persons with impairment like WC users is mandated in the Americans with Disability Act. This includes for instance: parking lot, restaurants and stores for all new buildings constructed after 1993. Further standards are set out in the Rehabilitation Act contained in the Federal Accessibility Standards

■ Even in the private sector, there are standards to follow like American National Standard Accessible and Usable Facilities

■ If the patient has detected the laws are being breached, an appeal can be lodged to relevant authorities such as the Architectural and Transportation Barriers Compliance Board

■ It is hoped that most countries in the world will follow the good example laid down by the US government to minimise the disability of our patients with physical impairment

6.8.5   Design Features Pertinent to Architectural Accessibility

6.8.5.1 Introduction

■ We will introduce the ideas of architectural adaptability and of universal design, which is gaining popularity in many countries

■ Although we need to remember that even given such versatile designs, home visits and home modification (e.g. light switches, bath handles, ramps, door handle adjustment, setting up of ECU, etc.) that are tailor made for our patient frequently need to be completed prior to the discharge of the patient from the rehabilitation centre

6.8.5.2 What Are the Preferred Designs?

■ Buildings in more and more countries besides the US are adopting the concept and use of "adaptable design"

6.8.5.3 What Are Adaptable Designs?

■ A type of housing design that can easily be altered for accommodation of occupants with impairments; usually this means the apartment will be made freely accessible to WC users; and that this "accommodation" process can be performed with as little cost and manual labour as possible

6.8.5.4 The "Universal Design" Concept

▓ This does not however mean that this type of housing is difficult to use for able-bodied occupants. Quite the contrary, another name for this design is called "universal design", meaning that this type of housing can freely be used by occupants with and without physical impairments freely and without hindrance. Hence, the design can freely accommodate, say, for instance one member of the family with physical impairment

6.8.5.5 Necessary Elements to Attain WC Accessibility

▓ As far as the patient's accommodation is concerned, minimum requirements for attaining WC accessibility include:
- WC transfer from bus-stop/car-park to the patient's home
- No hindrance at the lift and doorway
- Freely manoeuvre WC at home
- Freedom to access basic household facilities, e.g. bathroom, kitchen, storage area, etc.

6.8.5.6 Necessary Elements for Attaining Ready Access to Household Facilities

▓ Clear space for the patient's knees
▓ Reachable range
▓ Clear floor space
▓ Clear doorways
▓ Relevant adaptations in different areas, e.g. bathroom, kitchen, etc. (see Figs. 6.17, 6.18)

6.8.5.7 Other Public Areas

▓ Lift
▓ Passageways
▓ Presence of ramps

6.8.5.8 Accessibility with a View to Social Integration

▓ Combined general efforts of the government, employers and AT team members are needed to promote social integration of patients with physical impairments in order to ease:
- Return to community at large
- Return to work

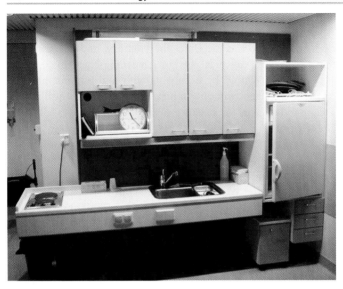

Fig. 6.17. Simple kitchen and cupboards designed specially for wheel-chair users

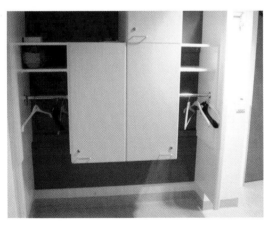

Fig. 6.18. Special wardrobe into which the patient can be wheeled for easy access

General Bibliography

Enders A (1990) Assistive Technology Sourcebook. RESNA Press, Washington
Trombly CA (2002) Occupational Therapy for Physical Dysfunction, 5th edn, Lippincott Williams & Wilkins, Philadelphia

Selected Bibliography of Journal Articles

1. Coggrave M, Wiesel PH et al. (2003) A specialist seating assessment, changing pressure relief practice. Spinal Cord 41(12):122–125
2. Mulvany R, Likens C et al. (1998) Cost analysis of adaptive seating system in a spe-
   cialty seating clinic. Health Care Superv 17(1):17–26
3. Borisoff JF, Birch G et al. (2006) Brain interface research for asynchronous application. IEEE Trans Neural Syst Rehabil Eng 14(2):160–164
4. Wolpaw JR, Birbaumer N et al. (2002) Brain-computer interfaces for communication and control. Clin Neurophysiol 113(6):767–791
5. Haik J, Tessone A et al. (2006) The use of video capture virtual reality in burn rehabilitation: the possibilities. J Burn Care Res 27(2):195–197

7 Neurophysiological Testing and Intraoperative Monitoring

7.1 The Basics in Neurophysiological Testing

7.1.1 Aim of Nerve Conduction Testing

▓ Aim:
  - Check motor/sensory responses of peripheral nerves
  - Check conduction velocity
  - Locate site(s) of compression or injury
  - Together with electromyography (EMG), may differentially diagnose denervation from myopathy
  - Other related studies, e.g. f-wave studies, etc.
  - Sometimes as base-line study for documentation before operative intervention and in medico-legal cases

7.1.2 Terminology

▓ Latency – time between stimulus onset and response
▓ Amplitude – size of response
▓ Velocity (V) – calculated by distance over time
▓ Motor response – elicited by neural stimulation over motor point after placement of ground electrode, point of stimulation is where the nerve is more superficial. Stimulator administered until CMAP (compound motor action potential) is obtained, later maximise potential
▓ Sensory response – the sensory nerve action potential (SNAP) has lower amplitude than motor potential, can either be anti- or ortho-dromic
▓ SSEP – refers to somatosensory evoked potential, elicited via stimulation of peripheral sensory nerves and recording on the scalp

7.1.3 Measuring Nerve Conduction Velocity

▓ Measures the time taken for the impulse to travel along the axon between the two sites of stimulation
▓ Velocity = distance between the two sites divided by the difference in latencies between the two sites of stimulation

7.1.4 Key Concept 1

▓ The measured conduction velocity represents the velocity of the fastest nerve fibres
▓ Hence, in order for velocity to diminish, almost all of the nerve fibres need to be affected

7.1.5   Key Concept 2

- Nerve conduction velocity can remain normal even in the face of only a few intact nerve fibres left

7.1.6   The H (Hoffman) Reflex

- Measured by stimulating the posterior tibial nerve, and checking the latency to complete the monosynaptic reflex arc from the Ia afferents to the a motor fibres of the S1 root
- Increased latency in the H reflex of the gastrocnemius-soleus muscle group can occur in S1 radiculopathy or peripheral neuropathy
- Can be absent in the elderly

7.1.7   The F Wave

- Elicited usually via a supramaximal stimulus during motor stimulation – via possible antidromic transmission of a handful of the stimulated motor fibres
- Latency may be increased in lesions at the proximal nerve fibres; f waves have been described most commonly for tibial nerve, peroneal nerve, ulna nerve, and median nerve
- It is not a reflex

7.1.8   Deductions from Compound Muscle Action Potential

- Compound muscle action potential (CMAP) amplitude: depends on the number of nerve fibres that are activated, decreased amplitude occurs in the face of axonal loss. The most significant end of the spectrum is conduction block (as occurs sometimes in segmental demyelination)
- CMAP duration: depends on the synchrony of conduction of individual nerve fibres throughout the nerve. Thus, increased dispersion or multiphase may be detected in the face of some fibres with much reduced conduction
- Both conduction block and dispersion can occur in demyelination

7.1.9   Generation of MAP

- Upon arrival of the action potential, an end-plate potential (EPP) is generated
- When EPP reaches the necessary threshold, a muscle action potential (MAP) will be generated, detectable by EMG as MUP

■ MUP as detected by our needle in EMG studies does not include the activity of all the fibres in the motor unit, but only the sum of the activity of muscle fibres in the neighbourhood of the needle electrode

7.1.10 Use of MUP in the Differential Diagnosis of Neuromuscular Disorders
■ Differential diagnosis is via MAP:
  – At rest and during insertion
  – During minimal voluntary contraction
  – By assessing the pattern of recruitment

7.1.11 EMG at Rest
■ In normal situations, should be silent at rest, though can be punctuated by miniature end plate potentials or end plate spikes

7.1.12 Selection of Needles
■ Concentric needles have the advantages of obviating the need for a reference electrode and less electrical noise. But have the disadvantages of less patient comfort and sensitivity for recording of spontaneous electrical activity
■ Monopolar electrodes therefore tend to be more popular

7.1.13 Insertional Activity
■ Some transient insertional activity is expected in normal individuals, duration <300 ms
■ Differential diagnosis of decreased insertional activity: myopathy, muscle fibrosis, paralysis
■ Differential diagnosis abnormal increase in insertional activity (>300–500 ms): can be seen in denervations, or myopathies, or normal variant

7.1.14 After Voluntary Contraction and Recruitment
■ Normally, the more voluntary contraction, the more motor units will be recruited
■ In muscles affected by axonal degeneration, the recruitment may become abnormal, for there may be very few motor units left

7.1.15 Factors Affecting Measurement

▪ Age: conduction velocity decreases at extremes of age. Adult value of nerve conduction velocity occurs at age 4, conduction velocity starts to decline > 60

▪ Temperature: velocity increases with increase in temperature and decreases in a cold environment. Reporting and performance of NCT should be done in a room shielded electrically from interference and with measured skin temperatures. Conversely, cool limbs need to be warmed before proper NCT measurements can be obtained

▪ Method of measuring the distance, such as proper positioning of body parts during measurement

7.2   Some Clinical Applications

7.2.1   Nerve Injuries

7.2.1.1 Nerve Anatomy

▪ Discussion of details of nerve anatomy is beyond the scope of this book, the reader is referred to standard neuroanatomy texts

7.2.1.2 What Happens After Nerve Injury?

▪ Retraction
▪ Inflammation + factors secreted to attempt to stimulate neurites
▪ Degeneration

7.2.1.3 What Happens After Injury – Microscopic?

▪ Distal part of severed nerve – Wallerian degeneration (according to Waller who first described the phenomenon) survival of nerve fibres occurs only if still remaining connected to nerve cell body – starts on day 3

▪ Proximal part of severed nerve – cell body becomes basophilic (chromatolysis), nucleus move to periphery, swollen (changes in proximal segment only as far as the next Ranvier's node)

▪ Activation of Schwann cells close to injured site – takes few weeks to clear debris + axonal sprouts start as early as day 1 (nerve growth factors help this process if the perineurium is disrupted)

▪ Self repair does not occur with gaps of > 2 mm

7.2.1.4 Outcome
- Sprouts make distal connection then nerve fibre matures, (increased axon and myelin thickness)
- Neurites that fail to make distal connection die back and lost → if the perineurium not disrupted, then the axons will be guided along the original path at 1 mm/day

7.2.1.5 Seddon Classes of Nerve Injury
- Neuropraxia – most are compressive in aetiology → local conduction block/demyelination – heal by repair of demyelination, especially of the thick myelin nerves
- Axonotmesis – mostly traction and/or severe compression cases, → Wallerian degeneration, prognosis not bad since will regenerate and not miswiring (sensory recovers better since sensory receptors live longer, especially more proximal injuries)
- Neurotmesis – complete cut, no recovery unless repaired – yet can miswire and hence reduced mass of innervation

7.2.1.6 Sunderland Classification
- Neuropraxia – no Tinel's sign
- Axon – both epi- and perineurium intact, Tinel's sign + progresses distally
- Axon – only epineurium injured, Tinel's sign + progresses distally
- Axon – perineurium injured, Tinel's sign + but Tinel's sign not progressing distally
- Neurotmesis
- Neuroma in continuity (i.e. partly cut nerve, the remainder can be 1st/2nd/3rd/4th degree of injury)

7.2.1.7 Feature of the Sunderland Classification
- Accounts for injuries between axonotmesis and neurotmesis – based on involvement of perineurium

7.2.1.8 Assessment After a Nerve Injury
- Motor – assess power + differential diagnosis level of injury
- Sensory – mapping and pattern recognition
- Autonomic – e.g. wrinkle test (RSD in 3%, featuring swelling, porosis, sweating, pain, etc.) Tinel's sign may be presen

▓ Reflexes – not good guide to injury severity → of course lost if afferent or efferent limb affected, but sometimes absent in partial injuries as well

7.2.1.9 Autonomic Changes After Nerve Injury

▓ Three major losses – vasomotor, sweat, "pilomotor"
  - Test pilomotor – loss of wrinkle of denervated skin when immersed in water
  - Test sweating – rub smooth pen against side of finger/ninhydrin test – due to diminished sweating
  - Vasomotor – observation: initial 2/52 pink, then pale and mottled skin

7.2.1.10 Checking for and the Importance of Tinel's Sign

▓ Start distally, proceed to proximal percussion when you test for Tinel's sign
  - Positive Tinel's sign = regenerating axonal sprouts that have not completed myelinisation
  - Distally advancing Tinel's sign = seen in Sunderland 2 and 3, good sign but does *not* indicate complete recovery alone
    (Note: Type 1 Sunderland with no Tinel's sign, types 4 and 5 Sunderland no Tinel's unless repaired)

7.2.1.11 Motor and Sensory Charting

▓ Motor
  - Grade 0 – NIL
  - Grade 1 – flicker
  - Grade 2 – not against gravity, can contract
  - Grade 3 – against gravity
  - Grade 4 – some resistance
  - Grade 5 – normal
    (Motor end plate lasts only 12 months after denervation)
▓ Sensory
  - S0 – nil
  - S1 – pain recovers
  - S2 – pain and touch returning
  - S3 – pain and touch throughout autonomy zone
  - S4 – as S3 + 2-point discrimination returning
  - S5 – normal

7.2.1.12 Investigations
■ Role of NCT/EMG in differential diagnosis of neurapraxia and axonotmesis
■ Presence or absence of a progressing Tinel's sign

7.2.1.13 Timing of NCT in Nerve Injuries
■ Ideal time after nerve injury = 2 weeks
■ Reason: needs 7–10 days to have absence of sensory conduction, (and 3–7 days to get an absent distal motor potential, or in other words, the distal motor response may still initially be intact in the immediate few days after nerve injury)
■ As from 2/52, usually can differentially diagnose axonotmesis from neurotmesis

7.2.1.14 What Happens to the Muscle After Denervation?
■ Increased excitability to Ach starts within 2 weeks
■ Increased response of the muscle to even smaller quanta of Ach

7.2.1.15 Key Concept
■ Excitability of nerves becomes abnormal around 72 h after a significant nerve injury

7.2.1.16 What are Fibrillation Potentials?
■ These represent the depolarisation of single muscle fibres

7.2.1.17 Summary of EMG Changes After Acute Nerve Injury
■ What changes do we expect after nerve cut?
■ Answer: at first normal then, positive sharp waves as from days 5–14; later, at 2 weeks, spontaneous denervation fibrillation
■ Implication: good sign if no denervation fibrillation at 2 weeks
■ Another important use of EMG: differential diagnosis of neuropathic muscle atrophy from myopathy

7.2.1.18 EMG Changes in the Face of Chronic Denervation
■ Expect to see long duration and high amplitude MUPs, since surviving muscle fibres in chronic denervation will increase fibre density and motor unit territory

7.2.2   Entrapment Neuropathy

7.2.2.1   Pathophysiology of Entrapment
- Mild – ionic block (recovers in hours)
- Moderate – myelin back-flow/myelin intussusception (recovers in ≤3 months usually), severe cases can have segmental demyelination
- Severe – axonotmesis (with Waller degeneration) takes longer to recover. Recovery related to distance between site of injury and motor end organs

7.2.2.2   More on Pathophysiology
- The more central fibres *spared* till late in compression process
- Proximal fusiform swelling of the nerve
- The only case of neurotmesis is that associated with fractures

7.2.2.3   Other Possible Contributing Factors Besides Compression
- Traction
- Excursion
- Tethering
- Scarring
- Ischaemia
  (Do not forget the "Double Crush" syndrome)

7.2.2.4   Physical Assessment
- Sensory symptoms sometimes not well localised and can be confusing
- Use provocative test to reproduce clinical symptoms if possible
- Accurate motor testing
- Refer to the indications for NCT (nerve conduction testing)

7.2.2.5   Typical NCT Findings
- Focal conduction block at the segment of entrapment with demyelination
- Evidence of axonal loss reflected more in the lowering of the amplitude.

7.2.2.6   CMAP Changes in Demyelination
- In general, both conduction block (or marked slowing of conduction velocity) and CMAP dispersion (with needling technique) can occur in demyelination
- In entrapment neuropathy, only focal demyelination occurs, unlike the more diffuse demyelinating neuropathies

7.2.2.7 CMAP Changes from Axonal Loss

- Here, conduction velocity is normal or slightly slowed, and reduced amplitude are the hallmarks of axonal loss
- The amplitude is most affected by axonal loss

7.2.2.8 Prognosis

- Age – worse in the elderly
- Chronicity
- Completeness of paresis – complete and >15 month much less likely to recover
- Underlying pathology
- If there is dissociated loss of motor or sensory function, prognosis sometimes better

7.2.3   Neuropathy, Myopathy and Neuromuscular Junction Disorders

7.2.3.1 Neuropathy

- Here, sensory fibres are usually affected earlier than motor fibres
- For this reason, the sensory nerve conduction changes are usually detected prior to motor nerve conduction changes
- The changes expected of demyelination have already been discussed. The loss of conduction velocity commences initially in the distal portion of the nerves (glove and stocking distribution)
- Assessing both UL and LL peripheral nerves are needed if polyneuropathy is suspected

7.2.3.2 Myopathy

- Here, the MUPs are of short duration and small amplitude as there is decreased fibre density and motor unit territory from degeneration of the muscle fibres
- In myotonia, there are high frequency discharges that wax and wane

7.2.3.3 Possible Faults at the Level of NMJ

- Presynaptic, e.g. botulinum toxin (see Chap. 11 on CP), and Eaton-Lambert syndrome – decreased presynaptic Ach release from antibody against calcium channel
- Postsynaptic: myasthenia – antibody binding to Ach receptor

7.2.3.4   Differential Diagnosis of NMJ Disorder – Repetitive Nerve Stimulation

▦ Pre- and post-synaptic disorders differential diagnosis by high rate stimulation at 10–50 Hz

7.3   Intraoperative Neural Monitoring

7.3.1   Indications of Intraoperative Neural Monitoring

▦ Real-time monitoring of function of neural structures (Figs. 7.1, 7.2)
▦ Help reduce intraoperative neural complications especially, e.g. at the time of deformity correction in spine surgery
▦ May aid in intraoperative identification of neural structures, e.g. brachial plexus surgery
▦ Adjunct in other advanced procedures like deep brain stimulation
▦ Also used in research

7.3.2   Main Goals of Intraoperative Neural Monitoring

▦ Detection of changes in neural function from say ischaemia and stretching
▦ And diagnose such changes early, before they become irreversible

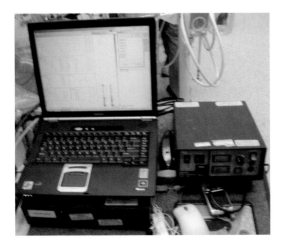

Fig. 7.1. A typical machine used for intra-operative neural monitoring commonly used in spinal operations. Picture shows the commercially used popular Axon System

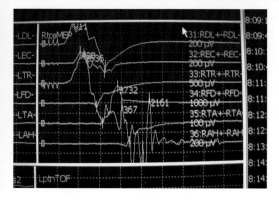

Fig. 7.2. Close-up film of the monitor screen of the system shown in Fig. 7.1

■ This requires knowledge of the possible changes in neural function, particularly early changes

7.3.3   General Categories of Methods
■ Non-electronic methods: wake-up testing; ankle-clonus test (less used, observed during induction of anaesthesia and these findings compared with the patient who is partially awake intraoperatively or post-operatively)
■ Electronic monitoring, e.g. SSEP/MEP

7.3.4   Wake-Up Testing
■ Advantage:
  – Safe when done properly
  – Excellent back-up test when comprehensive electrophysiological methods are unreliable or unavailable
  – Low cost
    (Procedure: the anaesthetised patient is awakened to a level that they can respond to verbal commands to move the hands. Once this has been performed, the patient is asked to move their foot and ankle)
■ Disadvantage:
  – The results are difficult to interpret in the context of global neurologic function
  – Delay in detecting adverse event

- Neurologic injury may have occurred hours before, especially if there is a delay in waking up after corrective manoeuvre. Best opportunity for timely intervention may be lost

7.3.5   Stimulation and Recipient sites for SSEP
▨ Stimulus:
  - Peripheral nerve
  - Skin dermatome – unreliable
  - Nerve root
  - Spinal cord
▨ Recording site:
  - Cranium scalp
  - Spine
  - Erb's point

7.3.5.1 Pros and Cons of SSEP
▨ Disadvantage:
  - Only indirect information of motor tract integrity
  - Crude global cord integrity
  - Not measure motor function
  - Owen (Spine 1991) documented SSEP alone detects 70% of spinal cord injuries, and motor loss can occur without SEP changes
▨ Advantage: sensitive to dorsal medial tracts of SC

7.3.5.2 Interpretation of SSEP
▨ Amplitude: depends on number of axons and synchrony; warning criteria – decrease in 50%
▨ Latency: depends on neuron conduction velocity. Changes early in compression; late in ischaemic warning criteria: >10% prolonged (but natural degradation only up to 5% when under anaesthesia)

7.3.6   Stimulation and Recipient Sites for MEP
▨ Site of stimulus: motor cortex, sometimes at cord
▨ Transcranial MEP more specific for cortico-spinal tract function
▨ Stimulus: electrical (magnetic not yet FDA approved)
▨ Advantage of electrical stimulus – less sensitive to anaesthesia, practical usefulness during operation

- Recording area:
  - SC (spinal cord evoked potential)
  - Muscle-myogenic: specific muscle function, useful for specific muscle group, e.g. polio surgery. More useful if already partial neurology preoperatively
  - Nerve-neurogenic, reflects global function of spinal cord and extremity, the waveform is mainly a backfire antidromic sensory potential, not a substitute for myogenic MEP

7.3.7 False-Positive and False-Negative for Nerve Monitoring

- False-positive: test abnormal, but wake-up/postoperatively normal
- False-negative: new neurology not detected intraoperatively by test; causes include inappropriate criteria, inappropriate test selected, equipment/personnel faults; notice SSEP cannot reliably detect motor function

7.3.8 Pre-Requisites for Proper Intraoperative Neural Monitoring

- Select the appropriate monitoring method
- Minimise interference
- Proper and secure positioning of electrodes
- Maximise quality of signals, e.g. in performing far-field SSEP, techniques like signal averaging and filtering are useful
- Trained personnel to run the monitoring devices, most having certification from ABNM (American Board for Neurophysiological Monitoring)
- Surgeon knowledgeable of basic neurophysiology and willing to take heed of intraoperative warnings voiced by the technicians

7.3.9 Selecting the Ideal Method

- Consider the anatomy at risk:
  - Spinal cord
  - Nerve roots
  - Level
  - Select appropriate procedure, e.g. SC at risk – MEP with stimulation at motor strip of cerebral cortex, SC, transcranial MEP
    (Or mixed nerve SEP with stimulation at median, ulna, posterior tibial, peroneal, femoral nerves)

7.3.10   Key Observations to Look for Intraoperatively

- Looking out for sudden changes (e.g. decrease in amplitude) in the neurophysiologic potentials rather than their absolute values
- The neurophysiologist must be able to diagnose quickly whether the change is likely to be genuine or represents interference

7.3.11   Typical Changes in Compression, Ischaemic and Traction Injuries

- Compression: less amplitude (fewer axons respond), increase latency (early)
- Distraction: less amplitude, increase in latency to as great as compression
- Ischaemic: less amplitude (fewer axons), change in latency occurs late
- Association with correction of deformity – slow deterioration multiple levels

7.3.12   Advantages of Spinal Cord Monitoring

- Easy to use
- Reliable
- Minimise significant changes in anaesthesia
- Not interfere with surgery
- Monitor continuously – not only during critical manoeuvre (P.S. ischaemic injury due to spinal distraction takes a while to become evident)

7.3.13   Disadvantage of Spinal Cord Monitoring

- False positives can occur: test abnormal, but wake-up/postoperatively normal
- False negatives can occur: neurological deficit not detected intraoperatively by test; causes include inappropriate criteria for what constitutes normality, inappropriate test selected, equipment/personnel faults; notice also SSEP cannot detect motor function. Owen (Spine 1991) documented that SSEP alone detects 70% of spinal cord injuries

7.3.14   Current Trend and the Future

- Simultaneous measure of various neurophysiological procedures since each with its own pros and cons
- Multiple recording sites – consider multiple permutation of stimulus and recording sites; multiple electro-physiological procedures

General Bibliography

Echternach JL (2003) Electromyography and nerve conduction testing, Slack, New Jersey

Selected Bibliography of Journal Articles

1. Lehman RM (2004) A review of neurophysiological testing. Neurosurg Focus 16(4):ECP1
2. Owen JH, Bridwell KH et al. (1991) The clinical application of neurogenic motor evoked potentials to monitor spinal cord function during surgery. Spine 16(8): S385–S390

8 Gait Analysis

Contents

8.1   Introduction

8.1.1   Traditional Definition of Gait
▪ A repetitive sequence of limb movements to safely advance the body forwards with minimum energy expenditure

8.1.2   Author's View
▪ The above definition of gait commonly found in most textbooks holds too simplistic a view of this complex yet seemingly simple neuromuscular task. For a detailed explanation please refer to the last chapter of this book
▪ A new, more suitable definition is hereby proposed

8.1.3   Revised Definition of Gait
▪ A repetitive sequence of limb movements to safely advance the human body forwards with minimum energy expenditure that requires higher cognitive neural function and a properly functioning neuromuscular system for its correct execution. It is far from being a simple automated task

8.1.4   Five Key Elements for Normal Gait (According to Gage)
▪ Stability in stance (foot and ankle)
▪ Clearance (of foot) in swing
▪ Pre-positioning of foot (terminal swing)
▪ Adequate step length
▪ Energy-efficient fashion (normal energy expended 2.5 kcal/min, less than twice that used for just standing or sitting). This requires the presence of efficient phase shifts

8.1.5   The Important Role of Energy Conservation
▪ The design of our LL is based on the bipedal gait
▪ Has to be energy efficient and equipped with methods of shock absorption

8.1.6   How is Energy Efficiency Achieved in Normal Gait?
▪ Muscles lengthen prior to contraction to maximise force generation
▪ Gait cycle designed to minimise the excursion of the CG during walking – through the intricate interactions of the segments of the LL via joint function, especially at the knee and pelvis

■ Bi-articular muscles like rectus femoris, psoas, hamstrings, gastrocnemius, are instrumental in aiding the transfer of energy between segments

■ Needs delicate neural control to effect efficient phase shifts

8.1.7 Shock Absorption

■ Especially important in the loading response:
  - Knee flexion during early stance
  - Eccentric tibialis anterior (TA) contraction
  - Change in orientation of the transverse tarsal articulation
  - Heel pad

8.1.8 Magnitude of Energy Expenditures

■ Brisk walking×60% more
■ Below knee brace×10% more
■ 15° knee flexion contracture×25% more
■ BKA × 60% more
■ AKA × 100% more
■ Crutches walking × 300% more

8.2   Nature of Gait Analysis

8.2.1   What is Gait Analysis?

■ An objective measurement of human locomotion (Fig. 8.1)

8.2.2   Common Patient Groups for Gait Analysis?

■ Children with CP: mostly diplegics, some hemiplegics
■ Some neuromuscular disorders, e.g. spina bifida, tiptoe walkers
■ Orthotic advice/comparison (see Chap. 11)
■ Prostheses advice/comparison, and investigate abnormal gait in amputees (see Chap. 10)
■ Investigate the cause of unsteady gait and frequent fallers (see Chap. 19)
■ As an objective outcome measure after, say, multi-level surgery in CP and other disorders (see Chap. 11)

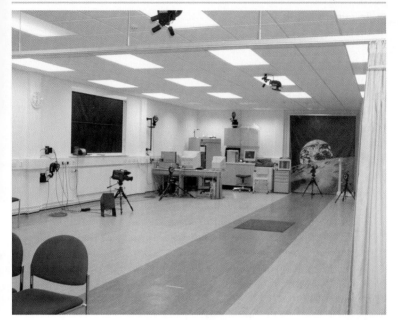

Fig. 8.1. Typical gait laboratory set-up. Shown here is the famous Oxford Gait Laboratory

8.2.3 Common Aims of Gait Analysis
- Understanding of complex gait patterns
- Assess and help differentiate dynamic vs static contractures
- Distinguish between primary problems and coping responses
- Analyse abnormal muscular firing patterns
- Objective comparison between preoperative and postoperative gait patterns
- Comparison between different prostheses or orthoses, etc.

8.2.4 The Gait Cycle
- Human gait cycle consists of the stance phase and the swing phase

8.2.4.1 Stance Phase (60%)
- Initial contact
- Loading response (0–10%)
- Mid-stance (10–30%)

- Terminal stance (30–50%)
- Pre-swing (50–60%)

8.2.4.2 Swing Phase (40%)
- Initial swing (60–73%)
- Mid-swing (73–87%)
- Terminal swing (87–100%)

8.2.4.3 Details of Components of the Gait Cycle
- The following discussion will be divided into different sections:
    - Sects. 8.3 and 8.4 detail the key events taking place in each phase of gait, the muscle activities, and the relevant kinetics (such as flexion or extension knee moments)
    - Sect. 8.4 details the typical kinematic data in 3D (based on tracings on Vicon systems, Fig. 8.2) with special emphasis on sagittal plane kinematics

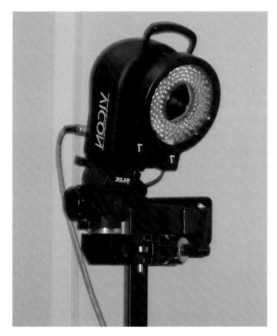

Fig. 8.2. Many gait laboratories utilise 3D gait analysis using the popular Vicon systems

- Sect. 8.5 details the relevant temporal parameters to be recorded in gait analysis
- Sect. 8.6 details the use of and need for EMG data; more discussion on the use of EMG will be found in the section on CP gait analysis in the last part of this chapter

8.3　Key Events in the Gait Cycle

8.3.1　Initial Contact
- Initiated by heel touching the ground
- Hip extensors decelerate thigh
- Passive knee extension due to anterior ground reaction force (GRF)
- Foot held in neutral by ankle dorsiflexors, and leg optimally positioned for progression to other stages

8.3.2　Loading Response
- Body weight transfer onto stance limb
- Knee flexor moment controlled by eccentric quadriceps activity
- Eccentric TA controls ankle plantar flexion (1st rocker)
- Hip extensors initiate hip extension
- Heel aids in shock absorption, other means of shock absorption will now be discussed

8.3.3　Shock Absorption During Loading Response
- During the loading response, the knee axis is orientated anterior to the line of the GRF, and the knee is subject therefore to a flexion moment
- Muscular forces are needed to overcome the tendency of the knee to buckle
- In the normal person, this is accomplished by the quadriceps
- But in normal gait, the knee is allowed a controlled amount of knee flexion, of up to $18°$ for better shock absorption

8.3.4　Mid-Stance
- Eccentric contraction of plantar flexors advances tibia over foot (2nd rocker)
- Knee extension assisted by "plantar flexion–knee extension couple"
- Progression assisted by momentum of swinging limb

8.3.4.1 Elaboration of the "Plantar Flexion–Knee Extension Couple"

- The knee flexion moment is diminished at mid stance by plantar flexion of the foot
- This will move the centre of pressure further anterior on the plantar surface of the foot. The result is moving the line of action of the GRF further anterior to the knee, thus explaining the so-called plantar flexion–knee extension couple

8.3.5   Terminal Stance

- Passive hip and knee extension allows forward progression of trunk
- Powerful contraction of plantar flexors assists forward acceleration (3rd rocker)

8.3.5.1 Key Event During Terminal Stance

- At terminal stance, the stance limb is stable because the ankle position is being regulated by an eccentric contraction of the plantar flexors. This move allows the foot to become a stable long-lever arm that generates a strong extension moment at the knee joint

8.3.6   Pre-Swing

- Body weight unloaded for transfer to opposite limb, stance limb unlocked for swing
- Plantar flexor activity decreases, and toes lift off
- Rapid initiation of knee flexion contributes to limb advancement in swing

8.3.7   Initial Swing

- Contraction of iliopsoas, short head of biceps and TA
- Momentum facilitated by hip and knee flexor activity

8.3.8   Mid-Swing

- Hip flexion and knee extension essentially passive, assisted by gravity
- Ankle continues to actively dorsiflex to neutral

8.3.9   Terminal Swing

- Transition phase between swing and stance
- Limb advancement completed by active knee extension to neutral
- Eccentric gluteus maximus and hamstrings decelerate hip and knee
- Neutral dorsiflexion maintained

8.4   Contribution of Ground Reaction Force Data

8.4.1   Introduction
Analysis of the magnitude and direction of GRF help us understand normal and abnormal kinetics such as momentum about the joints

8.4.2   Determinants of GRF Values
- Body weight
- Walking speed
- Cadence
- Other factors, e.g. amputees with "energy-storing" feet; energy release in terminal stance can affect GRF values (refer to the Sect. 8.8.1 on gait changes in amputees)

8.4.3   Determinants of Direction of GRF
- Alignment of body
- Alignment of LL segments during gait in particular
- Compensation mechanisms (if any) used by the individual

8.5   Kinematics Data Collection

8.5.1   Sagittal Pelvis (or Pelvic Tilt)
- In normal gait, no large fluctuations (Fig. 8.3)
- But significant change, e.g. in CP crouching as a compensation mechanism

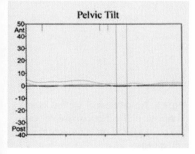

Fig. 8.3. Typical normal tracing of the sagittal pelvic kinematic profile. The limits of "normality" have to be found out for a particular population under study, however

8.5.2   Sagittal Hip (Flexion/Extension)

- Flexed at 35° at heel strike, then progressively extend in stance until a maximum of 6° in terminal stance (Fig. 8.4)
- Of course, flexion is seen in swing phase

8.5.3   Sagittal Knee (Flexion/Extension)

- Flex slightly in early stance to absorb shock (Fig. 8.5)
- Extended in terminal stance and pre-swing by the plantar flexion–knee extension couple
- Maximum knee flexion one third into the swing phase (to make up for the fact that the ankle has still at this time not recovered from its plantar flexion posture)
- After maximum flexion in swing, need to extend again to get adequate step length!

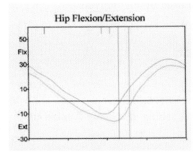

Fig. 8.4. Typical normal tracing of the sagittal hip kinematic profile

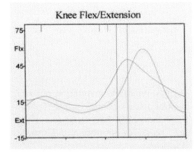

Fig. 8.5. Typical normal sagittal knee kinematic profile, notice maximal knee flexion at around one-third into the swing phase

8.5.4 Sagittal Ankle (Dorsiflexion/Plantar Flexion)

- Plantar flexion maximal in toe-off and early swing
- Amount of dorsiflexion increases as stance phase proceeds, ankle plantar flexors guide against excess dorsiflexion (Fig. 8.6)

8.5.5 Coronal Pelvis (or Pelvic Obliquity)

- Rises 4° during the loading response, due to eccentric contraction of the hip abductors
- Minor fall in swing phase sometimes seen (Fig. 8.7)

8.5.6 Coronal Hip (Abduction/Adduction)

- Adducted in early stance
- Late stance/swing, abducts and pelvis drops slightly
- Swing abduction eases foot clearance (Fig. 8.8)

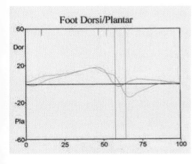

Fig. 8.6. Typical normal sagittal ankle kinematic profile. Notice that the amount of dorsiflexion increases as the stance phase proceeds, but excess dorsiflexion is prevented by the plantar flexors

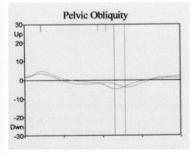

Fig. 8.7. Typical normal coronal kinematic profile of the pelvis

8.5.7   Transverse Plane Pelvis (or Pelvic Rotation)
- Only see slight internal rotation in early stance
- Needs 3D to ascertain any deviation

8.5.8   Transverse Plane Hip (Hip Rotation)
- Slight internal rotation in early stance, otherwise unremarkable (Fig. 8.9)

8.5.9   Coronal Knee (Varus/Valgus)
- This profile is not usually included on an ordinary computer print-out (Fig. 8.10)

8.5.10   Transverse Ankle (Foot Rotation)
- Most normal gait with around 15° external rotation of the foot (Fig. 8.11)
- This profile is not usually included on an ordinary computer print-out

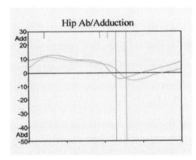

Fig. 8.8. Typical normal coronal kinematic profile of the hip

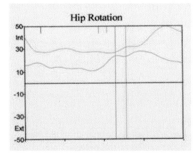

Fig. 8.9. Transverse plane kinematic profile of the hip, notice that there is some degree of internal rotation at early stance

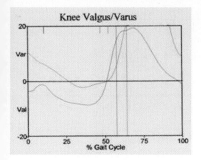

Fig. 8.10. Normal coronal kinematic profile of the knee

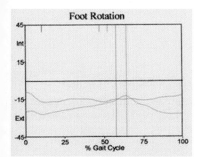

Fig. 8.11. Normal transverse plane kinematic profile at the ankle

8.6   Temporal Parameters (According to Sutherland)

Age	1	2	3	7	Adult
Single support (%)	32.1	33.5	34.8	36.7	36.7
Toe off (%)	67.1	67.1	65.5	62.4	63.6
Speed (cm/s)	63.7	71.8	85.5	114.3	121.6
Cadence (steps/min)	176	168.8	163.5	143.5	114
Step length (cm)	21.6	27.6	32.9	47.9	65.5
Stride length (cm)	43	54.9	67.7	96.6	129.4

(Fig. 8.12)

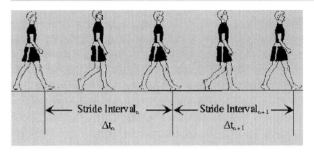

Fig. 8.12. Stride interval (courtesy of physionet.org). Other temporal parameters include speed, cadence, step length

8.7   Dynamic EMG Data

8.7.1   Electromyography
▥ Activation and control of muscles rely on electrical impulses
▥ Measuring electrical activity gives indirect indication of muscle action

8.7.2   Dynamic EMG
▥ Measures electrical activity of a contracting muscle (Fig. 8.13)
▥ Assesses timing, relative intensity and absence of activity
▥ Useful in isolating cause of particular abnormality, e.g. hindfoot varus

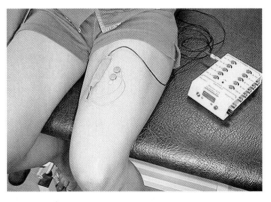

Fig. 8.13. Electrodes connected for testing of dynamic EMG

8.7.3   Surface Electrodes
▧ Easy to apply
▧ No discomfort to patient
▧ Good for assessing muscle groups
▧ Superficial muscles only
▧ Subject to cross-talk
▧ Signal attenuated by soft tissue

8.7.4   Fine-Wire Electrodes
▧ Good for isolating single muscle
▧ Used for deep muscles
▧ Requires skill to insert
▧ Some discomfort to patient
▧ Consider providing some distraction to patient to ease insertion

8.7.5   Assessing Kinetics and Joint Power
▧ Kinetics involves measurement of joint forces and moments (Fig. 8.14)
▧ Mechanical power = net joint moment×angular velocity
  – Gives an indication of net muscle power
  – Does not account for power produced in co-contractions

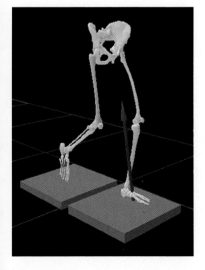

Fig. 8.14. Computer software animation of joint moment (courtesy of Vicon Motion Systems)

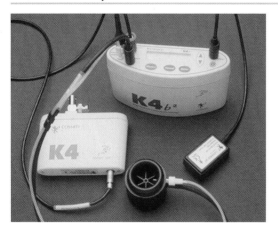

Fig. 8.15. Instrumentation for assessing oxygen consumption

8.7.6   Assessing Oxygen Consumption
- Physiological cost index (PCI) (Fig. 8.15)
- Heart rate and walking speed
- O_2 consumption and/or CO_2 production

8.8   Gait Anomalies

8.8.1   Amputee Gait Analysis

8.8.1.1 Uses of Gait Analysis in Amputees
- Gain knowledge of the adaptation strategies used and pattern of muscle firing and use
- Hence, designing better rehabilitation protocol for gait training in amputees
- Allows comparison between and testing of new prostheses (Rietman, Prosthet Orthot Int 2002)

8.8.1.2 Caution in Interpreting Gait Analysis Report of Amputees
- The gait of the amputee depends on:
  - The K-classification (see Chap. 10 on amputee rehabilitation)
  - Whether the alignment and fitting of the prosthesis is accurate
  - The type of prosthesis used
  - Whether the patient has adopted compensatory bodily manoeuvres

8.8.1.3 Contents
- Adaptive strategies in gait
- Influence of different parts of the prosthesis
- Pressure in the socket
- Influence of the mass of the prosthesis
- Energy considerations in gait

8.8.1.4 Adaptive Strategies in Gait

8.8.1.4.1 Transtibial Amputee
- Sound limb stance phase: near normal electrical activity in gait
- Affected limb stance phase: decreased energy-absorbing function of the quadriceps and the prosthetic ankle/foot unit → adaptation: increased work of the hip extensors, co-contraction to increased knee stability and/or in response to the increased activity of the hip extensors (according to Czerniecki)
- Sound limb swing phase: increased muscle work done at hip and knee muscles in deceleration phase of stance presumably will increase forward momentum of the weakened push-off on the affected limb (Czeriecki)

8.8.1.4.2 Transfemoral Amputee
- Sound limb stance phase: increased muscle work of both hip extensors and ankle flexors – to compensate for decreased push-off on affected limb (according to Seroussi)
- Sound limb mid-stance: increased higher than normal COM from increased plantar flexion work – creates a degree of vaulting to clear the other prosthetic leg
- Affected limb stance phase: adaptations needed since no sensory-motor function of knee and ankle/foot – increased firing of hip extensors (in a closed chain fashion) to prevent knee flexion in the first 30–40% stance, although knee stability will also be helped by correct prosthetic choice and alignment of knee and foot units (Seroussi)
- Affected side pre-swing: despite the prosthesis weighing only one third of the limb it replaced, the hip flexors activate the same extent as normal gait – to compensate for decreased push-off
- Dysvascular amputee tends to have worse gait performance, not because of speed, but from decreased push-off, and decreased ability of quadriceps and hamstrings to compensate for absent ankle/foot unit (Hermodsson)

▨ Running: obviously not all transfemoral amputees can run, for the very athletic subgroup who do "run", the kinematics of affected limb is much more abnormal than the transtibial amputee (Buckley)

▨ Affected limb swing phase: modern knee units are partly able to take over the energy-absorbing function of early and late swing phase of the quadriceps and hamstrings respectively

8.8.1.5 Influence of Different Prosthetic Parts

8.8.1.5.1 Influence of the Prosthetic Foot

ROM Issues

Many energy-storing feet (e.g. Seattle foot) have increased ROM more than conventional ones like SACH (Linden and Rao)

From a kinetic point of view, the most significant factor concerning prosthetic feet seemed to be presence or absence of a joint allowing plantar flexion (according to Cortes)

That said, balance in late stance is highly dependent on dorsiflexion mobility (Postema) in which significant late stance dorsiflexion may in fact provide a destabilising knee flexion torque

Too limited dorsiflexion mobility in late stance (e.g. SACH), although will provide a knee extension moment, but lacks a smooth third rocker roll-over

It is not surprising to find that:

– Older people not infrequently prefer feet like SACH that give them better stability at late stance

– Younger, more active amputees tend to prefer feet with some degree of dorsiflexion mobility

Energy Storage Release of Energy Storing Feet

Consider the three processes: energy absorption, energy storage and energy release

Heel strike: prosthetic feet will absorb energy at heel strike, but the stiffer the prosthetic foot the less energy is absorbed. Many energy-storing feet store part of the energy during stance in their spring mechanism, part of which is to be released later

Late stance:

– The amount of energy release reported in the literature by energy-storing feet varies a lot, from essentially no difference to significant differences, the study by Schneider for instance revealed that the Flex-Foot decreased energy cost of walking in childhood transtibial amputee more than conventional feet

- In fact, during push-off, there can be some energy storage – only this time by the forefoot, not the hindfoot, and again less if the forefoot is stiff
- Traditional SACH feet were found not to store energy from significant push-off activity

Choice of feet from the energy viewpoint:

- Heel-strike: feet with too stiff a heel will not absorb appreciable energy at heel-strike and will not be too comfortable to walk on since little shock absorption function. Decreasing the stiffness excessively is not good either, since too much energy gets absorbed and lessens the amount that might be stored or released later
- Push-off: contrary to popular belief, studies tend to show that energy release in energy-storing feet in fact occurs before push-off starts and does not coincide with push-off (Lehmann 1993)

Effect on Sound Limb Loading

Choice of feet from the viewpoint of the effect on the sound side; this has some bearing in dysvascular individuals and in those whose reason for amputation is very much DM-related. (High percentage of limb loss, especially in DM individuals on opposite side on serial follow-up studies). It was found that users of SACH feet cause a significantly higher loading response to the sound limb relative to Flex-Foot (Lehman). This may be partly due to lack of push-off from SACH feet, but also due to the lower centre of mass observed in late stance of energy-storing feet that have dorsiflexion mobility

8.8.1.5.2 Influence of Prosthetic Knee Unit

Knee Unit Influence

A comparison made between Otto Bock polycentric knee and pneumatic swing phase control knee found that the latter type ambulates at higher speed, but less ROM at swing and amputees seemed to favour the latter in terms of degree of comfort and speed (according to Boonstra)

Although literature here is not abundant, the important influence of the various types of knee units have been adequately discussed in the

Sect. 10.2.9.1 on prosthetic knee units in Chap. 10 on amputee rehabilitation

8.8.1.6   Pressure Measurements in the Socket in the Transtibial Amputee

▨ Most literature (concerning patella tendon-bearing socket) in this area was mainly case series and as such the level of evidence is not strong. There is some suggestion that:

– The variance in pressure differences with regard to variance in time seemed to be greater than that from subtle alignment changes. Also, fluctuations of stump volume appear to be an added confounding variable (according to Sanders)

– Another case series showed pressure concentration more in proximal-posterior aspect of socket in heel-strike, and shifting to proximal-anterior in mid-stance (according to Covery)

8.8.1.7   Effect of the Mass of the Prosthesis in the Transtibial Amputee

▨ The energy cost of (traumatic) transtibial amputees is 13% higher than that in healthy individuals (Gailey)

▨ Addition of weights to the prosthesis was found by Hillery to alter kinematics in transtibial amputees; ambulation with a lower mass prosthesis tends to have increased cadence, together with slight increase in hip flexion and extension, but not of the knee

▨ Addition of mass seems to increase the eccentric muscular effort of the hip extensors during deceleration in late swing (according to Halc)

▨ One additional similar study showed increased hip flexors with concentric firing to accelerate the prosthesis in early swing (according to Gitter)

▨ Overall, studies on adding weights evenly to the prosthesis have so far not revealed major kinematic changes

8.8.1.8   Energy Considerations

8.8.1.8.1 Transtibial Amputee

▨ A more heterogenous group of transtibial amputees studied by Gailey showed a 16% increase in energy and 11% increase in walking speed. No significant correlation of mass of prosthesis, stump length and cost of energy, although further data analysis did show the small advantage of longer stump length

8.8.1.8.2 Transfemoral Amputee
- One study comparing able-bodied individuals and transfemoral amputees revealed that the most comfortable walking speed in the former tends to be the most metabolically efficient. In transfemoral amputees, the comfortable walking velocity is lower than the most metabolically efficient walking velocity (according to Jaegers)

8.8.1.9 Gait Anomalies of Amputees

8.8.1.9.1 Causes of Stance Phase Problems

Excess Lordosis During Stance
- A poorly shaped post wall may cause a patient to forwardly rotate their pelvis with compensatory trunk extension. Other causes include insufficient initial flexion built into socket, hip flexion contracture, or weak hip extensors

Pistoning
- This is best seen in the coronal plane. Common causes include too loose suspension, inadequate prosthetic socks used, inadequate support under mediotibial flare or patella tendon in the transtibial amputee

Knee Buckling and Instability
- Causes include knee axis that is too far forward, insufficient plantar flexion, failure to limit dorsiflexion, weak hip extensors, hard heel, large hip flexion contracture, and posteriorly placed foot. Stability is achieved with a plantar flexed foot, a soft heel, or a more anteriorly placed foot

Lateral Trunk Bends to the Prosthetic Side in Mid-Stance
- Causes include a prosthesis that is too short, insufficient lateral wall, abducted socket, residual limb pain; leaning will reduce force on the prosthesis, abduction contracture, and foot is too outset

Vaulting
- Vaulting of the non-prosthetic limb may be due to prosthesis being too long, too much knee friction and poor suspension

8.8.1.9.2 Causes of Swing Phase Problems

Swing Leg in an Abducted Pose
> Causes include prosthesis being too long, abduction contracture, or medial socket wall encroaching on the groin

Circumduction
> Causes include prosthesis being too long, prosthetic knee joint with too much friction making it difficult to bend the knee during swing-through, or abduction contracture

Foot "Whips" Medially or Laterally in Initial Swing
> Causes include socket maybe being rotated medially or laterally relative to the line of progression, or cuff suspension tabs not aligned evenly

Prosthetic Foot Touching the Floor in Mid-Swing
> Causes include inadequate suspension, prosthesis being too long, limitation of knee flexion by the socket or suspension system, or weak plantar flexion of the non-prosthetic limb

Terminal Swing Impact
> Inappropriate selection of the type of prosthetic knee joint may cause the amputee to deliberately or forcibly extend the knee

Conclusion
> The above represents a summary of the latest research work on amputee gait
> One may argue against the applicability of findings in gait laboratory to real life, but it is one of the better objective measures at our disposal

8.8.2   Gait in Cerebral Palsy Patients

8.8.2.1   Timing of Gait Analysis in Children
■ Nearly all adult motions of walking are achieved in normal children by age 3 years. But the real adult pattern is not maturely formed until age 7. Thus, gait analysis is seldom performed prior to the age of 6–7

8.8.2.2 Causes of Gait Anomalies in CP
■ Spasticity
■ Dynamic or fixed muscle contracture
■ Lever arm dysfunction
■ Joint contracture
■ Impaired balance reactions and loss of selective muscular control and equilibrium reactions, e.g. difficulty stopping if walking quickly

8.8.2.3 Indications for Gait Analysis
■ Mainly in diplegia (e.g. from deteriorating gait, consideration for surgery, baseline for future management, orthotic management) and occasionally hemiplegia

8.8.2.4 Other Indications
■ Baseline to plan future management, e.g. physiotherapy, botulinum toxin
■ Consideration for surgery
■ Deciding the type of surgery
■ Orthotic management or comparison
■ Postoperative evaluation
■ Outcome measurement

8.8.2.5 Information Obtainable from 3D Gait Analysis
■ Information not always obtainable with 2D gait analysis, e.g. differentiating adduction from limb rotation when transverse plane analysis can help
■ Lever arm dysfunction
■ Coping responses
■ The exact abnormal muscle activity accounting for altered ROM of joints or motion of body segments
■ Information on muscle recruitment: notice that differences for balance control in children with spasticity are due to CNS deficits as well as mechanical changes in posture (Gait Posture 1998)

8.8.2.6 Summary of Limitations of 2D Observational Analysis
■ Descriptive not quantitative
■ No information on out-of-plane rotations
■ Easy to be visually deceived

8.8.2.7   Proper Physical Examination Before Gait Analysis

▦ Muscle tone (e.g. Ashworth scale)
▦ Muscle power and strength
▦ Assess any deformity or contracture
▦ ROM

8.8.2.8   What Other Data to Collect Clinically Besides Static Data

▦ Dynamic parameters like Tardieu scores and assess for the presence of selective muscular control

8.8.2.9   Measurements in Gait Analysis

▦ Motion (kinematics)
▦ Temporal parameters
▦ Forces causing motion (kinetics)
▦ Muscle activity (dynamic EMG – electromyography)

8.8.2.9.1 Kinematics

▦ A quantitative description of the motion of joints or body segments
▦ The normal kinematic tracings have been discussed. Here follows a few examples of abnormal tracings in CP patients

Crouch Knee
Characterised by:
- Increased stance phase hip flexion
- Persistent knee flexion >30° throughout stance
- Excessive dorsiflexion throughout stance (Fig. 8.16)

Jump Knee
Characterised by:
- Increased knee flexion at initial contact correcting to near normal in mid- to late stance
- Toe or flat foot strike
- Increased stance phase hip flexion

8.8.2.9.2 Kinetics

▦ Involves a study of internal and external forces involved in movement, and concerns the study of joint moments and powers. Figure 8.14 in this chapter illustrates the later use of force plate to demonstrate the

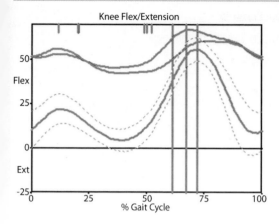

Fig. 8.16. Typical kinematic profile of crouch gait in a cerebral palsy patient

direction and orientation of dynamic knee valgus thrust on force plate analysis. Detailed discussion of kinetics is beyond the scope of this book. The reader is advised to read about the improved understanding of lower extremity joint moments based on the now popular 3D inverse dynamics model (Liu et al., Gait Posture 2006)

8.8.2.9.3 Temporal Parameters

- Cadence (steps/min)
- Speed (m/s)
- Stride/step length
- Stride/step time

8.8.2.9.4 Dynamic EMG

- Dynamic EMG was alluded to earlier (Sect. 8.7)
- Its use in decision-making in management of children with CP cannot be over-emphasised, e.g. to find the phase of gait where the muscle in question is active, presence of selective motor control, comparing the concomitant activities of the agonists and antagonists

8.8.2.10   Special Gait Patterns

8.8.2.10.1   Gait Patterns in Spastic Hemiplegia

Types of Spastic Hemiplegia Gait
  Gait types I–IV
  Type I: equinus in swing
  Type II: equinus in stance and swing, $2°$ knee hyperextension
  Type III: knee also involved with spastic rectus and hamstrings
  Type IV: hip involvement with spastic psoas and adductors
  Increased severity = increased proximal involvement (Winters et al., J Bone Joint Surg 1987)

8.8.2.10.2   Knee Patterns in Gait of CP

- Some experts believe that discreet descriptive patterns are recognisable in >80% of diplegics

8.8.2.10.3   Common CP Knee Patterns in Gait

- Crouch knee gait
- Jump knee gait
- Stiff knee gait
- Recurvatum knee gait (Sutherland et al., Clin Orthop Relat Res 1993)

Crouch Knee Gait
  Characterised by:
  – Increased stance phase hip flexion
  – Persistent knee flexion >30° throughout stance
  – Excessive dorsiflexion throughout stance
  Aetiology:
  – Weak ankle plantar flexors or over-lengthened TAs or from increasing height and weight
  – Overactive knee flexors (and/or rectus co-spasticity)
  – Overactive hip flexors
  Clinical examination – most have:
  – Hip flexion contractures
  – Knee flexion contractures
  – Severe hamstring tightness (popliteal angle >70°)
  Treatment:
  – Therapy – passive stretching and/or serial casting hamstrings

- Orthoses – but anterior GRF orthoses unsuccessful if high popliteal angle
- Botulinum toxin – but unsuccessful if fixed contractures
- Surgery – multilevel releases or transfers/osteotomies

Jump Knee Gait
- Characterised by:
  - Increased knee flexion at initial contact correcting to near normal in mid- to late stance
  - Toe or flat foot strike
  - Increased stance phase hip flexion
- Aetiology:
  - Overactive – hip flexors, knee flexors and/or rectus co-spasticity and/or plantar flexors
- Physical examination:
  - Usually associated with dynamic contractures
  - Moderate hamstring tightness (mean popliteal angle approximately 50°)
- Treatment:
  - Orthoses
  - Botulinum toxin
  - Multilevel surgery

Stiff Knee Gait
- Characterised by:
  - Delayed and reduced peak knee flexion in swing
  - Associated with compensations to aid clearance
  - Mainly a swing phase problem
- Physical examination:
  - Positive Duncan-Ely test
  - Reduced ROM in swing
  - Delayed and reduced peak knee flexion in swing
  - EMG = rectus co-spasticity in swing
- Treatment:
  - Rectus femoris transfer
  - Avoid isolated hamstring lengthening

Recurvatum Knee Gait

Characterised by:
- Toe or flat foot strike
- Recurvatum >2° in stance

Aetiology:
- Plantar flexor over-activity/contracture
- Weak dorsiflexors
- Overly aggressive hamstring lengthening

Physical examination:
- TA tightness
- Hip flexion contracture
- Some hamstring tightness (popliteal angle 40°)

Treatment:
- Passive stretching of TA contracture
- Serial casting
- Botulinum toxin to calves
- Leaf-spring ankle-foot orthosis (if drop foot in swing)
- Fixed ankle-foot orthosis (if equinus throughout)

General Bibliography

Kirtley C (2006) Clinical Gait Analysis – theory and practice. Churchill Livingstone, Elsevier, USA

Selected Bibliography of Journal Articles

1. Rietman JS, Postema K et al. (2002) Gait analysis in prosthetics: opinions, ideas and conclusions. Prosthet Orthot Int 26(1):50–57
2. Seroussi RE, Gitter A et al. (1996) Mechanical work adaptation of above-knee amputation. Arch Phys Med Rehabil 77(11):1209–1214
3. Hermodsson Y, Ekdahl C et al. (1998) Outcome after trans-tibial amputation for vascular disease. Scand J Caring Sci 12(2):73–80
4. Lehmann JF, Price R et al. (1993) Comprehensive analysis of energy storing feet: Flex Foot and Seattle Foot versus standard SACH foot. Arch Phys Med Rehabil 74(11):1225–1231
5. De Fretes A, Boonstra AM et al. (1994) Functional outcome of rehabilitated bilateral lower limb amputees. Prosthet Orthot Int 18(1):18–24
6. Gailey RS, Lawrence D et al. (1994) Energy expenditure of trans-tibial amputees during ambulation of self selected pace. Prosthet Orthot Int 18(2):84–91

7. Jaegers SM, Arendzen JH et al. (1996) An electromyographic study of hip muscles of transfemoral amputees in walking. Clin Orthop Relat Res 328:119–128
8. Patrick E, Ada L (2006) The Tardieu Scale differentiates contracture from spasticity whereas the Ashworth scale is confounded by it. Clin Rehabil 20(2):173–182
9. Winters TF, Gage JR et al. (1987) Gait patterns in spastic hemiplegia in children and young adults. J Bone Joint Surg Am 69(3):437–441
10. Sutherland DH, Davids JR (1993) Common gait abnormalities of the knee in cerebral palsy. Clin Orthop Relat Res 288:139–147

9   Principles of Sports Rehabilitation

Contents

9.1 Basic Principles in Sports Rehabilitation

9.1.1 Introduction

- We have already discussed the basic science of healing of soft tissues, and the various physical therapy techniques
- This short chapter serves to highlight the application of the principles discussed in sports rehabilitation
- A separate discussion has been included of the hot topic in sports medicine circles concerning the compatibility of simultaneous endurance and strength training for professional athletes

9.1.2 Cornerstones of Restoration of Proper Musculoskeletal Function

- Proper limb alignment and biomechanics
- Proper joint kinematics, stability and proprioception
- Proper neuromuscular control including sequence of firing (among individual muscles and between different functional groups)
- Proper length–tension relationships
- Proper force couples
- Proper pain management

9.1.2.1 Lower Limb Alignment

- Malalignment of the LL (e.g. bony deformity or malunion, or lever arm dysfunction) can adversely affect the biomechanics not only of the nearby joints, but of the whole kinetic chain and gait. Management of deformity and malunions was discussed in the companion volume to this book entitled *Orthopedic Traumatology, A Resident's Guide*

9.1.2.2 Joint Kinematics

- A very good example is the realisation in recent years that many ACL reconstructed knees may have residual abnormal kinematics as well as rotational instability

9.1.2.3 Illustrating the Importance of Joint Kinematics: Weak Point of Current ACL Single-Bundle Surgeries

- Normal knee kinematics not restored: most recent in vivo kinematics and high-speed stereo radiographic studies consistently show only antero-posterior stability is restored, but not rotational stability

- Under high loading conditions, the ability of brace to control pathological anterior laxity remains in question
- Delays voluntary muscle reaction time and muscular control
- Custom-made knee brace may be required in the setting of abnormal limb contour

9.1.2.5.2 Selecting the Ideal Knee Brace

▦ The ideal knee brace should allow normal rotation and translation to occur, preferably not increase (but decrease) the strain on ACL graft

▦ Important factors:
- Design – bilateral hinge-post-shell design most rigid; the 4-point fixation brace most effective in controlling anterior tibial translation
- Degree of fit between leg and brace
- Any axes mismatch
- Length – longer the brace, the more resistance it provides against anterior tibial displacement (balance between length and patient comfort)
- Some biomechanical studies did show a possible decrease in anterior tibial translation under low loads and/or having some restraint on axial rotation

9.1.2.5.3 Three Key Factors for Overall Brace Performance

▦ Mechanical feature of the brace – basic design and hinge

▦ Structure integrity of the design

▦ Brace limb interaction during loading. (On this point, a fine balance needed since brace–body interface being too rigid may accentuate effect of differences in axes between the knee and the brace)

9.1.2.6   Proper Length–Tension Relationship

▦ Example: the importance of length–tension relationship is exemplified by the observation that some athletes with ruptured Achilles tendon treated with casting may heal with the tendon lengthened

▦ This will cause weakened push-off, which may be reflected in a deterioration of sports performance, thus illustrating the importance of proper restoration of length–tension relationship in orthopaedic rehabilitation

9.1.2.7 Proper Force Couples

▓ Muscles around a joint are frequently designed to work as force couples; thus, under normal circumstances, the tone of agonist and antagonists around a joint work together to stabilise the joint

▓ An example of an area of the body where this principle of force couples needs to be particularly fine tuned and under delicate control are the rotator cuff muscles that help in stabilising the very mobile shoulder and centralise the humeral head in arm elevation

9.1.2.8 Management of Concomitant Pain

▓ The management of pain is so important that a separate chapter is devoted to pain (Chap. 15)

▓ Most literature on rehabilitation just mentions comments like "concomitant pain management is needed", etc. This is an understatement of the effects of pain

9.1.2.9 Key Concept: the Importance of *Early* Pain Management

▓ It cannot be over-emphasised that *early* pain management in the course of rehabilitation is most important, aiming at complete eradication of pain

▓ Pain, if persistent, will not only limit motion, it will limit flexibility, as is recorded in every standard textbook

▓ Pain, if persistent, causes prompt muscle wasting, e.g. pain after knee injury can quickly cause quadriceps shutdown and wasting if poorly managed

▓ Furthermore, if the patient is left with partially treated pain as well as the associated muscle weakness, the body tends to adopt an altered sequence of firing of muscles (Pathophysiology 2005) and rehabilitation of the wasted muscle group will be made even more difficult

▓ Persistent pain causes persistent spasticity and decreased relaxation of the affected muscle group. We know from our previous discussion that there is a narrow window for optimal sliding of muscle contractile units. Muscles persistently contracted and spastic from pain will affect performance and impair flexibility

9.2   Worked Examples: ACL Recent Advances and Rehabilitation After Acute Shoulder Dislocation in Sports

9.2.1   Introduction

■ Management of ACL injury was discussed in the companion volume of this book, including optimisation of surgical techniques in ACL reconstruction

■ Some recent advances include:

- The use of surgical navigation in improving the accuracy of tunnel placement is worthy of note (Fig. 9.1)

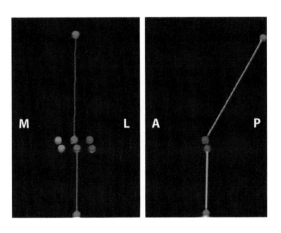

Fig. 9.1. Surgical navigation is now used in some centres to improve accuracy of tunnel placement in ACL reconstruction

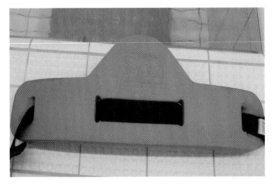

Fig. 9.2. Useful adjunctive equipment for performing under-water walking and other exercises popular in Scandinavian countries

- Incorporating the use of water sports in ACL rehabilitation programme (Fig. 9.2), such as underwater walking or running
- The growing need to document ACL outcomes with kinematic data
  instead of the usual KT-2000 measurements (see Figs. 9.3, 9.4)

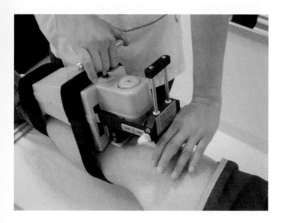

Fig. 9.3. Therapist performing the KT-1000 testing in a postoperative patient after ACL reconstruction

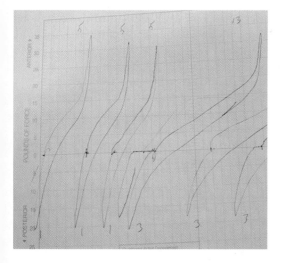

Fig. 9.4. KT-2000, which has superseded KT-1000, involves testing as in Fig. 9.3 together with objective machine testing with print-outs

9.2.2   Principles of Shoulder Rehabilitation After Acute Shoulder Dislocation

9.2.2.1 Introduction

▥ Acute shoulder dislocation is not uncommon in sporting events after rugby or other contact sports

▥ It is also a common question asked in professional examinations

▥ The following is a worked example of the use of the principles learned in rehabilitation of a patient after acute shoulder dislocation

9.2.2.2 Control of Pain and Inflammation

▥ Rest – in the case of shoulder dislocation, immobilise for ~3 weeks

▥ Pain-relieving modalities, e.g. ice, TENS, ultrasound, microwave diathermy

▥ Drugs, e.g. NSAID

▥ Soft tissue massage

9.2.2.3 Re-Establish Normal Activation Patterns of Kinetic Chain

▥ Rationale: the entire kinetic chain should be integrated into the rehabilitation process to minimise overload on the shoulder

▥ Assess and correct any breakdown and improper sequencing, e.g. poor shoulder and body stance posture, abnormal scapula positions, identify disorders of acromioclavicular joint (ACJ)/sternocostoclavicular joint (SCJ), muscular weakness and strength imbalances of UL/neck/trunk/LL

9.2.2.4 ROM Restoration

▥ Go gradually from passive, to assisted active, to active exercises

▥ Avoid movement in the direction that puts stress on the repair (e.g. if Bankart repair was done), or on the healing tissue for the initial period. Usually, soft tissue healing takes at least 6 weeks

▥ Establishment of full-shoulder ROM is essential, especially for professional athletes who perform overhead throwing

9.2.2.5 Restoration of Scapulothoracic and Glenohumeral Stabilisers

▥ A stable base for shoulder function is dependent on three main groups of muscles
  - The rotator cuff
  - Scapulothoracic stabilisers
  - Extrinsic muscles of the shoulder complex

9.2.2.5.1 The Rotator Cuff

- Important for the dynamic stability of the glenohumeral joint through the passive tension of the rotator cuff muscles and their action acting as humeral head depressor and stabiliser by compressing the joint surface and adjusting the tension of the static soft tissue restraints
- Especially important to restore the cuff function in cases of shoulder instability case

9.2.2.5.2 Scapulothoracic Stabilisers

- These consist of: rhomboids, trapezius, levator scapular, serratus anterior, pectoralis minor
- Important in stabilisation of the scapula. Normal scapula kinetics is important to elevate the acromion and avoid impinging the rotator cuff during arm elevation. Also, key role in subsequent sports-specific retraining, e.g. in professional throwers (e.g. scapula retraction during cocking, and protraction upon deceleration in the follow-through phase of throwing), swimmers

9.2.3   Neuromuscular Co-Ordination Training

- In later phase of rehabilitation: need to retrain deficits in proprioception and normal muscle co-ordination of the shoulder to avoid any impairment of functional stability and performance of complex activities especially in the athletic young patient
- Examples:
  - Stretch shortening drills to enhance neuromuscular coordination by combining strength with speed of motion
  - Proprioceptive neuromuscular facilitation adopts diagonal movement patterns that simulate normal functional planes of motion – can be used in enhancing neuromuscular control of the shoulder girdle by promoting co-contractions and facilitating muscular synergy and kinetic awareness

9.2.4   Sports-Specific Training

- In late rehabilitation, we may need to tailor the rehabilitation process to duplicate sport-specific dynamics and match individual needs
- Analysis of the biomechanical needs of specific sports is highly advisable. Illustrations of the biomechanical needs of common sports like tennis and the golf swing were discussed in Chap. 5

9.2.5   Cardiovascular Conditioning

▪ Total body aerobic conditioning should be initiated as early as possible after injury or surgery if this does not aggravate pain or impair healing

▪ This minimises effects of disuse and also has positive psychological impact on our patients

9.3   Concept of Strength–Endurance Continuum in Training for Professional Athletes

9.3.1   Introduction

▪ There has been much controversy among sports and athletic trainers as regards the compatibility of concomitant endurance vs strength training in high performance professional athletes

▪ The following discussion attempts to resolve the above controversy

9.3.2   Metabolic Pathway of Endurance Athletes

▪ Aerobic metabolism (the form used by endurance athletes) uses fat derived from triglycerides stored in muscles and glucose derived from glycogen stores. With endurance training, there is an adaptive increase in the enzymes for oxidation of lipids and relative sparing of glycogen stores

▪ An example of endurance athlete is a long distance runner

9.3.3   Physiological Adaptations After Prolonged Endurance Training

▪ Resting bradycardia (hence more heart rate reserve)

▪ Increased stroke volume, increased maximum cardiac output – that eases delivery of oxygen and substrates to tissues and quickens the rate of removal of unwanted metabolites from tissues

▪ Peripheral oxygen delivery is also aided by concomitant increases in total blood volume, red cells and haemoglobin

▪ Capillary density surrounding the types 1 and 2 muscle fibres also increases

▪ Increases VO_2 maximum by up to 30% with intensive training. Even when the increase in VO_2 maximum plateaus, endurance performance can sometimes increase further by mechanisms such as increased tol-

erance to the extent of exercise intensity before the onset of blood
lactate accumulation from more effective aerobic mechanism, and/or
more efficient removal of lactate from peripheral tissues

9.3.4　Metabolic Pathway of Athletes Needing "Strength and Speed"

■ These athletes use anaerobic metabolism with glucose as the major
fuel source. This results in lactic acid accumulation and an oxygen
debt. A transition to aerobic metabolism occurs as the sporting
event's duration exceeds 2–3 min
■ Sprinters are the typical examples of this type of athlete

9.3.5　Physiological Adaptations to Prolonged Strength Training

■ In response to resistance and strength training, there is mainly muscle
hypertrophy and the muscle cross-sectional area increases of both
slow- and fast-twitch muscle fibres depending on the training protocol. Slow-twitch fibres hypertrophy more with high-volume, low-intensity training; fast-twitch fibres hypertrophy more with low volume,
high-intensity training
■ On a microscopic scale, there is a decrease in "mitochondrial density"
or the number of mitochondria per volume of muscle tissue with increase in muscle mass, even though the number of mitochondria may
increase slightly. This change lowers aerobic capacity and is a phenomenon known as "mitochondrial dilution" – forms the basis of argument (by some) against concurrent strength and endurance training in professional athletes

9.3.6　Argument Against Concurrent Training

■ Loss of aerobic power can occur by the decrease in mitochondrial
density as muscle hypertrophy sets in with prolonged resistance training
■ Example: this explains why weight lifters for example refrain from endurance training, while do they take part in active strength training.
It has been shown in the literature in the past (Kraemer, J Appl Physiol 1995) that a short-term bout of high-intensity endurance exercise
inhibits performance in subsequent muscular strength activities

9.3.7   Argument for Concurrent Training

■ Unlike weight lifters for whom strength training forms the mainstay of their training programme. Other athletes such as sprinters who desire a well-rounded conditioning programme incorporating both aerobic and strength training should not be denied this opportunity; the same principle also applies to older athletes (Hurley, Exerc Sports Sci Rev 1998)

9.3.8   Use of "Circuit Resistance Training"

■ Newer regimens like "circuit resistance training" that de-emphasise the traditional, very brief intervals of heavy muscle strengthening in standard resistance training protocol are gaining in popularity. This is because this form of training provides a more general conditioning, with demonstrated improvements in body composition, muscle endurance and strength, as well as cardiovascular fitness (Haennel, Can J Sports Sci 1989)

■ In addition, circuit resistance training also provides supplementary off-season conditioning, even for sports that demand high levels of strength and power

9.3.9   Some Examples in the Sports Arena

■ Track and field: take the example of a runner who has had a hip injury that has lingered for some years, and who runs with a "seated" style due to his weak hip extensors. A strength training programme employing highly specific exercises designed to re-activate the hip extensors, as well as strengthen them, can make for more efficient and therefore faster running. Thus, strength training can sometimes be of benefit to endurance athletes

■ Rowing sports: take the example of the rower with weak low back muscles and poor core stability. Strengthening the weakened back and trunk muscles to improve core stability can correct the weak link and allow optimal connection between force generators and the oar. Again, this is an example of strength training benefiting an endurance athlete

■ Perhaps the best example of situations whereby strength training can become important even in endurance sports like the marathon one can think of is as follows. If one looks at the champion of an Olympic marathon and the champion of a wheel-chair marathon race for para-

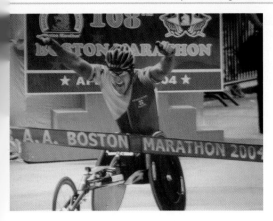

Fig. 9.5. Notice the well-built upper body of this gold medallist winning a marathon for wheel-chair users

athletes, one will make the following observation: many marathon champions have long thin non-muscular limbs. But the champions of wheel-chair races for paraplegics have strong muscular upper bodies (Fig. 9.5), in fact resembling athletes who do bench presses. In this scenario (the wheelchair endurance athlete), muscle strength of the upper body is key. Moreover, the wheelchair racer is depending on a much smaller total volume of muscle to do the work of the marathon race. The total volume of muscle is small enough so that the heart is no longer the limiting factor. In this situation, gaining muscle mass in combination with endurance training results in a more powerful endurance engine. In athletes such as these, strength training (of the upper body) is in fact a necessity in their training

9.3.10   Concept of "Strength–Endurance" Continuum

■ This implies that muscle strength and muscle endurance exist on a continuum, with muscle strength being 1 RM and muscle endurance representing the ability to exert a lower force repeatedly over time. Low numbers of repetitions (6–10 RM) are associated with increases in strength and high numbers (20–100 RM) are associated with in-creases in endurance. As repetitions increase, there is a transition from strength to endurance – thus the concept of a continuum

9.3.11 Importance of Specificity in Training in Endurance Sports

■ Example: cross-country skiing often requires the use of a lot of muscles simultaneously, making the heart the limiting factor and excess muscle mass wasteful. However, when it comes to double poling, the situation changes and adequacy of the upper body mass and muscular strength becomes very important. Double poling is important in cross-country ski racing. This is a good example of the frequent need for concomitant or concurrent strength and endurance training

■ This example also helps us to understand that the above statement should be qualified by the fact that strength training (in endurance athletes) should only be tailored to the particular type of sport, no more and no less

9.3.12 General Conclusions

■ Many sporting events involve both endurance and strength, and thus concurrent training may be more helpful than harmful

■ However, the above statement does have limitations. At one extreme end of the spectrum, we have weight lifting in which most coaches will still recommend a predominant strength training programme in preparation for competition rather than endurance training. At the other extreme end of the spectrum, we have marathon running in which most coaches will recommend a predominant endurance training protocol in preparation for competition for medals, although an occasional marathon runner with, say, weakness of hip extensors may benefit from some strengthening of these anti-gravity muscles

9.3.13 Practical Recommendation for Professional Athletes

■ Category 1: athletes whose sports involve mainly demands of strength and power: such as power lift, high jump, sprinting, shot putts – the main part of their training, especially when the competitive season is drawing near, is still strength training. For particular sports, we may wish to add speed and plyometric training. The role of circuit resistant training has been discussed and may be useful, but the author will shy away from its use when anywhere near the competitive season. Aerobic training for fitness can be considered off-season

■ Category 2: athletes whose sports involve both anaerobic power and endurance, such as the 200–400-m dash, 100-m swimming. The author recommends incorporating more aerobic as well as strength training into the programme. The muscle groups to be strengthened depend on the particular type of sport. Less intensive strength training occurs off-season to prevent the events of de-training, which can occur pretty quickly, as early as 2 weeks of de-training

■ Category 3: athletes whose sports entail mainly aerobic endurance involving oxidative phosphorylation pathways; the author recommends mainly endurance training. But early on between seasons, careful assessment of the different muscle groups of the athlete is important – the example given above of strengthening the weakened back muscles in an endurance rower has been referred to earlier, among many other examples. A good coach should spot these deficiencies early on and have the weakened muscle group(s) corrected before the competitive season arrives when predominantly endurance training (in the marathon runner, for example) holds the main key to getting the gold medal

General Bibliography

Anderson MK (2005) Foundations of Athletic Training, 3rd Edition. Lippincott Williams & Wilkins, Philadelphia, USA

Selected Bibliography of Journal Articles

1. Fabian S, Hesse H et al. (2005) Muscular activation patterns of healthy persons and low back pain patients performing a functional capacity evaluation test. Pathophysiology 12(4):281–287
2. Kraemer WJ, Patton JF et al. (1995) Compatibility of high intensity strength and endurance training on hormonal and skeletal muscle adaptations. J Appl Physiol 78(3):976–989
3. Hurley BF, Hagberg JM (1998) Optimizing health in older persons: aerobic or strength training. Exerc Sports Sci Rev 26:61–89
4. Petersen SR, Haennel RG et al. (1989) The influence of high velocity circuit resistance training on VO$_2$max and cardiac output. Can J Sport Sci 14(3):158–163

Contents

10.1 Introduction

10.1.1 Epidemiology

- There are slightly more than 1.5 amputees per 1,000 persons in the USA and Canada. Therefore, the present total in the USA is approximately 380,000
- Common indications include: perivascular disease (PVD), trauma, infection, tumour, trophic ulcerations and congenital anomalies
- The widely used K-classification gives a good idea of the functional abilities and potential of amputees

10.1.2 Functional K-Classification System

- Originated from HCFA: United States Health Care Financing Administration's common procedure coding system
- Gives a good description of functional abilities of amputees

10.1.3 Five-Level Functional Classification System

- K0 = unable to ambulate or transfer safely with or without assistance, a prosthesis does not enhance quality of life or mobility
- K1 = mainly household ambulator, may use a prosthesis for transfer or ambulation in level surfaces at a fixed cadence
- K2 = limited community ambulator, may be capable of using the prosthesis to negotiate low-level environmental barriers, e.g. curb, stairs and uneven surfaces
- K3 = community ambulator, with potential to achieve ambulation with variable cadence, negotiate most environmental barriers, may achieve prosthetic use beyond simple locomotion
- K4 = typical of prosthetic demands of the child, athlete, or very active adult. Having the potential to exceed basic ambulation skills, and participate in activities of high impact, stress and energy levels

10.1.4 Summary of K-Classification

- K0 = non-ambulator, not candidate for prosthesis
- K1 = household ambulator, consider fixed cadence prosthesis, non-dynamic foot
- K2 = limited community ambulation, fixed cadence prosthesis, non-dynamic foot
- K3 = community ambulator, consider variable cadence prosthesis, dynamic energy-storing foot

- K4 = high activity level; variable cadence prosthesis, dynamic energy-storing foot

10.2   Prosthesis Fitting for Amputees

10.2.1   Definition of Prosthesis
- A device designed to replace as far as possible the function (and sometimes the appearance) of a missing limb or part thereof

10.2.2   Common Terminologies
- Myodesis: direct suture of muscle or tendon to bone (via drill holes)
- Myoplasty: suturing agonist and antagonist muscles together
- Residual limb: remaining portion of the amputated limb
- Build-up: area of convexity designed for areas tolerant to high pressure
- Relief: area of concavity within the socket designed for high pressure bony prominence areas

10.2.3   Traditional vs Newer Componentry
- Traditionally prostheses were made in the form of exoskeleton, usually of wood or plastic
- Modern prostheses are endoskeletal
  - Constructed in a tube frame fashion
  - Flexible foam cover is used for the outer surface
  - Elements adjustable individually and detachable

10.2.4   Chief Goals of Prosthesis Fitting
- Limb substitution
- Cosmesis
- Locomotion (LL amputees)

10.2.5   Basic Principles of LL Amputation Surgery
- Preserve the knee joint whenever it is practical to do so and fashion the stump at the lowest practical level
- Very short stumps make fitting extremely difficult. However, very long transtibial stumps are prone to circulation problems in the elderly dysvascular patient

10.2.6   Elements to Consider in UL Prostheses

- The level of amputation
- Cognition
- Expected function required of prosthesis
- The job of the patient, e.g. sedentary vs. manual
- Patient's hobbies
- Cosmesis, importance can be increased if female or if the child grows up
- Other considerations: finance

10.2.7   Socket and Suspensions

10.2.7.1 Socket Fitting: Introduction

- No matter whether we are using an advanced or traditional prosthetic knee and foot, the socket remains an important component of a comfortable and well-functioning prosthesis
- It is the interface between the body of the amputee and the distal mechanical construction

10.2.7.2 Function of the Lower Limb Socket (According to Foort)

- To guide and link the residual limb to the prosthesis
- For transmission of support and control of forces
- The whole surface of the residual limb and its muscular system should be used for load transmission and guidance of the prosthesis
- Provides wearing comfort
- If possible to provide sensory information used in controlling the prosthesis
- Protect the stump from the environment

10.2.7.3 Biomechanical Principles of Socket (According to Hall)

- Proper contour and pressure relief for functioning muscles, allowance for dynamic changing contours
- Application of stabilisation forces to locations where no functioning muscles exist
- Functioning muscles need be stretched to slightly greater than length at rest to generate maximum power
- Pressure, if properly applied and evened out, can be exerted over neurovascular structures (such as the adductor canal in the case of transfemoral quadrilateral socket)

▨ Stress to tissues will be minimised if the force is applied over the widest possible area

10.2.7.4   Sockets for Transfemoral Amputee

10.2.7.4.1   Quadrilateral Socket

▨ Designed by University of California Berkeley

▨ "Quadrilateral" refers to the special shape of the four walls of the socket in axial view

▨ Ischial tuberosity and gluteal musculature are used as primary weight-bearing structures

▨ The design takes into account changing limb contours under dynamic conditions with provision of space to contracting muscles

Function of the Four Walls

Anteromedially: "Scarpa's Bulge" with its inward contour provides counterforce to maintain the ischium on the shelf

Anterolateral proximal convex contour to accommodate contraction and bulk of the quadriceps

Posterior shelf to support the ischial tuberosity and gluteal muscles

Medial wall to support medial adductor muscle mass with its adductor longus tendon

Design Rationale

The design is more than just working on pressure and counter-pressure of the muscle groups provided by the four walls, other rationales include:

– Lateral stabilisation

– Total contact

– Gluteal support

– Proper allowance for differences in residual musculature

Key to Success

Adequate lateral femoral stabilisation is needed to ensure an efficient gait (in transfemoral amputation)

To keep the femur in the adducted position, it is maintained by the angle of the lateral wall and the dimension of the medio-lateral wall

Femoral instability is exacerbated in mid-stance when the hip abductors need to contract to prevent drooping of the pelvis or Trendelenburg positioning

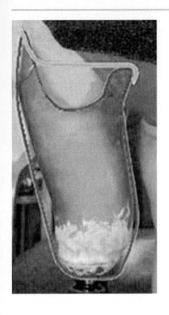

Fig. 10.1. Model showing the coverage offered by quadrilateral design as opposed to the older design

- Notice that failure of femoral stabilisation may result in walking with a wide base and truncal leaning laterally to the prosthesis side in the stance phase to minimise the force on the lateral side of the femur

10.2.7.4.2 Ischial Containment

- It was Long who came up with the idea of another type of socket with ischial containment after noting radiographically the not infrequent femoral malalignment and resultant lurch despite the use of the quadrilateral socket (Fig. 10.1)

Design Rationale

- Narrow the medio-lateral dimension in an attempt to better stabilise and control the femur, keeping it more adducted
- Containing the ischium may prevent the socket from moving laterally on weight-bearing
- Hence, the medial aspect of the ischium is now included in the socket to a varying extent
- Design rationale summary:
  - Provide more lateral stabilisation of the femur (Fig. 10.2)

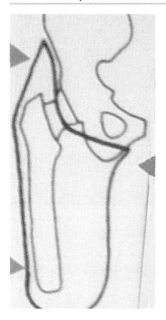

Fig. 10.2. Three-point pressure to attempt to keep the cut femoral bony stump in an adducted position

- Create "bony lock" between greater trochanter, ischium and femoral shaft
- Improve control of pelvis and trunk
- Better comfort for the perineum

ISO Recommendation for Transfemoral Socket

Maintain normal femoral adduction as far as possible to obtain more normal gait

Provide total contact

Enclose ramus and ischial tuberosity medially and posteriorly respectively. Thus, forces involved in the maintenance of medial lateral stability will be borne by the pelvic bone, creating a skeletal lock

Good distribution of forces along the femoral shaft

Decrease emphasis on maintaining narrow anteroposterior diameter to maintain ischial gluteal weight-bearing

Comparison Between Quadrilateral and Ischial Containment Sockets

- There is some suggestion of functional advantages of ischial containment over quadrilateral socket (Clin Orthop Relat Res 1989)
- This is in terms of:
  - Gait deviation
  - Metabolic demand and oxygen consumption
  - Possibly femoral shaft inclination

Some Recommendations (Reported in Prosthet Orthot Int)

- Quadrilateral sockets may be better for patients with firm adductor musculature and a long residual limb
- Ischial containment sockets may be better for more active amputees with short, fleshy residual limbs
- Successful users of quadrilateral sockets do not usually need to change socket type

10.2.7.4.3 Flexible Icelandic Scandinavian New York Socket

- Pioneered by Kristinsson
- Sometimes called Scandinavian Flexible Socket
- Featuring a flexible inner socket and outer rigid frames (see Fig. 10.3)

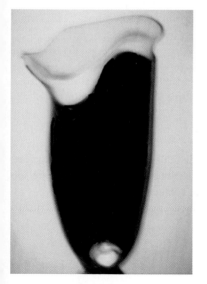

Fig. 10.3. Flexible Icelandic Scandinavian New York socket

- Some variations in design have windows cut out in the outer frame to provide pressure relief
- The challenge: to find the reasonably durable thermoplastic material offering the right amount of flexibility without expanding or permanent deformation

Design Rationale
   Improved sitting comfort
   Improved proprioception
   Possibly improved heat dissipation
   Improved muscle activity
   Less heavy
   Better suspension (if suction is used)
   Easily interchange without loss of alignment
   (The only weak point is that it may be less durable)

10.2.7.5   Sockets for the Transtibial Amputee

10.2.7.5.1 Total Contact Socket
- Previously sometimes called "patella tendon-bearing" socket
- This is a misnomer since the patella tendon does not bear high loads in this type of socket: weight distribution is quite even
- There are relief areas for pressure points like the fibula head, hamstrings, and a wide tibial flare to even out the pressure

10.2.7.5.2 Icelandic Scandinavian New York Socket
- Featuring an outer rigid and inner flexible frame, as just mentioned
- Windows are present in the outer frame to provide pressure relief
- Not very durable

Adjuncts
   Inserts like silicone gel may provide added protection for the dysvascular patient or one with abundant scars. These should not be too proud in case they decrease surface contacts
   A soft foam at the distal socket may decrease the chance of verrucous hyperplasia formation

10.2.8   Suspension Systems

10.2.8.1   Introduction

▨ Proper suspension is important in its contribution to the comfort and safety of the prosthesis

▨ For example, before World War II, many traditional suspension systems made of belts caused lots of vertical pistoning and inefficient gait, abrasions, and distal stump oedema, etc., thus demonstrating the importance of proper suspension

10.2.8.2   Transfemoral Amputee

10.2.8.2.1   Silicon Liner with Shuttle Lock

▨ Can be used for both transfemoral and transtibial amputees

▨ Can be used for all K-level users

▨ Popular since advantages include: good cushioning, torque control, total contact, less shear on the stump, lessens distal oedema build-up

▨ Prosthetic socks can be added as needed to accommodate stump volume fluctuations

▨ Good alternative for users with difficulty donning the full suction socket

10.2.8.2.2   Suction Systems

▨ Also popular means of suspension, works by negative pressure and surface tension

▨ Not usually used in transtibial amputees as the local anatomy is not very suitable for a tight seal

▨ Advantages include: good contact between residual limb and socket, good level of comfort and control

▨ Highly active amputees may need additional suspension belts

▨ Drawback: DM patients with weak hand intrinsics can have difficulty donning and doffing as well as those with poor standing balance

10.2.8.2.3   New Seal-In Liner by Ossur

▨ This new development is promising as the user simply rolls on the liner, steps into the socket, and an integrated hypobaric sealing membrane (HSM) automatically creates a firm suspension. To remove the socket, the user just pushes a button

▨ Pistoning is decreased by the full-length matrix; while the seal and distal pad enhance rotational control, the HSM can conform to the

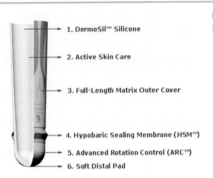

Fig. 10.4. New, very popular Seal-In liner by the company Ossur

1. DermoSil™ Silicone

2. Active Skin Care

3. Full-Length Matrix Outer Cover

4. Hypobaric Sealing Membrane (HSM™)

5. Advanced Rotation Control (ARC™)

6. Soft Distal Pad

shape of the socket wall creating a quick air-tight seal for easy donning (see Fig. 10.4)

10.2.8.2.4   Total Elastic Suspension
- Used sometimes in the elderly
- The total elastic suspension system is made of neoprene, usually equipped with a sleeve that attaches to the proximal prosthesis, then encircles the trunk to the waist line
- Can also be used as an auxiliary suspension method as well

10.2.8.2.5   Belt
- Still used especially sometimes in children
- Example: some children with congenital anomalies, e.g. proximal focal femoral deficiency (PFFD) and weak hip muscles, a belt may serve well in such cases (see Fig. 10.5)

10.2.8.3   Transtibial Amputee

10.2.8.3.1   Silicone Suction with Shuttle Lock
- The pin-and-lock system is equally very popularly used for transtibial amputees
- Details were just discussed, essentially features a stepless pin inside a unique locking mechanism, which results in a safe and non-pistoning suspension (see Figs. 10.6, 10.7)

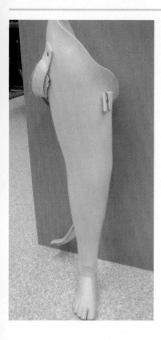

Fig. 10.5. Passive prosthesis tailor-made for a youngster with congenital proximal femoral deficiency

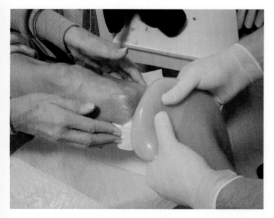

Fig. 10.6. Therapist helping the amputee to put on the popular silicon suction with locking pin

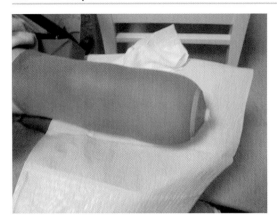

Fig. 10.7. Completion of fitting of silicon suction with shuttle lock

10.2.8.3.2 Suspension Sleeve

- Works by adherence to the skin via negative pressure, by using materials like neoprene. The other end is fitted to the proximal part of the prosthesis
- Again, DM patients with weak intrinsics can have donning difficulty

10.2.8.3.3 Supracondylar Cuff

- Used to be popular in the past
- The chief disadvantage is posing danger for the dysvascular patient from the constriction proximal to the knee
- Reserved mostly (very occasionally) for K1 amputees, especially those living in rural areas

10.2.9   The Prosthesis

10.2.9.1   Design of Prosthetic Knee Joints

10.2.9.1.1   Prosthetic Knees: Introduction

- Selection of prosthetic knee system depends on the patient's abilities, strength and balance
- Before we discuss the various designs, we need to recapitulate the gait difficulties facing the transfemoral amputation

10.2.9.1.2   Difficulties Concerning Gait Facing the Transfemoral Amputee

- Stance phase: quadriceps cannot provide sagittal knee stability after this amputation
- Swing phase: the knee with the prosthesis must provide stability and swing at appropriate rates to match the amputee's ability. An incorrect swing rate will result in the patient hopping on the good side, thus waiting for the knee unit to fully extend before weight can be transferred to the affected side

10.2.9.1.3   Selection Using the K-Classification

- K1 and K2 = constant friction type of swing phase control knee
- K3 and K4 = can prescribe variable cadence knee systems. As these more active amputees increase the cadence or velocity, the prosthesis is propelled forward more quickly – this requires greater resistance (to avoid excess knee flexion), thus necessitating fluid or hydraulic (sometimes pneumatic) control mechanisms

10.2.9.1.4   Constant Friction Swing Phase Control Knees

- Constant friction = simplest form of swing phase control
- Increased friction will decrease swing rate
- Degree of resistance set by prosthetist
- As the patient gets accustomed to the prosthesis, the prosthetist may need to readjust the swing rate
- Disadvantage: patient's cadence is limited to one speed (if the patient wants to ambulate faster, the knee will flex excessively)

10.2.9.1.5   Fluid (Hydraulic) Control Systems

- The fluid hydraulic system (Fig. 10.8) works on the principle that fluid is relatively incompressible, and forms the principle of many machines such as shock absorbers
- Similarly, if the patient has variable cadence, when his velocity increases, we also need to increase resistance in order to prevent excess knee flexion
- In short, adequate fluid resistance is needed for the prosthesis to keep up with the pace of the patient
- Similarly, we do not want the knee with the prosthesis to extend too rapidly either, because although some patients like this "feel" (from sensory feedback of the sudden jerk); this phenomenon may predispose to premature wear of the prosthesis

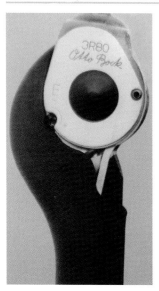

Fig. 10.8. Example of a prosthetic knee using the hydraulic system

- Hence, the hydraulic control knee unit needs to incorporate in its design both "flexion" *and* "extension" resistance
- The prosthetist then has to adjust the level of resistance to the range of velocities that will best suit our patient

10.2.9.1.6   Alternative: Pneumatic Units

- Can sometimes be used
- Since gas is more compressible than fluid, the range of resistance offered will therefore be smaller
- Another disadvantage is that the prosthetic response can be less smooth since as was said, gas is more compressible, although pneumatic units are lighter

10.2.9.1.7   New Improved Design: "Continuous" Resistance Adjustment

- These marvellous new advanced knee technologies were made possible only because of breakthrough microprocessor technology. Here, a closer match of the resistance needed by the active amputee is made possible – the microchip on board and sensors adjust swing resistance up to 50 times each second

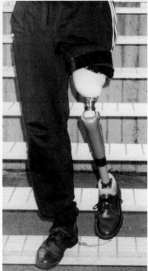

Fig. 10.9. Otto-Bock C-leg descending stairs

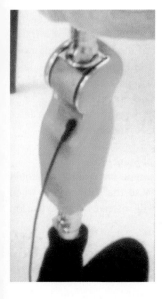

Fig. 10.10. Rheo leg by the company Ossur

Although these advanced systems have both pneumatic and hydraulic systems available; the hydraulic system (e.g. Otto Bock C-leg – Fig. 10.9, or Ossur Rheo Leg – Fig. 10.10) is more popular for obvious reasons

10.2.9.1.8   Microprocessor Technology
Benefits of microprocessor technology:
- Descent of ramp and stairs
- Cadence responsive
- Stumble recovery
- Stance flexion (better shock absorption)

10.2.9.1.9   Extension Assist
Many new amputees require the "extension assist" option, since it helps provide a sense of security as the knee approaches extension just prior to initial contact
- For constant-friction designs, this can be achieved by a spring-like mechanism
- Sometimes, the extension assist function can be incorporated into the knee system itself in other models

10.2.9.1.10 Problems at Initial Stance for the Transfemoral Amputee
It is common knowledge that the energy expenditure of the transfemoral amputee is much higher than that of the transtibial amputee

One of the reasons is that: at initial stance of normal gait, the knee flexion moment is countered by the quadriceps action. In the transfemoral amputee, there is no more quadriceps action

This results in the amputee needing to use the hip extensors to force the socket and thus the knee into extension voluntarily

How Can Prosthesis Design Help During Initial Stance?
Assuming we are to use a single-axis prosthetic knee unit, we should try to make the knee axis *slightly posterior* to the GRF so that when weight is borne on the prosthesis, there will instead be an extension knee moment

10.2.9.1.11 Mid-Stance Problems

■ We will recall from Chap. 8 on gait analysis of the "plantar flexion–knee extension couple" during this phase of gait
■ Plantar flexion of the foot in normal gait during mid-stance helps bring the GRF anterior to the knee joint, thus effecting an extension moment

How Can Prosthesis Design Help During Mid-Stance?

■ The traditional SACH foot has a soft foam keel allowing compression, thus simulating foot plantar flexion. This move helps move the GRF anterior to the knee
■ Many other prosthetic feet that allow a degree of plantar flexion can offer similar stability to the knee joint

10.2.9.1.12 Difficulties at Terminal Stance

■ In normal gait, recall that eccentric contraction of the plantar flexors will create a stable foot moment arm, creating an extension knee moment and stability
■ In the transfemoral amputee fitted with the traditional SACH foot, because of the rigid keel the distal end of the prosthesis provides an extension moment to the knee
■ The effect of other prosthetic feet varies in this stage of gait. Models allowing significant dorsiflexion will in fact have less stabilising extensor moment at the knee at terminal stance

Key Concept

From the above discussion, it will be obvious that finding ways to gain knee stability is important in transfemoral amputees; to summarise, the ways include:
– Making the knee axis more posterior
– Moving GRF anteriorly via plantar flexion (early stance)
– Moving GRF anteriorly by long toe lever
– Special knee design with multiple centres of rotation called "polycentric knee designs" (see discussion below)

10.2.9.1.13 Polycentric Knee Designs

■ A type of knee unit with multiple centres of rotation has evolved from four-bar linkage designs to the current complex linkages (Fig. 10.11)

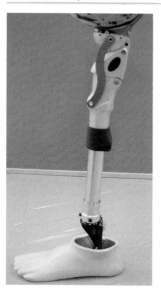

Fig. 10.11. Example of polycentric knee design

▓ The instantaneous centre of motion (ICOM) can be found by the intersection of lines from its linkages

▓ These systems are usually designed such that at full extension, the ICOM is posterior and proximal relative to the knee unit

▓ The posterior COM will add to the knee's stability, while the more proximal COM creates the mechanical advantage that less force is needed to initiate flexion or hold the knee in extension

10.2.9.1.14 Concepts of Stance Control

▓ Stance control mechanisms are intended to provide an added level of security for the new or active amputee

▓ This refers to a mechanism that prevents undesired knee flexion as the amputee loads the prosthesis, i.e. prevents knee buckle

▓ Common ways this was done in single axis knee system include:
  – Traditional obsolete locking mechanism that forces the amputee to walk with knee extension and unlock to sit is not popular
  – Friction-braking system – loading the prosthesis activates the system and flexion is halted. To flex the knee, the prosthesis needs to be entirely unloaded. Also, the prosthesis must not touch the

ground during swing phase since if flexion is suddenly halted, the amputee may stumble and fall
- There are systems where resistance is altered by the act of weight-bearing on the prosthesis
- Some are designed so that resistance to flexion automatically increases upon knee extension. This allows controlled knee flexion and even foot-to-foot stairs descent (e.g. Mauch SNS or Mauch S models, from Ossur)
- Others have special linkages allowing locking in extension at heel strike, and flexes easily upon toe loading near terminal stance (e.g. Otto Bock 3R60)

10.2.9.1.15 Option of Stance Flexion
- In normal gait, there is about 15–18° knee flexion to ease loading on the ipsilateral limb and prevent COM from fluctuating, thus ensuring gait efficiency
- It is deemed that building in 5–15° of knee flexion in stance in some prostheses may be good for the sound limb in dysvascular subjects. Whether this really works remains to be seen
- Example: Otto Bock 3R60 Knee

10.2.9.2 Design of Prosthetic Feet

10.2.9.2.1 Aim of Prosthetic Feet Designs
- Shock absorption
- Mobile yet stable
- Accommodate different surfaces

10.2.9.2.2 Advances in Design of Prosthetic Feet
- Newer materials allow prosthetic feet to be lighter and with better cosmesis
- Better able to control the dynamic load
- Memory return of the material once the load is removed
- May be better able to negotiate uneven surfaces or terrain

10.2.9.2.3 Typical Components of Prosthetic Feet
- The ankle block: the keel and ankle are *continuous* in conventional prosthetic feet

- The connection between the pylon and the foot is called the ankle attachment surface
- (Variant: can attach a multiaxial separate ankle system – in which case the pylon will then be connected to the top of the ankle system)
- The keel: at the plantar surface keel functions as the forefoot lever supplying stability in the second half of stance phase. Energy storage is effected by deflection of the keel, and provides a lively feel to the amputee when energy is released during push-off phase
- The shoe of the amputee: try to match the foot to the heel height of the shoe. If there is mismatch, malalignment can occur
- The angle that the tibia makes with the ground is also affected by the heel height of the shoe and foot
- In general, changes in the foot, i.e. the base of support, will result in corresponding changes in the joint angles higher up in the kinetic chain (e.g. increased dorsiflexion in transtibial prosthesis increases the flexion moment on the amputated side)

10.2.9.2.4   Key to Success of Prosthetic Feet
- Proper alignment
  - This means proper alignment in the coronal, sagittal and transverse planes
  - Important because this will make for the most energy-efficient and best-looking gait, and optimise pressure distribution, besides being less prone to wear
- Properly fitting choice of shoe wear as discussed

10.2.9.2.5   Adverse Effects of Poor Alignment
- Use up some of the ROM offered by the materials and components
- Difficulty for the amputee to meet the needed activity and terrain, and increased wear
- Can result in maladaptive compensatory gait pattern

10.2.9.2.6   Traditional SACH
- SACH = solid ankle cushioned heel
- The traditional SACH foot has a soft foam keel allowing compression, thus simulating foot plantar flexion
- This traditional design was found to be sometimes preferred by old folks as opposed to new "energy-storing" feet. One of the reasons may well be

because of the rigid keel; the distal end of the prosthesis provides an extension moment to the knee, thus affording greater knee stability

10.2.9.2.7 "Energy-Storing/Release Feet"

- Prototype: Seattle foot
- Forefoot keel deflects during weight-bearing, and springs back, thus creating an active push-off at the end of stance phase
- These energy-storing/release feet were found to increase self-selected walking speed, decrease the oxygen consumption and produce a more efficient gait (J Prosthet Orthot 1997)

Waterproof Feet

- An example is the SAFE-II feet
- SAFE = stationary ankle flexible endoskeletal foot
- A waterproof foot is useful in wet environment or if the individual has to wade through water

TruStep Foot

- Indication (K-level): 3
- Design rationale: attempt to replace the function of ankle and foot → equipped with subtalar, ankle and mid-tarsal joints. Ankle is multi-axis
- Material: carbon graphite
- Stability: normal foot tripod replaced by the heel and the two "toes", some coronal stability provided by the widely spaced "toes"
- Shock absorption: vertical shock absorption, some energy return possible
- Adjustability: interchangeable bumpers, ankle bushings, and mid-stance pads
- Company: College Park

Advantage Foot

- Indication (K-level): 3
- Design rationale: hybrid composite design (Fig. 10.12)
- Material: polyurethane elastomer in between two carbon plates
- Stability: supporting base offered by the lower carbon plantar plate
- Shock absorption: upper plate and polyurethane together help absorb vertical shock. Energy return by deflection of plantar plate, and partly by the properties of the polyurethane

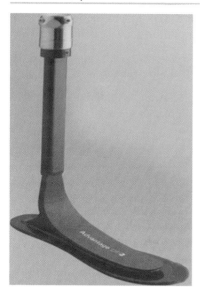

Fig. 10.12. Advantage foot; for details see text

Adjustability: newer model with an integrated pylon (Advantage DP foot)
Company: Otto-Bock/Springlite

Dynamic Response Foot

Indication (K-level): 3
Design rationale: offers a more responsive forefoot lever for more active patients with the keel ending distal to metatarsophalangeal joint (MTPJ) area
Material: adjustable carbon fibre keel
Stability and shock absorption: versatile since degree of stiffness and heel height adjustable
Adjustability: ankle stiffness of the multiflex ankle adjustable, as does the keel, and heel height
Company: Endolite (originated in UK)

Re-Flex VSP

Indication (K-level): 3
Design rationale: foot integrated with vertical shock-absorbing pylon. The system helps push the tibia forward at heel-strike and into swing at heel-off

- Material: carbon fibre foot with lateral springs
- Stability and shock absorption: active heel helps store energy, shock absorption both vertically and in the sagittal plane
- Adjustability: different foot modules and lateral springs available
- Company: Flex Foot (Ossur)

DAS-MARS Ankle
- Indication (K-level): 2–3
- Design rationale: multi-axial rotation ankle system that can be fitted to any variety of keel-only foot. The springs use tension and compression to mimic concentric and eccentric muscle activity
- Material: an anterior titanium spring and posterior rubber spring between two aluminium plates
- Stability and shock absorption: helped by the dynamic response of the springs mentioned
- Adjustability: each prosthesis is custom-made
- Company: Acadian Prosthetics

Dyna-Step Foot
- Indication (K-level): 3
- Design rationale: increased energy efficiency offered by an extended carbon keel and toe plate, and a reversed C-shaped carbon heel
- Material: carbon fibre, foot itself waterproof
- Stability: studies revealed more energy-efficient and may be more durable than SACH foot
- Shock absorption: reversed C-shaped carbon heel aids energy transfer to the pylon and propulsion of the tibia into mid-stance, while push-off aided by energy stored in the deflected carbon keel and toe plate
- Adjustability: can be attached to multi-axis ankle
- Company: originated in France

Genesis II Foot
- Indication (K-level): 2–3
- Design rationale: designed to approximate anatomic motion in all three planes, works on the assumption that walking is more brain driven than dependent on ground reaction forces
- Material: carbon graphite forefoot plates
- Stability and shock absorption: anterior and posterior bumpers. The deflected longitudinal arch releases energy at terminal stance to aid

push-off. Eases standing up from sitting since near normal dorsiflex-ion range

Adjustability: different bumpers allows for adjustability, as does heel height. So adjustable can be used in the growing child via changing to longer stiffer plates

Company: Jim Smith Sales

Master-Step Foot

Indication (K-level): 3

Design rationale: attempts to mimic more normal foot biomechanics, and coping better with uneven grounds

Material: carbon fibre plantar spring, toe plate, and reinforced tension cord

Stability: allows some inversion/eversion, can accommodate uneven terrain

Shock absorption: heel strike shock absorption by the spring, controlled plantar flexion offered by the cord; stored energy in spring released at toe-off

Adjustability: extremely adjustable, like heel height and resistance, spring stiffness, length of spring

Company: Cascade Orthopedic Supply

ADL Foot

Indication (K-level): 2

Design rationale: designed for the geriatric age group. Attempts to resemble a flat, pronated foot. Can be fitted to multi-axis ankle with low torque resistance for the elderly

Material: polypropylene keel

Stability and shock absorption: has anterior and posterior bumpers. The flexible keel stops short of the level of MTPJ

Adjustability: different levels of keel resistance available, low vs. medium torque resistance ankle to choose from

Company: Dycor

10.2.9.2.8   Athletes

Can request custom made foot and pylon system, and LL axis to suit the sport involved

10.2.9.2.9   Running-Specific Systems
▨ Aligned to desired running style
▨ No heel component

10.2.9.2.10 Prosthetic Feet: Current Status
▨ Not possible with the current state of technology for the prosthetic foot to imitate perfectly the human foot in form and function

10.2.9.2.11 Newer Prosthetic Feet for Children
▨ Newer stance-phase controlled prosthetic knee joint for children showed a decrease in the frequency of falls with the prototype, especially in active children in comparison to conventional knee joints (Trans Neural Syst Rehabil Eng 2005). Also, in general, energy-storing prosthetic feet like the Flex-foot produced significantly more energy (66% at comfortable walking and 70% at fast walking) than the SACH foot (21% at comfortable walking and 19% at fast walking). Thus, the Flex-Foot had a greater potential for reducing the energy cost of walking at comfortable and fast speeds for the below-knee child amputee (Schneider et al., J Biomech 1993)

10.2.10   Prostheses for Upper Limb Amputees

10.2.10.1   Commonly Used Upper Limb Prostheses
▨ Passive (see Fig. 10.13)
▨ Body-powered
▨ Myoelectric

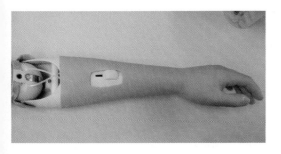

Fig. 10.13. An example of a passive upper limb prosthesis

10.2.10.2   Key Difference Between Body-Powered and Myoelectric Prostheses

- Myoelectric prostheses work by detecting the EMG activity of the contracting muscles of the residual limb
- Body-powered prostheses work by mechanical links and cable powered by the motion effected by the intact proximal musculature of the amputee (e.g. scapula muscle in the UL amputee)

10.2.10.2.1 Pros and Cons of Body-Powered Prostheses

- Moderate cost and weight
- Durable
- Higher sensory feedback
- Less cosmetic than myoelectric prosthesis
- Need more gross limb motion to activate

10.2.10.2.2 Pros and Cons of Myoelectric Prosthesis

- Expensive
- Heavy and need maintenance
- More cosmetic
- Less sensory feedback
- Works by transmission of electrical activity (that the surface electrodes receive from the residual limb muscles) to the electric motor

10.2.10.3   Types of Myoelectric Units

- One site, two functions:
  - e.g. one electrode for flexion and extension
  - Patient uses muscle contraction of different strengths to differentiate between flexion and extension. Example: stronger contraction to open the device, etc.
- Two sites, two functions:
  - e.g. separate electrodes for flexion and extension

10.2.10.4   Terminal Devices

- Passive
- Active

10.2.10.4.1 Passive Terminal Devices

▪ Advantages
  - Cosmesis
  - New materials can be made to closely resemble the natural hand
▪ Disadvantages
  - Expense
  - Less functional

10.2.10.4.2 Active Terminal Devices

▪ Advantages
  - More functional
  - Can be myoelectric or hooked prosthetic hand with cables
▪ Disadvantages
  - Less cosmetic

10.2.10.5   Upper Limb Prostheses by Region

10.2.10.5.1 Shoulder and Fore-Quarter Units

▪ Here, functional restoration is very challenging
▪ Reason:
  - High energy expenditure requirements
  - Weight of prosthesis
▪ (Because of the above, many patients selected a cosmetic passive prosthesis. But please refer to the Sect. 10.3 on prosthetic advances for exciting developments in this area concerning neuroprosthesis)

10.2.10.5.2 Above Elbow Prosthesis

▪ Design similar but:
  - Internal locking elbow substitutes for the elbow flexion hinge
  - Dual control cable instead of single control
  - No triceps and biceps cuff

10.2.10.5.3 Elbow Units

▪ Selection based on amputation level and amount of residual function

Rigid Elbow Unit

▪ A typical suitable candidate will be a patient with short transradial amputation, still with enough elbow flexion, but limited prono-supination

Flexible Elbow Units
>   A typical suitable candidate will be a patient with longer transradial amputation having adequate elbow flexion/extension, and prono-supination

>   In this situation, the flexible elbow unit will provide more function

10.2.10.5.4 Common Below Elbow Prosthetic Components (Body-Powered)

- Voluntary opening split hook
- Friction wrist
- Double walled plastic laminate socket
- Elbow flexible hinge – equipped with single cable system
- Triceps and biceps cuff
- Figure-of-eight harness

10.2.10.5.5 Wrist Units

- Commonly seen types include:
    - Locking wrist units: prevent rotation during grasping and lifting
    - Quick disconnect units: permit quick swapping of terminal devices with specialised function
    - Wrist flexion units: used on the longer residual limb in bilateral amputee; to allow ADL like buttoning, etc.

Voluntary Opening Hooked Active Terminal Devices
>   Device closed at rest
>   Proximal muscle contraction opens the device (via a system of cables and bands) – hook closes on relaxing the muscles
>   Voluntary opening mechanism is more popular

Voluntary Closing Devices
>   Voluntary closing mechanism tends to be heavier
>   Activation of residual flexor muscles effect grasping of objects

10.2.10.6   Upper Limb Prostheses for Children

10.2.10.6.1 Upper Limb Prosthetics: Principles

- Position hand in space
- Limb length and joint salvage are directly related to functional outcome
- Sensation important for function (see lower limb)
- Early fitting (85% if within 30 days, 50% with late fitting)

10.2.10.6.2 Fitting Principles
- Early fitting important for congenital amputees
- First 6–9 months fit with simple passive device
- Age-appropriate harnessing
- Education and complete discussion of prosthetic options with parents

10.2.10.6.3 Age 6 Months to 2 Years: Use Passive Arm
- Clenched fist type
- Open "doll's" hand
- "Easy feed"
- (Simple self suspension)

10.2.10.6.4 Later Conventional Body-Powered Prostheses
- Durable
- Powerful (especially the voluntary closing terminal device)
- Simple to repair
- Not too expensive
- Many choices of terminal devices

10.2.10.6.5 Mechanism of Body-Powered Systems
- Standard exoskeletal prosthesis with harness and self suspending socket
- Any motion that tightens the harness activates the terminal device:
    - Voluntary closing vs. opening
    - Scapular abduction (protraction)
    - Shoulder flexion

10.2.10.6.6 Myoelectric Prosthesis
- Fit early to increase the chance of the child using it in later life (Figs. 10.14, 10.15)
- Consistent wear
- Needs good team approach (orthopaedist, therapist, prosthetist)
- Although some centres report decreased use as child ages, the next section on new advances in neuroprostheses control and cutting edge technology will change this concept

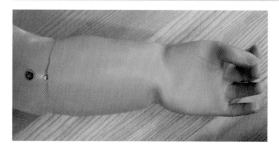

Fig. 10.14. Myoelectric prosthesis used for children

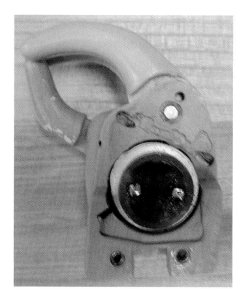

Fig. 10.15. Myoelectric wrist unit for the child amputee

10.3   Major Advances in Neuroprosthesis

10.3.1   The Basics
■ To understand some of the newer advances, we need some knowledge of artificial intelligence, and of artificial neural networks (ANN)

10.3.1.1 What Is Artificial Intelligence?

- Artificial intelligence (AI) is a broad field that focuses on the application of computer systems that exhibit intelligent capacities
- The term "intelligent" here means computer-based systems that can interact with their environment and adapt to changes in the environment
- One principal aim of AI is to produce machines that can function under adverse and unpredictable circumstances, and that are capable of human-like reasoning, decision-making and adaptation (according to Escabi)

10.3.1.2 What Type of Technology is Involved in Artificial Intelligence?

- AI can be built from a number of separate technologies, including:
  - Fuzzy logic
  - Neural networks
  - Others: probabilistic reasoning, genetic algorithms and expert systems
- We will talk a little more about fuzzy logic and artificial neural networks

10.3.1.2.1 Fuzzy Logic

- Fuzzy logic attempts to approximate human reasoning by the use of linguistic variables, instead of discreet numbers as in traditional computing
- Words tend to be less precise than numbers, e.g. when people talk about height, there are descriptions like very short, short, normal, tall, very tall, etc.
- Numeric sets in classic mathematics are called crisp sets; while those in fuzzy logic are called fuzzy sets
- Once fuzzy sets are established, rules will be constructed – fuzzy logic is in fact a rule-based logic

Clinical Application of Fuzzy Logic

- Fuzzy logic is especially useful when information is too limited or too complex to allow numeric precision since it can tolerate imprecision
- It finds important applications in analysis of biosignals like EMG signals, aids in the development of neuroprosthesis for locomotion using sensors controlled by fuzzy logic as in "intelligent prosthesis" for amputees or in neuroprostheses that aid SCI patients to walk

10.3.1.2.2 Artificial Neural Network

- Artificial neural networks (ANN) are the theoretical counterpart of real biological neural systems. ANN built to this date are much simpler than the human brain
- ANN are built to mimic and replicate the function of real brains. Some systems have learning, processing and adaptive capacities. ANN consist of multiple layers of "neurons" rather like real brain
- Example of its use in prosthetics for amputees: ANN systems can be used to learn to recognise certain inputs and to produce a particular output with certain input
- They are ideally used for pattern recognition and classification of bio-signals

10.3.2   Recent Advances and Successes

10.3.2.1   Myoelectric Prostheses: Current Status

- Current myoelectric prostheses are essentially terminal devices controlled non-intuitively by more proximal forearm, upper arm, shoulder, and chest musculature

10.3.2.1.1 How Can We Make Things Better for Upper Extremity Amputees?

- Possible improvements:
  - Current technology: only four degrees of freedom
  - New multifunction hands, humeral rotators, and shoulders are in development
  - Research is on-going on the possibility of prostheses control by intuition (see following discussion)

10.3.2.2   Summary of the Main Problem of Upper Limb Prostheses

- Amputees can operate only one joint at a time, even with body-powered or myoelectric prostheses

10.3.2.3   How Can We Improve This?

- Answer = by concomitant:
  - Development of multifunctional prostheses with many more degrees of freedom
  - Obvious need for enhanced channels of prostheses control, and also preferably intuition

▓ The latter is likely the more challenging of these two concomitant lines of development

10.3.2.4   Where Is the Information Needed to Control a Prosthesis?

▓ In the CNS
  – Difficult to obtain this information, but research in the use of brain waves and microchip brain implants is under way
▓ In the PNS (peripheral nervous system)
  – Difficult to amplify the information, but the following discussion will show ways of circumventing this problem
▓ In residual intact musculature
  – Data collection is difficult at this level because of too much background noise

10.3.2.5   Methods to Tap into the PNS

▓ Direct peripheral nerve recording (see subsequent discussion of Utah slanted micro-electrode arrays in Sect. 10.3.2.7.4)
▓ Surface peripheral nerve recording
▓ Nerve signal amplification (see the following discussion on "targeted re-innervation")

10.3.2.6   The First Strategy: Signal Amplification Via Targeted Re-Innervation

▓ Basic principle: the ideal nerve amplifier of neural signals is "local muscle re-innervated by peripheral nerve"

10.3.2.6.1 Concept of "Targeted Innervation"

▓ Via transferring peripheral nerves to otherwise functionless muscle segments in amputees
▓ Thereby developing the so-called myoneurosomes

10.3.2.6.2 Myoneurosome

▓ Definition: a muscle segment that can be isolated by EMG with a defined neurovascular anatomy
▓ Example: some conventional existing myoelectric prostheses are controlled by forearm flexors and extensors – we can consider these as two "native" myoneurosomes

10.3.2.6.3   Requirements for Successful Targeted Re-Innervation

▪ Good re-innervation
▪ Independent recording from targeted muscle segments
▪ Availability of multifunction arm and controller (Kuiken, Phys Med Rehabil Clin N Am 2006)

How to Ensure Good Re-Innervation

- In rats, nerve transfers are found to be more reliable when large proximal nerves are sewn to small distal nerves
- This phenomenon has been given the term "hyper-innervation" and reported in the literature
(Kuiken et al., Brain Res 1995)

Ensure Good Signal Detection

- Myoelectric signals must be independently recorded
- But what are the elements of good signal detection?

Elements of Good Signal Detection

- Adequate size: 3–5 cm across
- Adequate thickness: 1-cm thick muscle
- Surface electrodes need to be close to muscle – may need defatting surgery
- Physically separate the myoneurosomes

Ensure Good Prosthesis and Controller

- As mentioned, concomitant development of corresponding technologies of effector devices with the required degrees of freedom will be necessary. Newer advanced multifunctional effector prosthetic devices
- Examples:
  - Powered shoulders
  - Wrists with two degrees of freedom
  - Multifunctional hand
  - Greater microprocessor power
  - Sensory interfaces

10.3.2.6.4   Report of Initial Success (Chicago Rehabilitation Institute)

▪ One patient with bilateral shoulder disarticulation – successful motor and sensory re-innervation

▪ Three transhumeral amputations: two successful motor re-innervation, one unsuccessful (due to pathology in the peripheral nerve)
▪ One lady with humeral neck amputation: in effect functional shoulder disarticulation, four motor transfers and one sensory transfer performed with successful results

10.3.2.6.5 Role of Preoperative Cadaver Dissection
▪ Preoperative cadaver dissection prior to nerve re-routing in preparation for attempts at "targeted re-innervation" may be necessary

10.3.2.6.6 Example of Nerve Transfer Surgery in a Patient with Bilateral Shoulder Disarticulation
▪ Medial nerve used to control the "close hand" function
▪ Musculocutaneous nerve to control the "bend elbow" function
▪ Another portion of median nerve used to control "open hand" function
▪ Radial nerve to control "elbow extension"
▪ Ulna nerve attached to pectoralis minor
  (Kuiken et al., Prosthet Orthot Int 2004)

10.3.2.6.7 Functional Improvement
▪ New tasks the shoulder disarticulation patient was able to perform after nerve transfer surgery and fitting the new neuroprosthesis: self-feeding, opening small jar, throwing an object, shaving, etc.

10.3.2.6.8 Another Example of Nerve Transfer Surgery in Transhumeral Amputees
▪ Again, surgical creation of "myoneurosomes" involving transfer of major mixed nerves to specific muscles:
  - Median nerve – medial biceps
  - Musculocutaneous nerve – lateral biceps
  - Proximal radial nerve – triceps
  - Distal radial nerve – brachialis

10.3.2.6.9 Method of Prosthesis Control After Nerve Transfer Surgery
▪ Bending elbow: effected by using musculocutaneous → lateral biceps
▪ Extending elbow: effected by using proximal radial nerve → triceps
▪ Closing hand: effected by using median nerve → medial biceps
▪ Opening hand: effected by using distal radial nerve → brachialis

10.3.2.6.10 How Do Myoneurosomes Trigger Effector Arm Functions?

▓ Take the example of the patient with shoulder disarticulation, the different newly created myoneurosomes can trigger effector arm functions via the use of "high density surface electrode arrays"

10.3.2.6.11 High Density Surface Electrode Array

▓ Involves placement of large numbers of monopolar electrodes on the re-innervated area (e.g. on the chest or on the shoulder of the disarticulation patient)

▓ Can thus potentially perform multiple arm functions

10.3.2.6.12 How Is This Possible?

▓ Via a heuristic fuzzy logic approach to multiple electromyogram (EMG) pattern recognition for multifunctional prosthesis control (Weir et al., IEEE Trans Neural Syst Rehabil Eng 2005)

10.3.2.6.13 Other Facilitating Technology: IMES

▓ IMES = implantable myoelectric sensors (some have previously been called "Bion" – see Fig. 10.16)

▓ Functions by:
  – Allowing greater EMG data acquisition
  – More stable EMG recording
  – Some models are FDA-approved

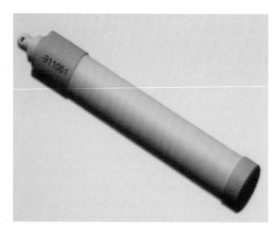

Fig. 10.16. "Bion"; for details see text

10.3.2.6.14 Summary of Initial Success of First Strategy (i.e. Targeted Re-Innervation)

- Targeted re-innervation can create new myoelectric control sites – known as "myoneurosomes"
- As such, multiple joints can be controlled with myoelectric signals
- Control will now be more physiologically appropriate: feels more natural, device easier and more intuitive to use
- Sensory feedback is possible

10.3.2.7 The Second Strategy: Development of Direct Neural Interface

- This technology will have the advantage of low current, yet high force output
- Patient needs simply to think about the task
- Multiple simultaneous motions possible
- Sensory feedback readily available

10.3.2.7.1 Problems Associated with Direct Neural Interface

- Will the brain still recognise signals from the nerve of an old amputee stump?
- Will the nerve stump function? And will the patient be able to intuitively control different effector functions at will?
- Problems of connecting the direct neural interface to nerves in the long-term?
- How do we prevent infections at the connection? Is the use of remote control and a totally implantable direct neural interface the answer?

10.3.2.7.2 Brain Plasticity

- Brain plasticity can be retrained even if the patient has a rather old amputation
- Use and availability of intact peripheral nerves are therefore viable options if we are planning a direct neural interface

10.3.2.7.3 Assuming a Still Functional Peripheral Nerve, How Can a Direct Neural Interface Control Different Functions

- One such successful "direct neural interface" was developed in Utah, USA (Branner et al., J Neurophysiol 2001)

10.3.2.7.4 The Utah Slanted Micro-Electrode Array
- An example of integrated neural interface (INI) technology
- Components:
  - Integrated circuitry with neural amplifier, signal processing, and radiofrequency telemetry electronics
  - Power receiving coil on polyimide with ceramic ferrite backing
  - SMD capacitor
  - Micro-electrode array itself made of bulk micromachined silicon with platinum tips and glass isolation between shanks
  - Entire assembly coated in parylene and silicon carbide

10.3.2.7.5 How Does USEA Work?
- It works via intra-fascicular multi-electrode stimulation (IFMS)

10.3.2.7.6 Intra-Fascicular Multi-Electrode Stimulation
- IFMS is made possible thanks to the invention of Utah Slanted Electrode Array (USEA) technology (McDonnall et al., Can J Physiol Pharmacol 2004)
- USEA can provide comprehensive coverage both in depth and in breadth of the nerve
- No proximity problem as a direct neural interface is established
- It is selective – hence activating only selected muscle fibres
- Multi-site – thus, can activate many different fibres independently

10.3.2.7.7 Main Advantages of USEA
- Force – highly controllable over a full dynamic range
- Selectivity – virtually no activation of other muscles, even at maximum forces
- Low frequency stimulation – reduces fatigue, potentiation, and hence can easily maintain the target force
- Wireless technology (by the use of radiofrequency technology)
  - Reduced infection risk
  - Reduced tether force
  - Improved stimulation
  - Cosmetic

10.3.2.7.8 Previous Cat Sciatic Nerve Stimulation Using USEA
- Nine different leg muscles selectively accessed via a single USEA implanted in the cat sciatic nerve
- Demonstrates:
  - Between muscle selectivity
  - Within muscle independence
  - With only low stimulation currents: of 1–10 µA
    (Branner et al., J Neurophysiol 2001)

10.3.2.7.9 Summary of the Second Strategy
- Graded, distally referred, tactile and proprioceptive sensory feedback can be provided by intra-fascicular stimulation of amputee nerve stumps
- Graded, distally referred, motor control signals can be obtained by intra-fascicular recording from amputee nerve stumps

10.3.2.7.10 Conclusion
- In summary, USEA provides an immediately functioning wireless interface
- Use of USEA to perform IFMS revealed that a direct neural interface is feasible – sensory and motor

10.3.2.7.11 Remaining Issues
- Body's response to implant over time
- Any interference with wireless technology
- Implant fixation issues

10.4 Optimising Surgical Technique and Perioperative Care

10.4.1 Pearls for Transfemoral Amputation
- The most commonly seen problem is inadequate or poor muscle or soft tissue stabilisation resulting in deviation of the residual femur into abduction, and flexion; together with an unstable medial soft tissue from the retracted and contracted adductors
- Proper myodesis and not myoplasty of the adductor magnus should be routinely done to stabilise and centralise the cut femur inside the soft tissue envelope

■ The level of bone cut should aim at 12–14 cm above the knee so as to allow adequate space for the placement of the prosthetic knee joint

10.4.2 Key Concept

■ Although lateral stabilisation of the femur in an attempt to maintain its adducted pose is one main goal of the socket, the socket itself cannot be relied upon to substitute for poor surgical technique

■ Previous teachings of myoplasty instead of performing myodesis of the adductor mass (especially magnus) is the cause of occasionally poor results with resultant femoral instability and poor gait. No socket types will correct this

■ Surgical technique has greater influence on femoral adduction than socket (Gottschalk)

■ Loss of the adductor magnus in the medial distal one-third of the femur significantly comprises 70% of adductor function; thus, myodesis of the adductor to the residual femur with the femur held in adduction is advised (Gottschalk)

10.4.3 Pearls for Transtibial Amputation

■ Level of bone cut: half to one-third length of tibia, in cases where short stump is mandated by local conditions, try to preserve up to tibial tubercle (or attachment of patella ligament)

■ Possible flap design:
  – Long posterior flap
  – Sagittal flap
  – Skew flap
  – Extended posterior flap if more distal tibial padding is deemed necessary

■ Myodesis to anterior tibia through drill holes is encouraged

■ Although bone-bridge technique (Fig. 10.17) proposed by some surgeons, arguing that it theoretically provides larger, more sturdy distal surface for end bearing, and prevents scissoring effect between tibia and fibula; in practice not commonly done since need to sacrifice 7–9 cm of bone, and contraindicated in PVD which forms the bulk of patients having LL amputations

■ (P.S. The novel technique of implanting a locking pin – for improved "feel" and security, to the cut end of the bony stump is described in some countries like Sweden, but not FDA-approved and will not be discussed)

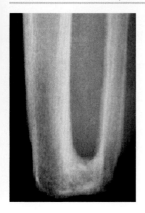

Fig. 10.17. Note the mature bone bridge between the tibia and fibula

10.4.4   Prediction of Healing of Amputation Wound
- Clinical assessment: checking pulses, soft tissue status and ankle brachial index
- Objective assessments:
  - Ultrasound Doppler and transcutaneous partial pressure of oxygen (assess vascular inflow)
  - General healing potential: healing affected if serum albumen < 3 g/dl, total lymphocyte count < 1,500

10.4.5   Key Elements of Postoperative Care
- Rigid vs. soft dressing
- Compression
- Avoid only proximal compression
- Early prosthetic fitting

10.4.5.1   Immediate Postoperative Care: the Options
- IPOP (immediate postoperative fitting prosthesis)
- Figure-of-eight elastic wrapping
- Rigid removable dressing

10.4.5.1.1 Figure-of-Eight Bandaging
- Quite commonly practiced, and sometimes patients are taught the technique
- For the average adult, one or two elastic bandages four inches wide are used. During the course of the wrapping, tension is used to main-

tain about two-thirds of the maximum stretch. The bandage should be changed every 4–6 h; it must not be kept in place for more than 12 h without re-bandaging

- The stump should be massaged actively for 10–15 min between sessions

10.4.5.1.2   Alternatives to Bandaging

- Special elastic "shrinker socks" are available for use instead of elastic bandages, while not considered by some to be as effective as a properly applied bandage
- A shrinker sock is better than a poorly applied elastic bandage

10.4.5.2   Prevention of Contractures

- Regardless of the type of dressing used, exercises are extremely important to prevent contractures
- Commonly seen contractures include hip flexion contracture (hence prone lying encouraged), hip abduction, and knee flexion contracture (knee extension splintage may be required)
- Postoperative immediate shoulder, elbow and wrist active ROM should be administered in LL amputee to prevent contractures

10.4.5.3   Advantages of Early Prosthetic Fitting

- Decreased oedema
- Decreased phantom pain
- Decreased postoperative limb pain
- Decreased hospitalisation period
- Improved rehabilitation

10.4.5.4   Common Postoperative Complications

- Poor stump preparation
- Infection
- Haematoma
- Wound necrosis
- Contractures
- Neuroma
- Verrucous hyperplasia
- Phantom pain (see Chap. 15)
- Terminal overgrowth (in children)

10.5   Miscellaneous Pearls for Amputations at Less Common Levels

10.5.1   General Treatment Goals

- Preserve length
- Preserve sensation
- Prevent neuromas
- Good coverage and padding
- Prevent nearby joint contractures
- Aim at early prosthetic fitting
- Early return to function and work

10.5.2   Shoulder Disarticulation

- Not common, only in some cases of tumour and trauma, or electric shock injury
- If possible keep the humeral head
- For there is difficulty in cloth wearing and lost shoulder contour after the disarticulation if the humeral head is absent

10.5.3   Proximal Humeral Amputations

- Very proximal humeral amputations behave like a shoulder disarticulation, but with better cosmesis and suspension

10.5.4   Transhumeral Amputation

- Preservation of bone length important
- Myodesis of triceps and biceps advisable not only for better strength, but for better control of prosthesis and myoelectric signals

10.5.5   Elbow/Distal Humeral Amputation

- Better suspension with elbow disarticulation, but poor cosmesis
- Better function with distal humeral amputation (3.5 cm proximal to elbow)

10.5.6   Transradial Amputation

- High functional level, good for myoelectric devices
- Rotation proportional to residual length, try to preserve length. Although distal radio-ulnar joint (DRUJ) is lost, there is a mild degree of retained prono-supination

- If there is a choice, the level is selected between junction of mid and distal third. Represents compromise between adequate wound healing and functional length
- The Krukenberg procedure is sometimes performed in some developing countries that lack prostheses

10.5.7   Transradial Amputation with Short Stump
- This is preferred to transhumeral there is a choice
- The biceps tendon is frequently reattached to proximal ulna to ease prosthetic fitting, and in such a way that its length is preserved; avoid attaching more distally as results in elbow contracture

10.5.8   Wrist Disarticulation
- May be preferable to transcarpal in children
- Preserves prono-supination and DRUJ, thus forearm rotation preserved
- Although the flare of the radial styloid is preserved for suspension, the styloid process itself needs some rounding off

10.5.9   Transcarpal Amputation
- Although lever arm is long, prosthetic fitting can be challenging
- The good thing is preservation of prono-supination as well as wrist flexion and extension

10.5.9.1 Word of Note
- Do not suture flexors to extensors
- These should be anchored to the remaining carpus in the line of their direction of insertion in order to preserve wrist motion
- Good padding can be obtained by full thickness long palmer and short dorsal flap created at a ratio of 2:1

10.5.10 Hand Amputations
- Preserve length, function, sensation
- Usually as salvage procedure or as primary amputation for irreversible loss of blood supply and tumours, etc.
- Salvage thumb as far as possible

10.6   Outcome Measures

10.6.1   Popular Outcome Measures

■ Previous popular outcome measure for the amputee population: functional independence measurement (FIM)
  - Validation: Dodds et al., Arch Phys Med Rehabil 1993
  - Criticism for the use of FIM in amputees: some studies found FIM not useful in predicting successful prosthetic rehabilitation in LL amputees (Leung et al., Arch Phys Med Rehabil 1996)

10.6.2   Other Instruments

■ Prosthetic goal and achievement test
■ Functional ambulation profile
■ SF-36

10.6.3   Newer Preferred Outcome Measurement and Predictor

■ Amputee mobility predictor (Gailey et al., Arch Phys Med Rehabil 2002)
■ Locomotor capabilities index (LCI; Franchignoni et al., Arch Phys Med Rehabil 2004)

10.6.4   Chief Advantages
of the Preferred "Amputee Mobility Predictor"

■ Ability to be performed with or without the use of a prosthesis
■ Not time-consuming: takes 10–15 min to perform, requires little equipment
■ Its simplicity allows personnel of different specialities like therapists, technicians and physicians to use it
■ High quoted inter- and intra-rater reliability
■ Overall, a good predictor of the distance an amputee can walk with a prosthesis

10.6.5   Paediatric Prosthetic Assessment Tools

■ PODCI: paediatric orthopaedic data collection instrument
■ UBET: unilateral below elbow test
■ Ped QL: paediatric quality of life
■ PSI: prosthetic satisfaction index

10.6.6 What Lies in the Future?

■ One of the drawbacks of current prosthetic limbs (e.g. upper limbs) is the weight, and is one reason for abandonment. The prosthetic industry is developing novel materials (electroactive polymers) that are not only light-weight and quiet, but potentially act as both sensors and actuators at the same time. One such material is the dielectric elastomer artificial muscle. If successful, use of these electroactive polymers can potentially offer a light-weight, pliable, yet soundless alternative to current prosthetics that are bulky, heavy, with sound-producing cams and gears. Research is under way in the Bloorview Macmillan Rehabilitation Institute in Toronto, Canada.

■ Traditional externally powered UL prosthesis only allows open/close function. One possible way being explored (besides targeted re-innervation) that will potentially allow different hand grips (hook grip, key grip, chuck grip, spherical grip) is via the use of a mechanomyogram (Alves et al., presented at RESNA 2005)

General Bibliography

Meier RH (2004) Functional Restoration of Adults and Children with Upper Extremity Amputation. Demos Medical Publishing, New York, USA

Seymour R (2002) Prosthetics and Orthotics – Lower Limb and Spinal. Lippincott Williams & Wilkins, Philadelphia, USA

Muzumdar A (2004) Powered Upper Limb Prostheses. Springer, Berlin Heidelberg New York

Selected Bibliography of Journal Articles

1. Gailey RS, Roach KE et al. (2002) The amputee mobility predictor: an instrument to assess the lower limb amputee's ability to ambulate. Arch Phys Med Rehabil 83(5):613–627
2. Pritham CH (1990) Biomechanics and shape of the above-knee socket considered in light of the ischial containment concept. Prosthet Orthot Int 14(1)9–21
3. Postema K, Hermens HJ et al. (1997) Energy storage and release of prosthetic feet, Part 1: Biomechanical analysis related to user benefit. Prosthet Orthot Int 21(1): 17–27

4. Postema K, Hermens HJ et al. (1997) Energy storage and release of prosthetic feet, Part 2: Subjective ratings of 2 energy storing and 2 conventional feet, user choice of foot and deciding factor. Prosthet Orthot Int 21(1):28–34

5. Schneider K, Hart T et al. (1993) Dynamics of below-knee child amputee gait: SACH foot versus Flex foot. J Biomech 26(10):1191–1204

6. Kuiken TA, Childress DS et al. (1995) The hyper-reinnervation of skeletal muscle. Brain Res 676(1):113–123

7. Kuiken T (2006) Targeted re-innervation for improved prosthetic function. Phys Med Rehabil Clinic North Am 17(1):1–13

8. Branner A, Stein RB et al. (2001) Selective stimulation of cat sciatic nerve using an array of varying length micro-electrodes. J Neurophysiol 85(4):1585–1594

9. McDonnall D, Clark GA et al. (2004) Selective motor unit recruitment via intra-fascicular multi-electrode stimulation. Can J Physiol Pharmacol 82(8/9):599–609

10. Ajiboye AB, Weir RF (2005) A heuristic fuzzy logic approach to EMG pattern recognition for multifunctional prosthetic control. IEEE Trans Neural Syst Rehabil Eng 13(3):280–291

11. Franchignoni F, Orlandini D et al. (2004) Reliability, validity, and responsiveness of the locomotor capabilities index in adults with lower-limb amputation undergoing prosthetic training. Arch Phys Med Rehabil 85(5):743–748

Cerebral Palsy Rehabilitation

Contents

Contents   289

11.1   Basic Concepts

11.1.1   Definition of Cerebral Palsy

- Group of non-progressive, motor (mainly) impairment syndromes secondary to lesions or anomalies of the brain from the foetus to around age 2
- (But its manifestations can change over time with growth, development and maturation)
- Can have defects in sensation, cognition, seizure, GI/GU problems, etc.

11.1.2   Aetiology

- Intrinsic abnormal CNS structure (e.g. chromosomal, metabolic disease)
- External insult (e.g. infection, ischaemia)

11.1.3   Classes

- Geographic classification (Gage)
    - Diplegic (30%)
    - Hemiplegic (30%)
    - Dyskinetic (15%)
      (All three types may walk)
    - Quadriplegic (25%)
      (Most will not walk)

11.1.4   General Problems in CP

- Loss of selective motor control: especially in the bi-articular muscles, and this loss tend to be more in the distal muscles although proximal affection can occur with enough severity
- Increased muscle tone and spasticity
- Imbalance of agonist/antagonist
- Faulty equilibrium reactions
- Sometimes dependent on primitive reflex patterns for walking

11.1.5   Primary Gait Abnormalities in CP

- Impaired tone/spasticity
- Impaired balance
- Loss of selective muscle control (but only spasticity can be treated)
  (N.B. So-called "secondary" gait abnormalities include muscular contractures and bony deformities and "tertiary" gait abnormalities refer to the coping mechanisms)

11.1.6   What Constitutes "Spasticity"

- Spasticity is defined as hypertonia in which one or both of the following signs are present, viz.:
    - Resistance to externally imposed movement increases with increasing speed of the stretch, and varies with the direction of joint movement
    - Resistance to externally imposed movement rises rapidly above a threshold speed or joint angle, i.e. spastic catch (R1 on Tardieu scale; after Task Force on Childhood Motor Disorders)

11.1.7   Gross Motor Function Classification System

- Level 1: walks with no restrictions, limited in more advanced gross motor skills
- Level 2: walks with no assistive devices, but limitations walking outdoors and the community
- Level 3: walks with assistive devices, limitations walking outdoors and community
- Level 4: self-mobility with limitations, children need transport or powered mobility in outdoors or the community
- Level 5: self mobility is severely limited even with the use of assistive technology
  (Palisano et al., Dev Med Child Neurol 1997)

11.1.8   Rationale Behind GMFCS

- This five-level classification system (gross motor function classification system) is based on self-initiated movement with emphasis on sitting (truncal control) and walking
- Differentiating between the five levels is based on the need for assistive technology, including crutches and canes, and wheelchair mobility, in addition to quality of movement

11.2   Importance of Goal Setting and Multidisciplinary Care

11.2.1   Introduction

- Management of CP patients is a typical example where a multidisciplinary team approach and goal setting (which we discussed in Chap. 1) is often absolutely essential

■ It is essential for every member of the team to know we are not managing spasticity (or deformity), but a patient with spasticity
■ The general aim of the rehabilitative team should be improvement in the level of function, with due regard to the patient's interest and goals

11.2.2   Essence of Health Care for Children with CP
■ "Multidisciplinary, community-based, aim or goal-orientated, and agreed amongst all interested parties" (Neville 1994)

11.2.3   Key Concept
■ CP involves a wide spectrum of disorders
■ As such, the goals for the ambulatory CP patients are vastly different from the non-ambulators
■ One implication of the above is that quality of life measures we employ should separately cater for the vast differences in the two ends of the spectrum of this disorder. One such measure under development at the famous Hospital for Sick Children in Canada is known as "CP Child"

11.2.4   Worked Example of Goal Setting
■ The following are examples of the use of goal setting in a hypothetical patient
■ Our hypothetical patient is a GMFCS level 3 with history of diplegic CP, but having some increase in difficulty lately in community ambulation despite the use of aids, after her recent adolescent growth spurt

11.2.4.1   Aim to Decrease Muscle Tone

11.2.4.1.1   Introduction
■ Importance of this goal:
  – Based on research in basic science: spasticity if left unchecked can cause lasting structural changes in the muscle, and thus patient will be more prone to secondary musculoskeletal deformity. Research in fact has found increased deposition of collagen in these spastic muscles (see later discussion in Sect. 11.2.4.2.4)
  – If even this level 1 goal cannot be reached, it will be difficult to move on to higher levels

11.2.4.1.2 Initial Physical Assessment
■ Relevant history and occupational assessment (see below)
■ Emphasis during physical examination:
  - Muscle tone and spasticity using Tardieu and/or Ashworth scale
  - Assessment of presence of selective motor control
  - Gross motor function measure
  - Other neurological assessment (sensation, cognition, perception)

11.2.4.1.3 Initial Occupational Assessment
■ COPM (Canadian Occupational Performance Measure, discussed in Chap. 1)
■ Goal attainment scaling
■ FIM (Functional Independence Measure)
  - The above are some of the most frequently used measures in the initial assessment and will aid the multidisciplinary team to set goals for our patient. (N.B. the younger the patient, the more important it is that the goal needs to be agreed with the parents as well)

11.2.4.1.4 Potential Problems Created by UMN Spasticity
■ Limited mobility
■ Gait alterations
■ Limitation of ROM and/or contractures/subluxations
■ UL dexterity sometimes affected (e.g. hemiplegics, and some total body)
■ Pain (more in total body)
■ Skin complications

11.2.4.1.5 General Management for Increased Tone
■ Must understand the nature of UMN spasticity, and its complications
■ Understand and treat common aggravating factors of spasticity (Sect. 11.2.4.1.6)
■ Role of botulinum toxin (Sect. 11.3.1)
■ Role of physiotherapy (Sect. 11.3.4)
■ Role of intrathecal baclofen (Sect. 11.3.2)
■ Role of dorsal root rhizotomy (Sect. 11.3.3)

11.2.4.1.6   Common Factors That May Aggravate Spasticity

- Bowel problems (e.g. constipation)
- Skin ulceration
- Poor fitting shoes
- Undetected occult fracture
- Urinary tract incontinence
- Others: e.g. ingrown toenails, etc.

  (N.B. Factors differ between patients, the factors that may trigger spasticity in each particular patient need to be recorded)

11.2.4.2   Aim of Muscle Strength Training and Regaining ROM

11.2.4.2.1   Introduction

- Importance of this goal:
  - Helps avoid contractures and deformities
  - It will be very difficult for the patient to regain function if the two components of this level 2 goal cannot be achieved

11.2.4.2.2   Input from Basic Science That May Help Achieve Level 2 Goals

- This is dependent in the first place on an understanding of the elements essential for more normal movement in CP:
  - Postural tone
  - Reciprocal innervation
  - Sensory-motor feedback and feed-forward
  - Balance reactions
  - Biomechanical properties of muscle

Postural Tone

  Posture in CP also depends on factors like severity and distribution of spasticity

  Besides measures to decrease tone previously discussed, other measures may help, e.g. widening the base of support sometimes help decrease tone; some patients have increased postural tone lying flat and better positioning including WC positioning that may decrease tone can be considered

Reciprocal Innervation

- Normal reciprocal inhibition is essential for balance and maintaining centre of gravity within the base of support, as well as providing stability through postural adjustment, which occur prior to and during performance of a movement
- A commonly seen problem in CP is increased contraction of antagonistic muscle or static co-contraction with possible failure or attenuation of normal reciprocal inhibition
- Since some techniques of PNF (proprioceptive neuromuscular facilitation) make use of this principle, PNF is a potential method of strengthening in CP patients. Discussion of PNF will thus be included later in this chapter (Sect. 11.3.4)

Sensory-Motor Feedback and Feed-Forward

- The established pattern of spasticity and the underlying weakness create new (cerebral) motor programs that are dictated by the stereotyped activity. The resultant effort and compensatory strategies, which are adopted to counteract the dominant spastic posturing and the underlying weakness, produce an abnormal sensory input to the brain (Edward, 1996)
- The role of the physiotherapist is to modify this stereotyped response by facilitation of a more normal pattern
- Prolonged use of a limited repertoire of movement patterns creates a dominant abnormal response, which becomes increasingly difficult to reverse
- Once established, re-education can sometimes only be achieved after botox intervention to weaken dominant spastic muscles (Shumway-Cook, 1995)

Balance Reactions

- Patient with altered postural control are often apprehensive of losing balance, movements tend to be slower with increase in background muscle tone, especially in standing and walking, in anticipation of potential falls (Edward, 1998)

Biomechanical Properties of Muscle

- Prolonged spasticity can produce both intrinsic and extrinsic changes in muscle structure (that can affect its function even further)

11.2.4.2.3   Extrinsic Structural Changes
- Changes in connective tissue structure can occur, which may contribute to stiffness

11.2.4.2.4   Intrinsic Structural Changes
- Accumulation of collagen demonstrated in these spastic muscles (Booth, 2001)
- Over-representation of slow-oxidative type of muscle fibres occurs
- Decreased number of sarcomeres in those muscles held shortened (Ada, 1990)
- Possible increased elastic and plastic resistance in the face of long-standing spasticity (Mauritz, 1986)
- Reversal or abnormal sequence of firing of motor units

11.2.4.2.5   Recent Studies on the Effect of Muscle Strengthening in CP
- Task-specific closed chain strengthening programmed training seemed effective in children: a recent study with spastic diplegic children who are not cognitively impaired found group training in a circuit class is effective, feasible and even enjoyable for CP children (Blundell et al., Clin Rehabil 2003)

11.2.4.3   Improvement in ADL

11.2.4.3.1   Introduction
- The input of the occupational therapist of the rehabilitation team is indispensable here

11.2.4.3.2   Examples of Possible Intervention
- Provision of assistive technology
- Wheeled mobility
- Adjuncts to wheeled mobility like wheelchair glove, ramps
- Home modification
- Provision of splints and orthoses to improve function

11.2.4.4   Performance of Specific Functional Tasks: Elements Needed to Achieve Level 4
- Achieve control and strength of antagonists and agonists
- Reciprocal activities in muscles
- Active voluntary movement and control of the joint and limb

■ Specific functional tasks will need specific training pertaining to the task to be successful

11.2.4.5 Increased Independence and Improved Quality of Life

11.2.4.5.1 Common Measures Used to Measure Quality of Life

■ Child Health Questionnaire (CHQ)
■ Paediatric Outcomes Data Collection Instrument (PODCI)
■ Health-Related Quality of Life (HRQL)
■ Measures that help assess the relationship between environment and participation and quality of life, e.g. Parenting Stress Index, Strength and Difficulties Questionnaires, Kidscreen (Colver et al., BMC Pub Health 2006)

11.2.4.5.2 Pitfalls of Current Measures

■ It is common knowledge that CP involves a very wide spectrum of disorders from those with minimal impairment to the total body quadriplegic
■ Most of the popular questionnaires do not take account of this very wide spectrum

11.2.4.5.3 Towards a New Quality of Life Measure: from HSC in Canada

■ Quality of life measures we employ should separately cater for the vast differences amongst CP patients at the two ends of the spectrum of this disorder. One such measure under development at the famous Hospital for Sick Children in Canada is known as "CP Child"; detailed discussion is beyond the scope of this book, but a multicentre assessment of this new QOL measure is on-going

11.2.4.6 Monitoring Progress

11.2.4.6.1 Of Muscle Strength

■ Strength testing
■ Use of myometry – which is a more objective measure of muscular strength (see Fig. 11.1)

11.2.4.6.2 Of Motor Function

■ Most will recommend measures of gross motor functioning that are validated: use of GMFM-88 (now revised to GMFM-66)

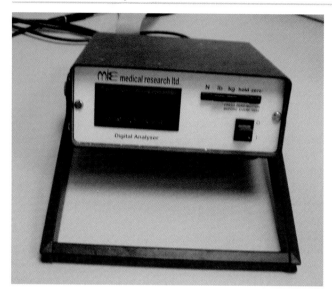

Fig. 11.1. Machinery needed for myometry

■ GMFM means gross motor function measure – it originally consists of 88 items, now changed to 66 items

11.2.4.6.3 Use of Gait Analysis in CP
■ Refer to the section on gait analysis (Sect. 11.5.2)
■ Mainly for those CP patients who are ambulatory (mostly diplegics, some hemiplegics)

11.2.4.6.4 Community Integration
■ Assessment and monitoring of any residual problems of community integration can be followed using "Community Integration Questionnaires"

11.3   Major Therapeutic Modalities Used in Management of CP

11.3.1   Botulinum Toxin

11.3.1.1   Introduction

- Botulinum toxins are neurotoxins produced by some strains of clostridia
- There are types A to G, but only A and B, particularly type A, are in general use
- There are two commercial brands in use, but are not interchangeable as the dosing is very different as is possibly bioavailability
- The use of botulinum toxin is now regarded as an established method of management of spasticity in cerebral palsy patients in many countries
- There are many randomised controlled clinical trials supporting its efficacy given the right indications, especially for the lower extremities (Ubhi, Arch Dis Child 2000; Barwood, Dev Med Child Neurol 2000, Koman, Paediatrics 2001), but also for the upper limbs (Boyd, Eur J Neurol 2001; J Pediatr 2000)

11.3.1.2   Mechanism of Action

- Reversible, highly specific blockade of presynaptic cholinergic nerve terminals
- Toxin is then internalised into the nerve terminal and inhibits the release of Ach at the NMJ
- The result is reduction in tone and local muscle weakness

11.3.1.3   Goal of Therapy

- Reduction of spasticity
- Decrease in painful spasms
- Improvement in motor function
- Promotion of longitudinal muscle growth (Fehlings, Paediatr Child Health 2005)
- Improvement in quality of life (Clin Neuropharmacol 2004)

- Weakening of nearby muscle (diffuse along muscle fascia)
- Aspiration can occur if neck muscles injected
- Systemic toxicity not common if we abide by the usual maximum dose with due regard to the weight of the child

11.3.1.16 Causes of Unresponsiveness
- There are many causes of lack of response besides presence of neutralising antibodies – estimated incidence 3.5% of cases only (Graham et al., Gait Posture 2000)
- Further research needed on the mechanism of progressive diminishing response, especially in cases without neutralising antibodies

11.3.1.17 Key Concept
- Do not attempt to increase dose of toxin as a treatment for botulinum toxin unresponsiveness

11.3.1.18 The Problem of Neutralising Antibodies
- One test said to be able to help differentiate a general cause of the unresponsiveness (e.g. presence of antibodies) from a local cause is via injection to the frontalis muscle. If it is a general cause, the efficacy of the toxin on the frontalis may also be affected. This differentiating test was reported in the Japanese Literature

11.3.1.19 Adjuncts to be Used with Botulinum Toxin Therapy
- Physiotherapy, e.g. involves stretching, strengthening of antagonist, attempt increase excursion of agonists
- Orthosis, e.g. use of ankle/foot orthosis (AFO)
- Short-term casting

11.3.1.20 Clinical Examples
- In the LL:
  - Spastic equinus: treatment with injection to the gastrocnemius
  - Hip subluxation: treatment with injection to iliopsoas, medial hamstrings and adductors
  - Multilevel in spastic diplegics with frequent injections to gastrocnemius, soleus, medial hamstrings, adductors and iliopsoas
- In the UL: occasionally in spastic hemiplegics, quadriplegics

11.3.2   Intrathecal Baclofen

11.3.2.1 Why Use Intrathecal Baclofen?
▥ Via the oral route it gets metabolised by the liver; chronic use also induces hepatic enzymes (Figs. 11.2, 11.3)
▥ Does not readily cross the blood–brain barrier, which is the main site in which we want the drug to act

11.3.2.2 Mechanism of Spasticity Reduction with Baclofen
▥ Potentiates central inhibitory neurons by its GABAb Agonist action
▥ As exemplified in previous animal (rat) experiments

11.3.2.3 Suitable Condidates
▥ Need to be very selective in patient selection
▥ Mostly for CP children with global spasticity
▥ Most children are seen in combined clinics in the presence of both neurosurgeons and orthopaedic surgeons
▥ Note: while spasticity is usually reasonably well controlled, dystonia is much more difficult to handle

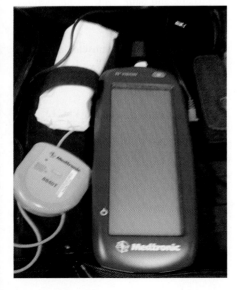

Fig. 11.2. The baclofen pump and its accessories

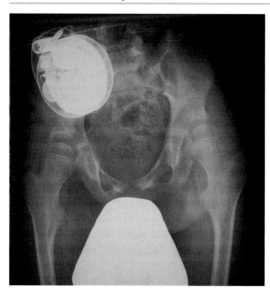

Fig. 11.3. A radiograph showing the baclofen pump in situ

11.3.2.4 Complications
■ Uncommon but serious: severe spasms and pain, even myoglobulinae-mia and death on sudden withdrawal (rebounds), such as in catheter breakage
■ Progressive increased scoliosis in some children (muscle tone keeps the spine from collapsing in some)
■ Infection near the pump
■ Pump malfunction, wrong programming, etc.

11.3.2.5 Mode of Administration
■ Most will be given a trial infusion for 3–4 days to assess patient toler-ance and possible side effects
■ If patient tolerates and is responsive, the pump can then be interna-lised
■ Pump refilling every 3 months

11.3.3   Dorsal Root Rhizotomy

11.3.3.1 Indications
- Difficult to control (often global) spasticity with no contractures
- Some centres reserve rhizotomy for the total body with significant spasticity, while others only consider its use in patients still with some potential for ambulation

11.3.3.2 Technique
- Involves laminotomy L1–S1
- Intraoperative electrical stimulation
- Around 20–40% posterior root division

11.3.3.3 Goal of Treatment
- Improved function/tone
- Improved velocity and joint ROM
- One long-term study found a reduction in the number of subsequent orthopaedic surgical procedures

11.3.3.4 Complications
- Persistent tone/dystonia
- Spinal deformity
- Long-term: weakness and crouch

11.3.4   Physiotherapy for CP Children and Role of PNF

11.3.4.1 Role of Physiotherapy
- The methods and the underlying rationale of muscle stretching have been discussed in Chap. 4. Improved mobility can sometimes be achieved by the combined use of techniques like hydrotherapy (Fig. 11.4), and Snoezelen techniques either at the bedside or combined with music in an under-water pool (Fig. 11.5). The former needs careful supervision by trained therapists in the presence of the child's parents, while those interested in the Snoezelen techniques can visit the relevant website at www.isna.de
- But the role of stretching in patients with CP, particularly of bi-articular muscles, as well as immobilisation in a stretched position, cannot be over-emphasised

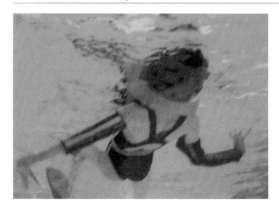

Fig. 11.4. Hydrotherapy is sometimes given to CP children, but strict supervision is required

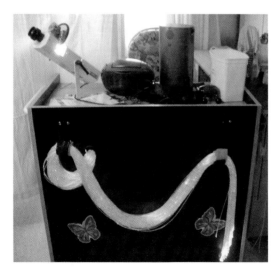

Fig. 11.5. An example of machinery needed for bed-side Snoezelen technique

11.3.4.2 Role of Immobilisation in a Stretched Position

▨ Normal muscle determines its length by the number of sarcomeres and its adaptation to different lengths appears to involve the production and removal of sarcomeres

▨ Previous experimental work has confirmed that immobilisation in a stretched position leads to muscle lengthening resulting from the increase in the number of sarcomeres

■ Consequently, joint mobility may be closely associated with daily opportunities for muscle stretching, particularly in bi-articular muscles (Kuno, Gait Posture 1998)

11.3.4.3   Role of PNF
■ We introduce here a time-honoured technique described by Knott and Voss, known as proprioceptive neuromuscular facilitation (PNF)
■ Although PNF is now widely used in increasing flexibility, the traditional indication is in the management of neuromuscular disorders

11.3.4.4   Proprioceptive Neuromuscular Facilitation

11.3.4.4.1   Definition
■ A therapeutic approach used mostly by physiotherapists to obtain functional improvement in motor output or control, via proprioceptive, cutaneous and auditory input (according to Knott and Voss)

11.3.4.4.2   History of PNF
■ More popularly employed methods of PNF include those proposed by the following workers:
  – Bobath (published in Physiotherapy 1955)
  – Voss and Knott (published in their popular text *Proprioceptive Neuromuscular Facilitation Patterns and Techniques*, 1968)

11.3.4.4.3   Relevant Anatomy
■ Skeletal muscle stretch reflex involves two types of receptors:
  – Golgi organs – sensitive to tension
  – Muscle spindles – sensitive to length changes, and rate of length changes
■ Muscle stretch → increased firing of muscle spindles → message relay to SC → increased motor nerve impulse and increased resistance of muscle to stretching
■ But if too much tension → Golgi organ fires → inhibits motor impulse and muscle relaxes

11.3.4.4.4   Rationale of PNF (in Producing Muscle Relaxation)
■ Application of muscle stretching for an extended period can potentially cause muscle relaxation as the inhibitory signals (from Golgi) override the excitatory ones (from spindles)

▦ Another mechanism used in PNF makes use of reciprocal inhibition of the agonist/antagonist muscle couple. (In normal circumstances, receipt of excitatory afferent impulses of motor neuron from agonist will cause concomitant inhibition of motor neurons of the antagonists)

11.3.4.4.5   Rationale of PNF (in Producing Strengthening)
▦ Our brain cannot recognise individual muscle firing, as the brain only detects gross joint motion
▦ It therefore pays to maximise the number of motor units being stimulated and firing to get as much strength as we can

11.3.4.4.6   Clinical Applications
▦ Improvement in neuromuscular control
▦ Improvement in strength, flexibility and motion

11.3.4.4.7   Techniques in Favour of Facilitation
▦ The principle of strength gains in PNF technique is based on the principle of maximising the number of motor units stimulated in order to strengthen whatever remaining muscle fibres are available after injury

11.3.4.4.8   Examples of Strengthening Techniques Employed
▦ Progressive passive, then slowly progressing to active motion against resistance
▦ If there is weakness at a certain point of a ROM, concentrate on repeated isotonic contraction exercises in that motion arc
▦ If more joint stability is desired, can resort to isometric contraction of the agonist, followed by isometric contraction of the antagonist

11.3.4.4.9   Technique in Favour of Inhibition, Causing Relaxation
▦ When there is tightness on one side, i.e. either the agonist or antagonist; begin with isometric contraction of the muscle group to be stretched, then concentric contraction of its opponents coupled with pressure by the therapist to stretch out the tight muscle group
▦ If both agonist and antagonist are tight, proceed by isotonic contraction of each muscle group in turn with resistance by the therapist, the muscle group is then relaxed and the therapist passively effects as much ROM as can be attained to effect muscle stretch

11.3.4.4.10 Word of Note

- There are different varieties of techniques within the arena of PNF that are outside the scope of this book, e.g.:
  - Hold–relax method
  - Slow reversal hold-relax
  - Contract-relax, etc.

11.4   Use of Ankle Foot Orthoses in the Management of Ambulant Children with Cerebral Palsy

11.4.1   Aims of Orthotic Intervention for Children with Cerebral Palsy

- To prevent deformity (e.g. mid-foot break in spastic planovalgus in diplegics)
- To correct deformity (e.g. milder cases of spastic equinus)
- As an adjunctive measure in correcting deformity (e.g. used with botulinum toxin in more spastic equinus)
- To provide a stable base of support (e.g. may help in crouch gait)
- To facilitate training in skills (e.g. walking skills)
- To improve the efficiency of gait in selected cases

11.4.2   Prescription Criteria

- Diagnosis
- Physical examination
- Gait pathology assessment
- Review therapeutic objectives
- Need for associated interventions

11.4.3   Prerequisites for Normal Gait (According to Gage)

- Stability in stance phase
- Clearance in swing phase
- Foot pre-positioning in swing
- Adequate step length
- In an energy-efficient manner and efficient phase shift
  (The reader is assumed also to be familiar with the three rockers concept in stance phase ankle kinematics according to Perry)

11.4.4   Common AFO Options for CP

▪ Rigid AFO
▪ Anterior ground reaction AFO
▪ Hinged AFO
▪ Leaf spring AFO
▪ Dynamic ankle foot orthosis (DAFO)
▪ Supra-malleolar orthosis (SMO)
▪ University of California Biomechanics Lab (UCBL) orthotic heel cups

11.4.4.1 Rigid AFO

▪ Prevents equinus and knee hyperextension and may increase hip extension and step length (Meadows, 1984; Butler et al., 1992; Fig. 11.6)
▪ Stretches gastrocnemius when knee is extended

11.4.4.2 General Indications for AFO

▪ Helps maximise stability of ankle, subtalar and midfoot joints in all planes in swing and stance
▪ To prevent knee hyperextension in stance (since changes the direction of GRF and knee moments in patients with spastic equinus)

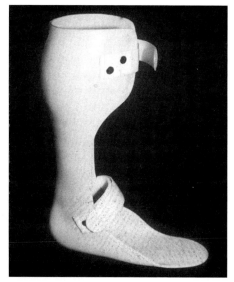

Fig. 11.6. An example of a "rigid ankle foot orthosis"

- To help prevent crouch (where moderate to severe loss of knee and hip extensors are present)
- For moderate to severe spasticity
- To protect an unstable midfoot from the closed chain effects of ankle dorsiflexion when a spastic triceps sura is active in stance (i.e. to prevent spastic equinus causing or worsening any pre-existing midfoot break)
- Post-surgical applications or after botulinum toxin injection

11.4.4.3 Rigid AFO: Other Functional Indications
- Child is ready to stand, but unable to balance on feet, which are in a pathological position (equinus, equino-valgus, varus, equino-varus)
- Child stands on heels, but walks on toes

11.4.4.4 Anterior Ground Reaction AFO
- Design features (Fig. 11.7):
  - Donning: posterior entry; or proximal entry
  - Anterior shell

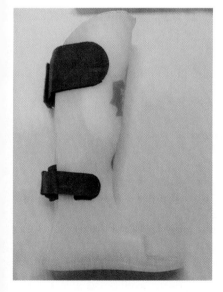

Fig. 11.7. Posterior entry "ground reaction force ankle foot orthosis"

11.4.4.4.1 Function of Anterior Ground Reaction AFO (According to Harrington)

- Creates a knee extension moment during stance phase
- Orthosis dorsiflexion angle:
  - Can be decreased to protect weak quadriceps, promote knee extension
  - Can be increased to accommodate knee flexion contractures
- Suitable for mild crouch (with excessive knee flexion)
- Intervention to hamstrings or gastrocnemius may be necessary

11.4.4.4.2 Anterior Ground Reaction AFO: Other Functional Indications

- Overactive hamstrings with weak quadriceps leading to overflexed knees
- Surgically overcorrected heel cord
- Over-extended heel cord due to poor postoperative protection
- Over-lengthened heel cord from long-term flexion pattern
- Contraindicated: whenever ankle motion increases function

11.4.4.5 Articulated (Single Axis) AFO

- Design features (Fig. 11.8):
  - Mechanical joint types
  - Free motion
  - Dorsiflexion assist
  - Plantar flexion stop
  - Dorsiflexion stop

11.4.4.5.1 Articulated AFO Indication

- When it is deemed that variable ankle motion allows a more functional gait pattern:
  - A plantar flexion stop prevents plantar flexion in toe walkers in stance, knee hyperextension from foot flat to toe-off (GRF control) and plantar flexion in swing
  - A dorsiflexion stop helps resist knee flexion for a mild crouch gait pattern (GRF control)
  - Free motion in dorsiflexion will encourage normal tibial excursion over the foot with stretching of soleus (not gastrocnemius) during stance

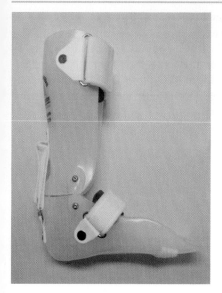

Fig. 11.8. An example of an "articulated ankle foot orthosis"

- Use requires 5–10° of passive ankle dorsiflexion (without compromising neutral subtalar joint [STJ] and musculotendinous junction [MTJ] positions)
- Can control moderate to severe spastic deformity at the subtalar joint
- Can control mid-foot instabilities including:
  - Forefoot abduction or adduction
  - Forefoot valgus or varus
  - Forefoot dorsiflexion

11.4.4.5.2 Contraindications

- Hamstring contractures and/or moderate to severe loss of ankle, knee and hip extensors resulting in crouch gait
- When ankle dorsiflexion is completely restricted by severe triceps sura spasticity
- Fixed plantar flexion contractures
- Excessive fixed equinovarus deformity
- An unstable mid-foot occurs when subtalar joint put in neutral
- The increased range of dorsiflexion allowed must not be achieved through compensatory pronation of the STJ

- Good control of the STJ should be secured before increased motion in ankle dorsiflexion is permitted
- As the tibia rotates forward in stance, a spastic triceps sura will block ankle dorsiflexion and transfer the forces and moments of weight-bearing to the mid-foot. The hinged AFO allows this motion, resulting in collapse of the unstable mid-foot against the orthosis, producing unacceptable interface pressures

11.4.4.6 Posterior Leafspring AFO

- Design: dynamic dorsiflexion assist (Fig. 11.9)
- General indications:
  - Flaccid foot drop (Type 1 and 2 hemiplegia)
- Contraindications:
  - Moderate to severe spasticity
  - Excessive plantar flexion
  - Medio-lateral deformity

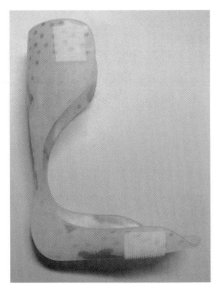

Fig. 11.9. Posterior "leafspring ankle foot orthosis"

11.4.4.7   Dynamic Ankle Food Orthoses: Tone-Influencing Orthoses?

- Evidence of tone reduction achieved using below-knee casting only (Watt, 1986)
- DAFO controls valgus/varus, providing a stable base only if there is no equinus
- DAFO is appropriate as part of an intensive, progressive therapeutic programme
- Different designs

11.4.4.8   Supra-Malleolar Orthosis

11.4.4.8.1   Indications

- Excessive inversion/eversion in stance
- Forefoot abduction/adduction
- Forefoot valgus/varus
- Localised high plantar pressure (Fig. 11.10)

11.4.4.8.2   Contraindications

- Moderate to severe spasticity
- Excessive plantar flexion

11.4.4.9   UCBL Heel Cup

- Control of mild medio-lateral calcaneal deviation
- Assisted by intrinsic/extrinsic posting
- Unsuitable for moderate/severe deformity or spasticity (Fig. 11.11)

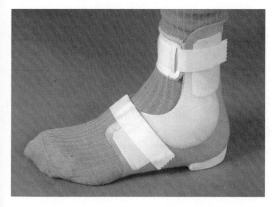

Fig. 11.10. A supra-malleolar orthosis

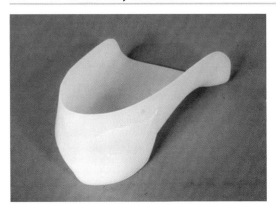

Fig. 11.11. A University of California Biomechanics Lab (UCBL) heel cup

11.4.4.10   A Word on Shoe Selection (When an Orthosis is Used)

- Heel height – can affect direction of GRF and knee moment
- Heel shape and material – affects initial contact, or first rocker
- Shape of the shoe – affects the interface with AFO
- Sole profile and material – affects fulcrum position and third rocker
- Upper design – foot entry affects containment, thus AFO function
- Other aspects – flexibility and rigidity

11.4.5   Recent Studies Comparing Different Orthoses

11.4.5.1   AFO vs DAFO

- The DAFOs allowed a significantly larger total ankle ROM than the AFOs. However, AFOs significantly reduced the median frequency of EMG signals (MF) while DAFOs did not. The reduced MF seen when wearing AFOs suggested an improvement in walking endurance. The DAFO had the advantage of less restriction on ankle movement, which avoids muscular atrophy and improves orthotic compliance (Lam et al., Gait Posture 2005)

11.4.5.2   Hinged AFO Use in Hemiplegic CP

- The peak activity of the tibialis anterior muscle was reduced by 36.1% at initial contact and loading response phase and by 57.3% just after toe-off when using a hinged ankle foot orthosis (HAFO). The decrease in activity was thought to result from the change in gait pattern from a toe gait to a heel-toe gait as well as the use of a HAFO. The HAFO also slightly decreased muscle activity in the proximal leg muscles, mainly during swing phase, improved stride length, decreased cadence, improved walking speed, increased peak hip flexion, improved kinematics in loading response phase at the knee, and reduced the excessive ankle plantar flexion (Romkes et al., Gait Posture 2006)

11.4.5.3 Rigid vs Hinged AFO in Diplegics

▓ Both orthoses increased stride length, reduced abnormal ankle plantar flexion during initial contact, mid-stance and terminal stance, and increased ankle plantar flexor moments closer to normal during TST. Hinged AFOs increased ankle dorsiflexion at TST and increased ankle power generation during pre-swing compared with solid AFOs, and increased ankle dorsiflexion at loading compared with no AFOs. No other significant differences were found for the gait variables when comparing these orthoses. Either AFO could be used to reduce the excessive ankle plantar flexion without affecting the knee position during stance. The hinged AFO would be recommended to produce more normal dorsiflexion during TST and increased ankle power generation during PSW in children with spastic diplegic CP (Radtka et al., Gait Posture 2005)

11.5   Role of Surgery

11.5.1   Introduction

▓ The role of surgery in CP has been discussed in great detail in the companion volume of this book *Orthopaedic Principles, A Resident's Guide*

▓ Here, we will briefly review how surgery can sometimes improve the gait of the patient. Finally, we will briefly discuss the pros and cons of multilevel surgery in CP

11.5.2   Information Obtainable from 3-D Gait Analysis

▓ Information not always obtainable with 2-D gait analysis, e.g. differentiating adduction from limb rotation when transverse plane analysis can help

▓ Lever arm dysfunction

- Coping responses (does not need treatment)
- The exact abnormal muscle activity accounting for altered ROM of joints or motion of body segments
- Information on muscle recruitment: notice that differences in balance control in children with spasticity are due to CNS deficits as well as mechanical changes in posture (Gait Posture, 1998)

11.5.3 Examples of the Use of Surgery to Improve Gait

- Improve stability in stance, e.g. correction of contractures
- Correcting lever arm dysfunction, e.g. osteotomies to correct femoral anteversion or tibial torsion
- Stiff knee gait with clearance problems, e.g. rectus femoris transfer
- Dynamic equinus, e.g. gastrocnemius recession
- But remember to do no harm:
    - Avoid tensioning spastic muscles
    - Avoid weakening accelerators
    - Avoid correcting normal body's coping responses

11.5.4 Advantages of Multilevel Surgery in CP

- Doing the corrections at all levels in one go avoids the need for subsequent repeat surgery, refer to the "birthday syndrome" of Mercer Rang
- Literature abounds in support of multilevel surgery

11.5.5 Literature in Support of Multilevel Surgery

- One-session surgery for correction of lower extremity deformities in children with CP (Norlin et al., J Pediatr Orthop 1985)
- One-session surgery for bilateral correction of lower limb deformities in spastic diplegia (Brown et al., J Pediatr Orthop 1987)
- A functional assessment of simultaneous multiple surgical procedures to assist walking (Nene et al., J Bone Joint Surg 1993)
- Rectus femoris surgery in children with cerebral palsy: a comparison of the effect of transfer and release of the distal rectus femoris on knee motion (Ounpuu et al., J Pediatr Orthop 1993)
- Alterations in surgical decision-making in patients with CP based on 3-D gait analysis (DeLuca et al., J Pediatr Orthop 1997)
- The effect of rectus EMG patterns on the outcome of rectus femoris transfers (Miller et al., J Pediatr Orthop 1997)

11.5.6 Summarising the Advantages

■ Improved kinematics confirmed with preoperative and postoperative gait analysis
■ Improved mobility level and sometimes GMFCS class
■ Improved higher level functional skills

11.5.7 Disadvantages of Multilevel Surgery

■ Decreased muscle strength:
  - Muscle strength return can take up to 18 months (according to research done in Oxford)
  - Some experts suggest the optimal time to assess outcome is 3 years after multilevel surgery (Saraph et al., J Pediatr Orthop 2005)
  - Animal studies revealed muscle or tendon surgery produces a temporary loss of strength, which recovers in 6–12 weeks (Brunner et al., 2000)
■ Decreased GMFM scores (according to research done at Nuffield Orthopaedic Centre, Oxford)

General Bibliography

Miller F (2005) Cerebral Palsy. Springer, Berlin Heidelberg New York

Selected Bibliography of Journal Articles

1. Palisano R, Rosenbaum P et al. (1997) Development and reliability of a system to classify gross motor function in children with cerebral palsy. Dev Med Child Neurol 39(4):214–223
2. Booth CM, Cortina-Borja MJ et al. (2001) Collagen accumulation in muscles of children with cerebral palsy and correlation with severity of spasticity. Dev Med Child Neurol 43(5):314–320
3. Blundell SW, Shepherd RB et al. (2003) Functional strength training in cerebral palsy: a pilot study of a group circuit training class for children aged 4–8 years. Clin Rehabil 17(1):48–57
4. Boyd RN, Morris ME et al. (2001) Management of upper limb dysfunction in children with cerebral palsy – a systematic review. Eur J Neurol 8 (Suppl 5):150–166
5. Ubhi T, Bhakta BB et al. (2000) Randomized double blind placebo controlled trial of the effect of botulinum toxin on walking in cerebral palsy. Arch Dis Child 83(6):481–487

6. Barwood S, Bailieu C et al. (2000) Analgesic effects of botulinum toxin A: a randomized placebo-controlled clinical trial. Dev Med Child Neurol 42(2):116–121
7. Koman LA, Brashear A et al. (2001) Botulinum toxin type A neuromuscular blockade in the treatment of equines foot deformity in cerebral palsy: a multicenter, open-label clinical trial. Pediatrics 108(5):1062–1071
8. Jankovic J, Fehlings D et al. (2004) Evidence-based review of patient-reported outcomes with botulinum toxin type A. Clin Neuropharmacol 27(5):234–244
9. Fehlings D, Rang M et al. (2000) An evaluation of botulinum A toxin injections to improve upper extremity function in children with hemiplegic cerebral palsy. J Pediatr 137(3):331–337
10. Graham HK, Aoki KR et al. (2000) Recommendations for the use of botulinum toxin type A in the management of cerebral palsy. Gait Posture 11(1):67–79
11. Baker R, Jasinski M et al. (2002) Botulinum toxin treatment of spasticity in diplegic cerebral palsy: a randomized double-blind placebo-controlled dose-ranging study. Dev Med Child Neurol 44(10):666–675
12. Kuno H, Suzuki N et al. (1998) Geometrical analysis of hip and knee joint mobility in cerebral palsied children. Gait Posture 8:(2):110–116
13. Butler PB, Thompson N et al. (1992) Improvement in walking performance of children with cerebral palsy: preliminary results. Dev Med Child Neurol 34(7): 567–576
14. Lam WK, Leong JC et al. (2005) Biomechanical and electromyographic evaluation of ankle foot orthosis and dynamic ankle foot orthosis in spastic cerebral palsy. Gait Posture 22(3):189–197
15. Romkes J, Hell AK (2006) Changes in muscle activity in children with hemiplegic cerebral palsy while walking with or without ankle foot orthoses. Gait Posture, doi:10.1016/j.gaitpost.2005.12.001
16. Radtka SA, Skinner SR et al. (2005) A comparison of gait with solid and hinged ankle-foot orthoses in children with spastic cerebral palsy. Gait Posture 21(3): 303–310
17. Norlin R, Tkaczuk H (1985) One-session surgery for correction of lower extremity deformities in children with cerebral palsy. J Pediatr Orthop 5(2):208–211

Contents

12.1   Introduction

- Epidemiological data indicate that spinal cord injuries (SCI) most often occur in young males, especially between 16 and 30 years of age
- New cases: 30–50/million (US data) per annum
- The study of SCI is especially important since it frequently affects individuals in the prime of their life in our society
- Most are the results of high-energy trauma such as traffic accidents and fall accidents, or being struck in sports
- Despite the initial enthusiasm with hyperacute administration of high-dose steroids that have allegedly shown benefit, there is increasing scepticism about the original publications from the scientific world, and in some places like Alberta, surgeons have forsaken their use for want of better evidence

12.1.1   Key Concept
- Most damage to cord done at the time of injury

12.1.1.1 Concepts of Primary and Secondary Damage to the Spinal Cord
- Primary injury:
  - Sustained at the time of impact
  - From compression and cord contusion
  - Involves neuronal damage, disruption of axonal membrane and blood vessels
- Secondary injury:
  - Involves a cascade of auto-destructive processes lasting hours to days expanding the injury zone
  - Details of the cascade discussed under pathophysiology (Sect. 12.2)
  - Limiting the extent of secondary injury is part of our goal of management in acute spinal cord injury

12.1.2   Spinal Shock
- Spinal shock occurs mostly after significant cervical cord injury; characterised by a state of flaccid paralysis, hypotonia and areflexia (e.g. absent bulbocavernosus reflex)
- The sensory and motor symptoms usually resolve by 4–6 h, but autonomic symptoms can persist for days or weeks

■ Most typical signs include bradycardia despite hypotension, flaccid paralysis and lack of painful sensation to the limbs affected; other signs that can be present depend of the level of injury

12.1.3   End of Spinal Shock
■ Characterised by the return of the bulbocavernosus reflex
■ This reflex is elicited by a gentle squeeze of the glans penis in men; and a gentle tug of the Foley catheter in ladies
■ In most of the cases, this reflex returns within 24 h at the end of spinal shock
■ If there is no evidence of sacral sparing or spinal cord function distal to the level of injury when spinal shock is over, we can diagnose complete cord injury with a much graver prognosis. Never comment on the completeness of cord injury during the period of spinal shock

12.1.4   Diagnosis of Level of Injury in Unconscious Patients
■ Diagnosis of level involves careful clinical neurological testing in a conscious patient
■ If the patient is not conscious, we can resort to the use of SSEP (somatosensory evoked potentials)
■ Notice SSEP are unaffected by spinal shock

12.1.5   Frankel's Grading of Injury Severity
■ Frankel A: complete motor and sensory loss
■ Frankel B: motor complete, sensory loss incomplete
■ Frankel C: some motor power left, but not useful
■ Frankel D: some motor power left, and useful
■ Frankel E: normal motor and sensation

12.1.6   ASIA Scale
■ ASIA A = no motor or sensory preservation, even in the sacral segments S4–S5
■ ASIA B = sensory, but no motor function preserved below the neurological level including the sacral segments (S4–S5)
■ ASIA C = motor function is preserved below the neurological level, and more than half of the key muscles below the neurological level have a muscle grade less than 3 (voluntary sphincter contraction, sparing of motor function more than three segments below)

- ASIA D = motor function is preserved below the neurological level, and at least half of the key muscles below the neurological level have a muscle grade of 3
- ASIA E = motor and sensory functions are normal

12.1.7 Points to Note
- Motor level: most caudal level grade ≥3, and rostral muscles are grade 5
- Sensory level: most caudal level with intact grade 2 sensation
- Neurological level: the most caudal level where both motor and sensory modalities are intact bilaterally

12.1.8 Key Motor Points to Be Tested in ASIA Scale
- C5: elbow flexors
- C6: wrist extensors
- C7: elbow extensors
- C8: flexor digitorum profundus, third digit
- T1: finger abductors
- L2: hip flexors
- L3: knee extensors
- L4: ankle dorsiflexion
- L5: big toe dorsiflexion
- S1: ankle plantar flexion

12.1.9 Key Sensory Points to Be Tested in ASIA Scale
- C2: occiput protuberance
- C3: supraclavicular fossa
- C4: ACJ superior aspect
- C5: lateral antecubital fossa
- C6: dorsal proximal thumb
- C7: dorsal proximal middle finger
- C8: dorsal proximal little finger
- T1: medial antecubital fossa
- T2: hip flexors
- T4: medial to nipple
- T10: umbilicus
- T12: inguinal ligament
- L2: medial anterior thigh
- L1: between T12 and L2

- L3: medial anterior knee
- L4: medial malleolus
- L5: medial dorsal foot
- S1: inferior part of lateral malleolus
- S2: popliteal fossa
- S3: ischial tuberosity
- S4–S5: mucocutaneous part of the anus

12.1.10 Incomplete Spinal Cord Syndromes
- Central cord syndrome
  - Mainly affects the upper extremities
  - Association with elderly with pre-existing cervical spondylosis
  - Hyperextension injury
  - Buckling of ligamentum flavum causing compression to medially placed arm fibres in the corticospinal tract
  - Subsequent elective laminoplasty or laminectomy with lateral mass plating commonly required
- Anterior cord syndrome
  - Aetiology: anterior spinal artery territory ischaemia, e.g. from axial loading or hyperextension injuries, teardrop fractures
  - **Loss:** motor function and pain, and temperature sensation
  - Prognosis: 10–20% muscle recovery, poor muscle power and coordination, worst prognosis among the forms of incomplete spinal cord syndrome
- Posterior cord syndrome
  - **Aetiology:** rare
  - Posterior spinal artery damage
  - Diffuse atherosclerosis: deficient collateral perfusion
  - Loss: position sense
  - Rule out B12 deficiency
  - Prognosis: better than anterior syndrome
  - Poor ambulation prospect: since proprioceptive deficit
- Brown Sequard Syndrome
  - **Aetiologies: penetrating** trauma
  - Radiation
  - Ipsilateral weakness and position sense loss
  - Contralateral pain and temperature loss
  - **Prognosis:** 75–90% ambulate on discharge

- 70% independent ADL
- 89% bladder- and 82% bowel-continent
- Conus medullaris syndrome
  - Epiconus: L4–S1
  - Sparing of sacral reflex: bulbocavernosus, micturation
  - Conus: S2–S4
  - Sacral reflex loss
  - Detrusor weakness and overflow incontinence
  - Loss of penile erection and ejaculation
  - If root escapes: ambulatory, ankle jerks normal
  - Symmetric defects: small size of conus
  - Pain: inconstant; perineum and thighs
  - Weakness: sacral
  - Sensory loss: saddle in distribution
  - Prognosis: limited recovery

12.2   Pathophysiology of Spinal Cord Injury in General

- Most texts focus on mechanism of secondary injury to the spinal cord
- But to think of the body's inflammatory and other responses as a purely detrimental entity is an over-simplification of the state of affairs
- There is in fact simultaneous initiation of neuroprotective + injurious mechanisms provoked by the injury

12.2.1   Role of the Inflammatory Response: a Blessing or a Curse?
- Thanks to well-designed studies by workers like Bethea; we now know that there are both sides to the coin
- Bethea pointed out in Prog Brain Res 2000 the concept of a "dual-edge sword": thus, the inflammatory process that occurs in response to spinal cord injury can have both deleterious and neuroprotective effects

12.2.2   Pathophysiology in Detail
- Pathogenetic mechanisms we know of are based mainly on animal models, they include:
  - Lipid peroxidation and free radical generation
  - Abnormal electrolyte fluxes and excitotoxicity
  - Abnormal vascular perfusion
  - The associated inflammatory and immune response

12.2.2.1 Lipid Peroxidation and Free Radicals

- Free radicals are frequently released in spinal cord injury
- They cause damage by:
  - Disruption of the cell membrane
  - Mediated by oxidation of fatty acids in cellular membrane (lipid peroxidation). This peroxidation process resembles a chain reaction, generating more active lipid-derived radicals
  - Free radicals also damage mitochondrial enzymes inside cells such as ATPase, which produces cell death
- Many therapeutic interventions employ agents that help prevent lipid peroxidation, e.g. methylprednisolone, antioxidants such as tirilazad mesylate (used in a treatment arm in NASCIS study)

12.2.2.2 Abnormal Electrolyte Fluxes and Excitotoxicity

- Glutamate is a prevalent neurotransmitter in the CNS. Its receptors include NMDA (N-methyl-D-aspartate) among others that allow ions to pass such as calcium and sodium. (P.S. high cytosolic calcium is lethal to cells)
- Accumulation of glutamate occurs after cord injury, and over-excitation of these receptors can occur, i.e. excitotoxicity; causing abnormal ionic fluxes. Methods of blocking NMDA receptors have been used as a treatment method to prevent further cellular damage

12.2.2.3 Abnormal Vascular Perfusion

- Normal blood flow to the spinal cord is under auto-regulation
- Impaired vascularity of the cord in spinal cord injury includes:
  - Loss of autoregulation
  - Spinal shock and hypoperfusion
  - Shock due to blood loss from associated injuries
    (One needs to avoid hypotension and decreased oxygenation at all costs, most need ICU care)

12.2.2.4 Abnormal Intracellular Sodium Concentration

- Normal intracellular sodium is kept at a low level, and is kept low by ATPase ionic pumps
- Abnormal Na^+ fluxes affect especially the white matter glial cells
- Neuroprotection especially to white matter can be achieved by blocking abnormal sodium fluxes by pharmacologic agents

12.2.2.5   Associated Inflammatory and Immune Response

- Details of interactions between inflammatory mediators are not fully known, but key players include:
  - Tumour necrosis factor: said to have both neuroprotective and neurotoxic properties
  - Arachidonic acid metabolites: these are formed from phospholipase at cell membranes; the accumulation of which is metabolised via cyclo-oxygenase to prostaglandins, which can affect vascular permeability, etc.
- Note that in secondary spinal cord injury, cell death can occur either through cell necrosis or apoptosis

12.2.3   Planning of Treatment Strategies Based on Pathophysiology

12.2.3.1   Acute Intervention Part 1: Pharmacologic Interventions

12.2.3.1.1   Pharmacologic Strategy 1: Steroids

- Steroids mainly act by prevention of lipid peroxidation by free radicals, and membrane stabilisation. It may help prevent apoptosis by checking calcium fluxes, improving vascular perfusion, etc.
- Methylprednisolone was selected from among the different steroids because it is more effective at preventing lipid peroxidation

NASCIS 1 Trial
- Reported in JAMA by Bracken in 1984
- Less often quoted of the NASCIS trials
- This trial showed that late administration within 48 h of a relatively lower dose of methylprednisolone (than the high dose used in NASCIS 2 and 3 trials) showed little significant neurologic recovery

NASCIS 2 Trial
- Found that higher dose of methylprednisolone given <8 h later causes neurological improvement (not beyond 8 h)
- Paraplegics recovered 21% of lost motor function relative to 8% among controls
- Patients with paraparesis recovered 75% of lost motor function relative to 59% among controls
- Dose of steroid: 30 mg/kg bolus over 1 h, followed by 5.4 mg/kg/h for 23 h

NASCIS 3 Trial

- Further studies based on the findings in NASCIS 2
- Recommend:
  - The dose mentioned in NASCIS 2 for 24 h if patient presents < 3 h after injury
  - If between 3 and 8 h, give the above steroid infusion for total of 48 h
  - Tirilizad mesylate (an antioxidant) has a similar effect to that of steroids if given in hyperacute phase

Criticism of the NASCIS Trials

- Many criticisms have been lodged against especially NASCIS 2, e.g. the conclusion of a small but significant statistical benefit in those having steroids after < 8 h only occurred in a post hoc analysis – the primary outcome analysis of neural recovery in all randomised patients was in fact negative
- The very high dose of steroids was not without significant side effects

Pharmacologic Strategy 2: Naloxone

- Naloxone is an opiate receptor. Included in one treatment arm in the NASCIS study
- Found to be effective in the subgroup of patients with incomplete spinal cord injuries (J Neurosurg 1993)

Pharmacologic Strategies 3: Gangliosides

- They are glycosphingolipids at outer cellular membranes at the central nervous system
- There is some evidence that gangliosides may have a neuroprotection action, with more speedy recovery of motor and sensory function in partial cord injuries
- Although a large multicentre study failed to show obvious beneficial effects of GM 1 ganglioside at 26 weeks relative to placebo
- The multicentre study reported in Spine did show a more rapid neurological recovery when used with IV methylprednisolone vs steroid alone. However, the two groups had similar outcomes at 26 weeks (Geisler, Spine 2001)

Pharmacologic Strategies 4: Calcium Channel Blockers

- Thought to work by improvement in blood flow via vessel dilatation

Pharmacologic Strategies 5: Antagonists of Glutamate Receptors

Work by prevention of excitotoxicity as a result of glutamate accumulation – help preventing abnormal sodium and calcium fluxes that may prove lethal to cells

Pharmacologic Strategies 6: Others

BA-210 (Rho antagonist) – discussed later (Sect. 12.2.3.3.7)

Inhibition of cyclo-oxygenase

Minocycline

Sodium channel blockers

Erythropoietin

Cyclosporin

12.2.3.2   Acute Intervention Part 2: Role of Decompression

- Persistent compression of the cord from any structure is a potentially reversible type of secondary injury
- Abundant animal studies show beneficial effects of early cord decompression (J Neurosurg 1999)
- Clinical studies in the past with varied results:
  - Some show little benefit of "early" surgery (Spine 1997)
  - Some show beneficial effect (Clin Orthop Relat Res 1999)
  - But note wide variation of definition of "early" between animal and clinical studies; and between clinical studies
- In general, recent papers tend to propose early interventions as the adverse results of older studies are now partly circumvented by improvements in anaesthesia and critical care
- In the setting of conus medullaris injury, no correlation between the timing of surgical decompression and motor improvement was identified. Root recovery was more predictable than spinal cord and bladder recovery (J Spinal Cord Med 2006)

12.2.3.2.1   Decompression in Incomplete Spinal Cord Injury

- Most experts will agree nowadays to aim at either early (< 24 h) or urgent decompression of partial cord injuries
- Extreme care, however, needs to be exercised in achieving stable haemodynamics and adequate oxygenation, especially since the patient may be suffering from polytrauma
- Also, when the spine is stabilised, intensive physical therapy can be initiated to decrease other complications related to spinal cord injury

12.2.3.2.2   Decompression in Complete Spinal Cord Injury

- Despite the fact that the NASCIS study was not designed to assess timing of surgery; systematic data analysis of the raw data did reveal improved outcome from early surgery, which included both complete and incomplete cord injuries (except may be central cord syndromes)
- Also, even in the face of complete cord injury, early spinal stabilisation (if indicated) eases nursing and prevents complications like decubitus ulcers and pulmonary complications

12.2.3.3   Experimental Intervention: Prospects of Cord Regeneration

- Progress has also been made in this field, there has been much enthusiasm concerning stem cell research and we will look into this subject in Sect. 12.2.3.5
- This section is important as it will talk about many new and interesting advances in spinal cord injury

12.2.3.3.1   Introduction

- Significant advances and some very interesting observations have been made in the following fields in recent years
- We will take a look first at the interesting major advances, and explore the remaining challenges that still await us on the topic of barriers of regeneration and possible ways to overcome them

12.2.3.3.2   Space Physiology vs SCI (Findings of NASA)

- The National Aeronautics and Space Administration (NASA) recognises that astronauts exposed to microgravity suffer from physiological alterations that resemble those experienced by patients with SCI: including muscle atrophy, bone loss, disruption of locomotion and coordination, and impairment of functions regulated by the autonomic system. Although astronauts suffer from a mostly reversible and milder degree of the symptoms, the similarities are significant enough to suggest that both areas of research could benefit from each other's findings and therapeutic developments (Vaziri, J Spinal Cord Med 2003)
- Opportunities for cross-fertilisation between studies of SCI and space physiology are now being explored subsequent to the National Institute of Neurological Disorders and Stroke Meeting in 2000

12.2.3.3.3   Discovery of Oscillatory Circuitry in the Spinal Cord: CPG

- The spinal cord harbours a "central pattern generator" (CPG), a group of neurons that generates oscillatory patterns of activity and coordinates movements required for locomotion
- The CPG is not simply a hard-wired clock or pacemaker that sets a fixed pace for locomotion, it is modulated by sensory feedback, which plays a key role in triggering successive movements
- In addition, the spinal cord appears to contain collections or modules of neurons that activate specific groups of muscles, and allow the CPG, as well as supraspinal and reflex pathways, to translate their signals into actions
- In amphibians and some mammals, different combinations of these modules, also known as "primitives", appear to be capable of generating a large range of complex movements

Further Research on the "CPG"

These endogenous pacemaker circuits in the cord and CPG were further investigated by special optical imaging by Lea Ziskind-Conhaim (J Neurophysiol 2005)

Initially, both sides of the cord fire are in synchrony early in development, but begin to fire in alternating bursts at the time when descending fibres arrive from the brain and when afferent, sensory inputs arrive from the periphery

These inputs from the periphery have a profound influence on the formation and development of the endogenous pacemaker circuits in the spinal cord

Locating these circuits and determining how they are regulated by sensory and supraspinal inputs will be necessary for developing appropriate feedback devices for musculoskeletal rehabilitation

Weight-loading and sensory feedback highlight the spinal cord's adaptability and its capacity for re-training

12.2.3.3.4   Neuroplasticity of the Spinal Cord

- Spinal cord is now known to harbour the ability to adapt to change, and, when appropriately harnessed, it has the potential to overcome functional disruptions caused by SCI
- Even when completely disconnected from the brain, the spinal cord is capable of learning and storing memories. Although the cellular and

biochemical mechanisms underlying this "plasticity" or ability to change are not well understood, recent studies have shown that spinal cord neurons can undergo long-term potentiation, and long-term depression, two mechanisms believed to underlie memory and learning in the brain

▧ In addition, it is believed that growth factors may be instrumental in mediating some of the adaptive changes in the spinal cord. The topic of growth factors will be further explored later (Sect. 12.2.3.4.3)

12.2.3.3.5   Concomitant Neuroplasticity of Higher Cortical Brain Centres

▧ Imaging studies of the brain reveal changes in the cortical maps of patients with SCI indicating a functional reorganisation of their primary sensorimotor cortices. Their clinical significance is uncertain

▧ These same changes can occur in patients having limb amputation in the relevant sensorimotor cortex of the body part amputated

12.2.3.3.6   Use of Olfactory Ensheathing Cells for Neural Regeneration

▧ Almudena Ramon-Cueto found that neurons in the mammalian olfactory bulb are able to elongate and connect with their targets in adulthood (Santos-Benito et al., Anat Rec B New Anat 2003)

▧ She then transplanted olfactory ensheathing glial cells to promote regeneration in the cord. In contrast to peripheral grafts, the olfactory glia allowed axons of injured central neurons in rats to elongate for long distances well into the segments of the cord caudal to the lesion, accompanied by a striking recovery of function

▧ Experimental paraplegic rats regained locomotor and sensorimotor reflexes and were able to move their hind limbs voluntarily, and respond to touch and proprioceptive stimuli applied to their hind limbs with this technique

12.2.3.3.7   On the Topic of Neuroprotection and Apoptosis Cascade

▧ New clinical drug trials include the use of BA-210 (Bioaxon Therapeutics), essentially a recombinant protein with possible neuroprotection action (found in animal studies) via acting as Rho antagonist – thus attempting to abort the apoptosis cascade

▧ In practice, it is applied at the surface of the dura and used with a fibrin sealant. The trial is carried out at Thomas Jefferson's Delaware Spinal Cord Injury Center

12.2.3.3.8   Importance of Ambient Conditions in Cord Recovery

- Cohen discovered that the coupling of oscillatory activities between segments of the cord and cord recovery after artificial severing the cord in larval lampreys (with relatively simple neural circuitry) was greatly affected by even minor difference in ambient conditions
- The outcome underscores the difficulty in predicting the response to injury in higher vertebrates with more complex networks of coupled oscillators

12.2.3.3.9   Towards Better Sphincter Control

- Electrical prostheses to directly stimulate bladder and sphincter muscles, or their motor neurons, can provide some control for micturition. Although the prostheses cannot coordinate the timing of contractions as precisely as uninjured neural circuits, they can generate out-of-phase contractions that allow voiding or emptying of the bladder (Johnston et al., Spinal Cord 2005)
- William Agnew, for instance, showed that micturition can be induced with a single, unilateral electrode implanted near the central canal in sacral levels of the spinal cord in normal anaesthetised cats
- To tackle the drawback of electrodes, such as associated tissue damage, and problems of anchorage, is the discovery and the development of microelectrode arrays

12.2.3.3.10 Micro-Electrode Arrays

- McCreery, using photo-lithographic technologies adapted from the semiconductor industry, was able to create microelectrodes with stimulation radii as small as 10 µm that are capable of stimulating single neurons (IEEE Trans Neural Syst Rehabil Eng 2004)
- Also, since the probe he created can hold multiple electrodes, a single array can stimulate several sites simultaneously, and the number of wires can be drastically reduced. Because of their increased stability, the arrays are also better than conventional electrodes for long-term applications, thus tackling the two common drawbacks of electrode placement

12.2.3.4   Obstacles to Regeneration

12.2.3.4.1   Challenges

- We need to know more about strategies for harnessing natural mechanisms of plasticity and repair and circuitry of the CNS
- Need to overcome the inhibitory environment inside the CNS
- Relative lack of regenerative capacity of CNS neurones
- Neurotropic factors to support axonal sprouts
- Bridging strategies across the zone of injury
- Presence of navigation molecules to let the axons grow into proper targets
- Finally, the re-grown axons must be functional and develop a synapse at the target tissue

12.2.3.4.2   Advances in the Understanding of CNS Circuitry

- Circuitry maps describing functional connectivity within the normal spinal cord are greatly needed if we are to understand how the spinal cord is altered by injury
- The use of neurotropic viruses (e.g. herpes simplex and pseudorabies viruses), which invade permissive cells, replicate, and move to infect other neurons trans-synaptically (from one neuron to the next connected by active synapses) is a promising tool. The viruses act as self-amplifying tracers that light up specific pathways or circuits

Elucidating of Neurocircuitry by Neurotropic Viruses

- To actually map the circuit, the use of viral strains is helpful. Viral strains vary in their direction of motion – retrograde or anterograde – and in their ability to infect different classes of neurons. By choosing the appropriate viral strains, it is possible to map a wide variety of neuronal circuits – a promising technique used by scientists like Reginald Edgerton

Other Techniques to Map Out the Location of CPG

- We have alluded to the CPG in the spinal cord. Research is under way by scientist Lea Ziskind-Conhaim to identify the regions of the spinal cord where oscillations originate by optical imaging techniques involving voltage-sensitive dyes and large arrays of photo detectors to monitor the simultaneous activities of large groups of neurons in real time. If successful, attempts to pinpoint the individual neurons involved in the process will be feasible

On the Neuroplasticity Front: Natural Protection Mechanism

The topic of neuroplasticity has just been discussed

But it is interesting to note that scientists recently observed the formation of gap junctions between lumbar spinal motor neurons in the adult cat following injury to the peripheral nerve. This electrical coupling may be a compensatory or protective mechanism that helps keep motor neurons alive until they re-establish synaptic connections

12.2.3.4.3   Central Nervous System Inhibitory Environment

- The first question to ask is what is the cause of the inhibitory environment in the CNS
- It was found that although cut nerve fibres in the CNS often sprout spontaneously, they fail to elongate along their original pathways
- Inhibitory factors on the surface of glial cells and in the extracellular matrix both contribute to an environment that is inhospitable for regeneration

Use of Neurotropic Growth Factors

Mark Tuszynski investigated the use of growth factors (e.g. NT-3) – powerful tools for repairing the nervous system because they:
- – Protect neurons against death
- – Induce them to sprout or regenerate

But the key question is how to ensure that the growth factors act only on the site we want, while leaving the non-target neural areas unaffected to prevent unwanted sprouting

Limiting Growth Factor Action on Target Areas

The answer is that use of growth factors needs to be combined with genetic engineering to control local expression of growth factors, or conversely, to downregulate growth factor receptors in non-target areas. Although the development of increasingly small, hollow microelectrodes for the targeted delivery of minute volumes may also help localise the effects of specific growth factors, as well as technology to effect timed delivery of growth factors

12.2.3.4.4   Lack of Regenerative Capacity of CNS Neurons

Animal studies have shown that multipotent neural progenitors and stem cells can integrate into the CNS and restore function. For example, stem cells have been used to replace damaged cerebellar Purkinje neurons in mice. Multipotent cells can also be used to replace genes and provide neuroprotective molecules, such as growth factors

- Electrodes offer a potentially safer alternative for restoring lost function because they can be controlled more easily. The time, place, magnitude, and polarity of stimulating currents can be regulated with great precision. This forms a second strategy to circumvent the limited regeneration capacity of CNS neurons

Stem Cell Research

- Using genetic engineering, it is possible to create stem cells that package and produce vectors carrying specific genes, or create cells that synthesise and secrete the products of inserted genes

Strategically Placed Electrodes for Stimulation and Feedback

- The success of this strategy relies very much on our understanding of CNS neural circuitry just discussed
- Better understanding of the location and circuitry of CPG (just discussed) will open the door to control and produce a variety of complex motions, including those involved in locomotion via placement of both stimulating electrodes and electrodes for sensory feedback purposes

Role of Neurotrophic Factors

- Several growth factors, including brain-derived growth factor (BDNF), neurotrophin-3 (NT-3) and neurotrophin-4/5 (NT-4/5) are synthesised by neurons in the adult spinal cord, which may play a role in its neuroplasticity (Lu et al., J Neurosci 2004)
- When stimulated by the glutamate agonist, kainic acid, subsets of these neurons show specific increases in their expression of BDNF and NT-4/5, suggesting that signalling between neurons controls the availability of these factors, which, in turn influence the properties of local circuits within the cord

12.2.3.4.5 Bridging Strategies and Use of Neurons from PNS

- In contrast to CNS neurons, it is well known that neurons in the peripheral nervous system are capable of re-tracing their paths and restoring proper connections

- This has led researchers to attempt to repair injured spinal cords by transplanting segments of peripheral nerve or Schwann cells cultured from peripheral nerves as scaffolding or paths for axons to use
- The difficulty with this method is that although efforts such as these have allowed cut nerve fibres from the spinal cord to regenerate into the transplants, the fibres fail to leave the transplants and re-enter the host nervous system
- This has led to the stress on stem cell research and the works of Almudena Ramon-Cueto just discussed

12.2.3.4.6 Use of Reconnection and Re-Routing Strategies

- This technique was tried in China and Italy
- Involves re-routing of the peripheral nerve emanating from the spinal cord above the level of injury. Re-routing and reconnection was performed to re-establish a "functional connection" from the brain to the motor and sensory system below the site of the injury
- The rationale behind this type of strategy stems from the fact that the muscle wall of the bladder contracts at a slower, but more sustained rate than the sphincter, which prevents release; presence of a somatic nerve reflex can be used to achieve voluntary control of voiding
- As an example, the somatic efferent is surgically connected to the bladder to trigger micturition by a voluntary act, such as scratching a limb
- There are occasional successful reports from surgeons in China such as Shanghai

12.2.3.4.7 Navigation Molecules

- For successful regeneration to occur following spinal cord injury, damaged nerve cells must survive or be replaced, and axons must regrow and find appropriate targets
- Scientists are in search of navigational molecules, which may well be one of the growth factors alluded to earlier (Sect. 12.2.3.4.3)

12.2.3.4.8 New Synapse Formation

- Assuming we have the technology for neural regeneration, the new axons and their targets still need to interact to construct synapses, the specialised structures that act as the functional connections between nerve cells
- This forms another arena of active research

12.2.3.5   Appendix: Stem Cell Research

12.2.3.5.1   Stem Cell Research: the Obstacles

- Because a person's body does not have spare neurons for transplantation, efforts are being made to find other cells that can be transformed into neurons. One potential source is "stem" cells from human embryos
- Early in the life of an embryo stem cells have the potential to differentiate into the more than two hundred types of cells in a human body
- Using embryonic stem cells for transplantation is controversial because it is necessary to first create human embryos to produce the stem cells and then kill the embryos in the process of "harvesting" the stem cells, thus creating ethical issues
- Another obstacle is the body's immune system
- One is to find a transplant donor who has genetic markers (HLA) that are similar to those of the person receiving the transplant. The more similar the markers, the less likely it is that the immune system will reject the transplant. The other strategy is to administer drugs to transplant recipients that suppress the ability of the immune system
- One potential solution to the problem of transplant rejection would be to create a transplant with markers identical to those of the person; this involves human cloning and even more ethical issues
- Even if cloning were successful, researchers would still need to learn how to stimulate an embryonic stem cell to produce a neuron rather than a skin cell or some other type of cell. Transplanting undifferentiated stem cells runs the risk of creating a tumour

12.2.3.4.2   More Practical Source: Olfactory Ensheathing Cells

- These are found in one of the nasal sinuses. These cells are already part of our nervous systems and function in our sense of smell. The olfactory cells include neurons, progenitor stem cells that can differentiate into neurons, and OEG cells (olfactory ensheathing glia cells; also sometimes referred to as OEC). OEG cells normally surround and protect neurons that are part of the olfactory system and assist those neurons in first developing and then repairing themselves if needed. They can secrete "growth factors" that stimulate neuronal growth. OEG cells also provide a track or framework on which the neuron grows. The fact that olfactory neurons, unlike neurons in the central nervous system, can repair themselves is one reason why researchers are studying them

12.2.3.4.3 Latest Development

▨ Olfactory cell transplants have been started in Portugal by Dr. Lima. There has been improvement with many, but not all, patients

▨ Improvement ranges from increased sensation or decreased pain to improved motor abilities or bowel and bladder function. Dr. Lima's team is now collaborating with the Detroit Medical Center in treating American spinal cord injury survivors (procedure not yet FDA-approved)

12.2.3.6   Need for Special Spinal Cord Injury Centres

12.2.3.6.1 Setting up

▨ Setting up of more specialised spinal cord injury centres in which specialised care can be commenced in the emergency department is the modern tendency to manage these significant, devastating injuries. There are 16 such specialised centres in the US, for instance

12.2.3.6.2 Team Approach Care

▨ Acute care team typically consists of orthopaedic surgeons, neurosurgeons, rehabilitation physiatrists, spinal cord injury nurses and anaesthetists

▨ An SCI co-ordinator who is on-call 24 h is important

▨ Most acute SCI patients in such settings will be admitted to specialised neurosensory ICU. An example will be the Delaware Valley Spinal Cord Injury Center in USA serving Jersey and Philadelphia

▨ Periodic team meetings are necessary for progress

12.2.3.6.3 Early Commencement of Acute Rehabilitative Care

▨ Acute rehabilitation commences after initial resuscitation by physiotherapists, occupational therapists, psychologists, speech therapists and case managers, who will be in charge of following progress, even after subsequent discharge to a rehabilitation hospital

12.2.3.6.4 Aspects of Acute Nursing Care

▨ Bladder management depending on type of injury – see subsequent discussions (Sect. 12.5)

▨ Bowel management depending on type of injury – see subsequent discussions (Sect. 12.6)

- Pressure relief techniques, preventing decubitus ulcers (see also Chap. 6)
- Wound care

12.2.3.6.5 Physiotherapy

- Chest physiotherapy
- ROM maintenance
- ASIA scores charting and serial monitoring
- Sitting balance
- WC mobility and use, including weight shift techniques
- Early locomotor training – see later discussion
- Muscle strengthening then ensues, improvement in muscle grades is expected especially in partial injuries
- Familial support
- Occupational therapy training and AT use will be discussed

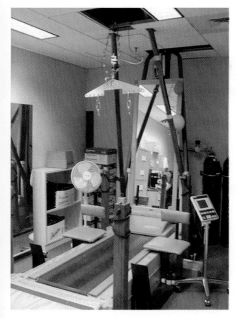

Fig. 12.1. Typical set-up for the performance of bodyweight-supported treadmill training for SCI patients

Early Locomotor Training (Weight-Supported Treadmill Training)

One such protocol works by suspension of the patient in a parachute-like harness attached to overhead bar and beginning walking movement on a treadmill (Figs. 12.1, 12.2)

Therapists will help break the spasticity and attempt to optimise sensory inputs to LL during treadmill training

Treatment Rationale

Using the parachute suspension system enables a person to use weak muscles by counteracting the gravitational pull

This system can be used with treadmill training, and the upright posture will aid sphincter function, and help prevent contractures while maintaining ROM

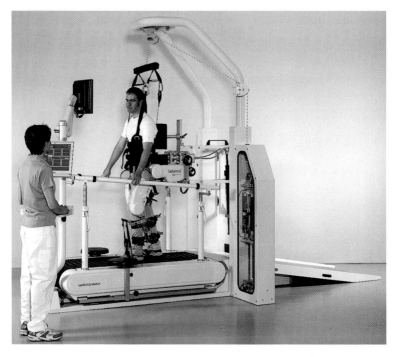

Fig. 12.2. Similar parachute-like harness together with adjunctive robotics (the Loko-mat system) was developed by Swiss company, Hocoma

Control of Spasticity
- The current classification system of spasticity is not perfect, but most use the Ashworth scale
- Proper control of spasticity such as by medications is needed before the above-mentioned locomotor training can be commenced
- Detailed discussion of spasticity control is beyond the scope of this book, the reader is referred to a recent Cochrane Review on this subject

12.3 Rehabilitative Phase Management

12.3.1 Physiotherapy Pearls in SCI
- Identify muscles with low but measurable potentials
- Commence by attempting reduction of the degree of hyperactivity and spasticity
- Attempt recruitment of weak but important muscles
- Also, look for types of reflex-induced movements that can produce measurable neuromuscular activity, or that can be put to good use
- Evaluate improvement in muscle strength, periodic review and documentation important
- Use of biofeedback devices to give feedback to patient and therapist during exercise
- Attempt to incorporate feedback with strengthening exercise and gait training if possible

12.3.2 Use of Biofeedback in SCI
- Since many of the physical training techniques were described in Chap. 4, they will not be repeated here
- However, a few comments will be added on the use of biofeedback in SCI

12.3.2.1 Indication and Efficacy
- Have been tried in both adults and children
- Occasional reports of success (Goldsmith, JAMA 1985)
- Mostly for those with partial cord lesions

12.3.2.2 Key Points

- Identification of remaining neuromuscular function in the individual
- Promote neuromuscular control of important muscles and/or inhibit antagonists
- Setting of functional goal, e.g. an initial goal may be to gain control of amplitude of the spasms, a later functional goal can be, say, reduction in assistive devices and improved speed of ambulation in those with partial SCI
- Requires lots of motivation

12.3.2.3 Biofeedback Pearls

- When we examine a specific muscle group, dual-channel monitoring should be used so that both the spastic muscle as well as its antagonist can be observed
- Goldsmith et al. described the strategy of controlled reversal of antagonists during functional upper or lower extremities during later stage of training

12.3.2.4 Word of Note

- Some centres had attempted to apply skin electrodes early on after SCI both to monitor voluntary muscle activity around hip and knee, as well as to allow the chance to maintain isometric contractions during periods of immobilisation

12.3.2.5 Limitations and Contraindications

- Not for patients who are not motivated, and with poor psychological strength
- Unlikely to benefit chronic SCI patients with little/no remaining neuromuscular activity left
- Not always successful, and improvements attained may sometimes disappear upon removal of feedback

12.3.3 Occupational Therapy Assessment: Key Elements

- Checking patient's life history and priorities
- Assessing basic ADL
- Assessing instrumental ADL
- Motor testing
- Sensory testing
- Psychosocial and perceptual skills

- Pre-discharge preparation and post-discharge supports
- Vocational outcome
- Use of special illness models in special cases

12.3.3.1   Checking Patient's Life History and Priorities
- COPM can be used (Canadian Occupational Performance Measure)
- Usually coupled with the use of "goal attainment scaling" to aid in proper goal setting

12.3.3.2   Assessing Basic ADL
- Assessment by FIM (functional independence measure) is used by most centres
- Alternatives include: performance assessment of self-care skills (PASS), or Klein-Bell daily living scale, etc.

12.3.3.2.1   Teaching Transfer Techniques (WC users)
- Discussion about WC hardware can be found in the chapter on assistive technology (Chap. 6) and subsequent sections of this chapter
- WC use can be considered if the patient's spine and vital signs are steady, and tolerates progressive sitting up in beds of up to around $60°$

12.3.3.2.2   Techniques to be Learned by WC Users
- Learn the types, basic components and use of WC (see also Chap. 6)
- Learning the use of weight shifts
- Learning WC transfers

12.3.3.2.3   Learning Weight Shifts
- Weight shifts are needed every 20 min to provide pressure relief
- Involves the following manoeuvres:
  - Push-ups
  - Forward weight shifts
  - Lateral weight shifts
  - Backward tilts, etc.

12.3.3.2.3   Learning WC Transfers
- Basic golden rules:
  - Minimise height difference between transfer surface
  - Minimise distance between transfer surface
  - Transfer done in a manner that reduces shear

- Lock the bed and WC before transfer
- Ensure Foley not get caught by WC
- If arm-rest or other removable components blocking the way, remove them
- Balance and steady the patient before transfer
- If patient has one UL and/or LL that is stronger, transfer using the strong side
- If electric WC used, turn power off prior to transfer
- Before transfer to a car/van, recline the seat

▓ Different types of transfers:
- WC to bed and vice versa
- WC to commode and vice versa
- WC to shower-commode and vice versa
- WC to vehicle and vice versa
- WC to bath and vice versa

▓ Learn the use of "wheelies" by patient and assistant

▓ The concept of tilt vs recline of a WC is illustrated in Figs. 12.3 and 12.4

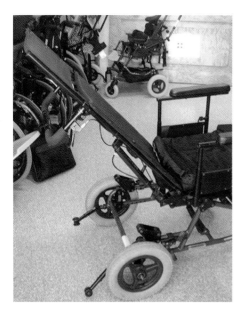

Fig. 12.3. Reclining wheelchair

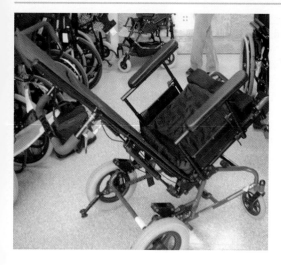

Fig. 12.4. Tilting wheel-chair

12.3.3.2.4 What is the Meaning of "Wheelies"

▨ Refers to the method of pushing the WC through rough or uneven terrain, manoeuvre steps, or curbs by maintaining the WC in the tipped back profile

▨ This is done to ensure added safety and at the same time conserves energy

12.3.3.3 Training IADL

▨ Equipment to aid ADL and IADL can be found in Sect. 12.3.4 on assistive technology

12.3.3.3.1 Assessing Instrumental ADL and Community Integration

▨ Commonly use Rabideau Kitchen Evaluation-Revised (RKE-R) assessment or Assessment of Living Skills and Resources (ALSAR)

▨ An alternative is Kohlman Evaluation of Living Skills, or use the "Community Integration Questionnaires"

12.3.3.4 Motor Testing

▨ Check:
  - Passive ROM
  - Muscle tone and manual muscle testing

- If ambulatory, assess gait, functional reach and Tinetti
- Test of UL coordination, e.g. nine-hole peg test

12.3.3.5   Sensory Testing
- Somatosensory screening
- Sensitivity to cold and hot water during bathing should be noted

12.3.3.7   Psychosocial and Perceptual Skills
- Psychosocial problems if detected should be brought up in multidisciplinary team meeting and proper referral to psychiatrist and/or social service workers
- If brain function possibly altered, use mini-mental state testing and/or Lowenstein occupational therapy cognitive evaluation

12.3.3.6.1 In the Presence of Psychosocial Elements
- Further assess by:
    - Allen Cognitive Level Test-90 (ACLS-90)
    - Occupational Case Analysis and Interview Rating Scale (OCAIRS)

12.3.3.7   Pre-Discharge Preparation and Post-Discharge Supports
- Pre-discharge home visit
- Meeting of the team with the family
- Pre-discharge home leave during weekends to assess coping level
- If return to work planned, assessment by the Worker's Role Interview
- Home modification as required

12.3.3.8   Vocational Outcome
- In a recent review in a Dutch Rehabilitation Centre from 1990 to 1998, the authors found that questionnaire with items related to vocational outcome, job experiences, health and functional status
- It was found that of 49 patients who were working at the moment of SCI, 60% currently had a paid job. Vocational outcome was related to a higher educational level. A significant relationship between the SCI-specific health and functional status and employment was not found. The respondents who changed to a new employer needed more time to resume work, but seemed more satisfied with the job and lost fewer working hours than those who resumed work with the same employer. In spite of reasonable to good satisfaction with the current work situation, several negative experiences and unmet needs were reported

▨ Thus, despite a reasonable participation in paid work following SCI in this Dutch study, the tremendous effort of the disabled worker to have and keep a job should not be underestimated. Constant and adequate support should be given (Clin Rehabil 2005)

12.3.3.9   Use of the PLISSIT Model to Handle Sensitive Issues on Sexuality

▨ As pointed out rightly by Laflin, sexual health is an integral part of enablement and should form part of rehabilitation (Top Geriatr Rehabil 1996)

▨ This is particularly true in the often young SCI patients

▨ In addition, the article by McBride is particularly useful for nurses caring for SCI patients on this aspect (SCI Nurs 2000)

12.3.3.9.1   Introduction

▨ The PLISSIT is quite a popular model that can be used by health professionals (not only by occupational therapists) when it comes to sensitive issues like sexuality

▨ The model was designed by an American psychosexual therapist Annon in 1976 (Annon, J Sex Edu Ther 1976)

12.3.3.9.2   What does "PLISSIT" Stand for?

▨ P = permission

▨ LI = limited information

▨ SS = specific suggestions

▨ IT = intensive therapy

12.3.3.9.3   Ideas Behind PLISSIT

▨ Step 1 involves giving permission for patients to talk about matters relating to sex, the team member should remain non-judgmental, respect the patient's privacy and be professional

▨ Step 2 of the process involves giving preliminary information to the patient pertaining to the subject, be it verbal or written, like an information leaflet

▨ Step 3 involves, where needed, the provision of additional, more specific information by for instance a fertility expert such as on problems of conception or contraception

▨ Step 4 involves "intensive therapy" where needed, such as referral to the proper speciality, like psychiatrists or urologists with a view to intervention

12.3.4   Use of Assistive Technology

12.3.4.1   Specially Designed Powered Wheelchair
for High Cord Lesions

▓ Very high lesions need breath controls (sip and puff) and mouth sticks
▓ Other controls include:
   – Chin controls
   – Hand controls (flap-like) – Fig. 12.5
   – Voice activation

12.3.4.2   Other Modifications or Adjustments
for Powered Wheelchairs

▓ Special pressure mapping to ensure adequate pressure relief
▓ Also, avoidance of pressure concentration during position shifts is important
▓ Some chairs can be reclined by head activation switches to make allowance of pressure relief

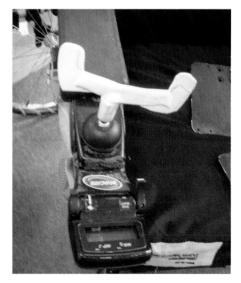

Fig. 12.5. Flap-like control paddle for SCI patient

12.3.4.3   Voice Recognition Software
- Very useful for high cervical cord lesions
- Many companies produce voice recognition software, e.g. United Research Lab, Microsoft Dictation Buddies, Neumemo by NeuVoice, etc.

12.3.4.4   "Voice Command Software" While Patient Not at Home
- Microsoft's new Voice Command (version 1.5) can transform the patient's Pocket PC into his own virtual personal assistant
- By using his voice, the patient can look up contacts (including resources for emergency medical assistance) and place phone calls, get calendar information, play and control his favourite music, and start programs, etc.

12.3.4.5   Speech-Enabled Web Browsing Technology
- Very promising in this field and already in the market are like IBM's ViaVoice Pro Millennium line of products; other similar software

12.3.4.6   Text-to-Speech Software
- These useful software programs are provided by major companies, e.g. IBM, Cisco, Microsoft

12.3.4.7   Electrically Powered Page Turner with Switch
- See Fig. 12.6, discussed in Chap. 6 already

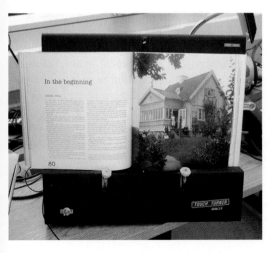

Fig. 12.6. Electric-powered page turner

12.3.4.8   Environmental Modifications at Large
▦ Examples:
- Special vehicles that are designed for patients with limb weakness
- Special public transportation adaptation platforms that allow easy access by wheelchair-bound patients
- Lifts specially designed for wheelchair-bound individuals

12.4   Regaining Mobility and Sometimes Ambulation

12.4.1   Ambulation and Stepping Training Based on Concepts of CPG

12.4.1.1   Recapitulating the CPG: Cat Spinal Cord Transection Experiments

▦ Concepts of oscillating spinal circuits including CPG have been discussed earlier in this chapter

▦ After experimental spinal cord transection, an adult cat was able to step independently with the hind-limbs after weeks of training, which provides phasic sensory information associated with locomotion and loading (Lovely et al., Exp Neurol 1986)

▦ The cat whose spinal cord had been transected was initially suspended in the quadruped position over a treadmill. Manual assistance was given to the hind-limbs to ensure rhythmic loading and unloading of the limbs (Conway et al., Exp Brain Res 1987)

▦ The cat was able to step independently after weeks of training, and the trunk support and assistance were no longer necessary; implying the neural circuits in the lumbosacral cord caudal to the lesion responded to the peripherally mediated information to produce a co-ordinated, adaptable locomotor pattern in the absence of supraspinal influence (Barbeau et al., Brain Res 1987)

12.4.1.2   The Case for Weight-Supported Human Locomotor Training
▦ Initial successes were obtained (mainly case series) in humans with mainly partial to complete thoracic cord injuries given weight-supported locomotor training over a treadmill. Experts like Harkema and Behrman believe the human lumbosacral spinal cord has the capacity to respond to sensory information related to locomotion. (Harkema and Behrman, Phys Ther 2000)

12.4.1.3   Key Basic Assumptions
of Weight-Supported Locomotor Training

- The cord has the ability to respond to appropriate afferent information to generate stepping (Edgerton et al., Adv Neurol 1997)
- Activity-dependent plasticity occurs in the neural circuitry responsible for locomotion at both spinal and supraspinal levels (according to the marvellous works of Harkema, Edgerton, etc.)

12.4.1.4   Further Evidence from Space Travel

- Edgerton's recent space flight studies suggest that alterations that occur during spaceflight may also occur in SCI. He found that control of motor pools changes in response to changes in weight-bearing activity
- Thus, the physiology of the human body adapted to the bipedal gait is that continuous LL loading and sensory input are needed for the established oscillatory circuitry and CPG to work
- After exposure to microgravity for 14 days, rhesus monkeys showed adaptations in the tendon force and electromyographic amplitude ratios of different muscles, indicating that their patterns of muscle recruitment were reorganising. Since SCI also involves changes in weight-bearing activity, it is possible that motor output in SCI is affected by similar reorganisations of muscle recruitment

12.4.1.5   Keys for Success with Human Weight-Supported
Locomotor Re-Training

- Proper loading and unloading to increase extensor motoneuron activity
- Aim at obtaining normal walking speed with serial treadmill training
- Step training with proper body weight support to ensure safety
- Ensure adequate hip extension and unloading of the limb at the end of stance phase
- Reciprocating arm swing is encouraged, but concomitant weight bearing of the UL using, say, parallel bars is not advised (according to Harkema)

12.4.1.6   Prospects of Better Prediction of Future Walking Ability of Partial SCI Patients Using New Neurophysiological Techniques

- Recent study by Hansen revealed that it is possible to obtain information about the synaptic drive to motoneurons during walking by analysing motor-unit coupling in the time and frequency domains, and comparing motor-unit coupling during walking in healthy individuals and patients with incomplete spinal cord lesions to obtain evidence of differences in the motoneuronal drive that result from the lesion

- It was found that supraspinal drive to the spinal cord is responsible for short-term synchrony and coherence in the 10- to 20-Hz frequency band during walking in healthy individuals. Absence or reduction of these features may serve as physiological markers of impaired supraspinal control of gait in SCL patients. Such markers could have diagnostic and prognostic value in relation to the recovery of locomotion in patients with central motor lesions (J Neurophysiol 2005)

- The reader is assumed to be accustomed to the popular Walking Index for Spinal Cord Injury (WISCI II) proposed by Dr. Dittuno (past president of ASIA), revised in 2001

12.4.2   Retraining of Ambulation Via Functional Electrical Stimulation

12.4.2.1   Principle of the Use of FES

- Different types of functional electrical stimulation (FES) share the common principle of applying bursts of electrical stimuli to selected peripheral nerves. These stimuli trigger action potentials in the stimulated nerve fibres, and effect contractions of the corresponding muscle groups

- However, to be successful, the sequence of firing has to be correct. This is helped by modern microprocessor technology as well as the use of fuzzy logic technologies before a meaningful functional task can be performed

12.4.2.2   Aim of FES in SCI patients

- Ambulation
- Standing
- Some companies have FES systems fitted to bicycle ergometers (that can effect cardiovascular conditioning) – Fig. 12.7

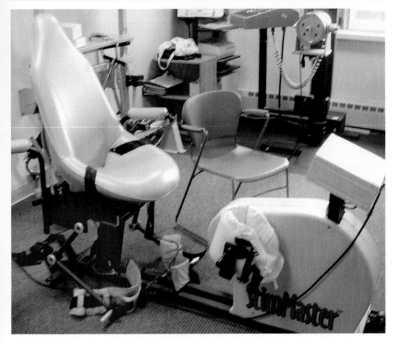

Fig. 12.7. Bicycle ergometer equipped with functional electrical stimulation (FES) capabilities

12.4.2.3   Potential Candidates

- Mostly for complete or near complete thoracic cord injury patients at T4–T12

  (T1–T3 cases may have too much truncal instability; lower than T12 implies either conus or cauda equina and represent lower motoneuron lesions)

12.4.2.4   Exclusion Criteria

- Not usually for partial cord lesions – for patients who cannot voluntarily extend their legs
- If lesion incomplete, *pain* may result from the electrical stimulation
- Not for lumbar levels since these cases are lower motoneuron (LMN) lesions, not upper motoneuron (UMN) lesions

- Not usually for cervical cord lesions since associated UL weakness and truncal weakness making ambulation unlikely to be achieved and cannot hold on to the walker

12.4.2.5   Advantages of FES
- May produce reduction in spasticity
- Improve LL blood flow
- Reduced chance of decubitus ulcers
- Cardiovascular conditioning
- Improved depression scores
- Selected patients achieve ambulation with a walker (Parastep) or with assistance of orthosis like reciprocating gait orthosis (RGO) (hybrid FES/body orthosis systems)

12.4.2.6   Disadvantages of FES
- Donning and doffing (especially RGO systems)
- Cost of equipment

12.4.2.7   Types of FES to Be Discussed
- The Parastep system (FDA-approved)
- Hybrid FES/body orthosis systems using RGO
- Other systems (e.g. percutaneous, totally implantable systems)

12.4.2.7.1   Parastep

Introduction
    A popular system and only system that is FDA-approved, commonly distributed by Sigmedics (Fig. 12.8)

Mechanism of the Parastep System
    The Parastep is a non-invasive system and consists of the following components (Fig. 12.9):
    – A microcomputer-controlled neuromuscular stimulation unit
    – A battery-activated power pack with recharger
    – The Paratester, a unit for pretesting main system operation and electrode cables
    – Surface applied skin electrodes
    – Power and electrode cables
    – A control and stability walker with finger-activated control switches

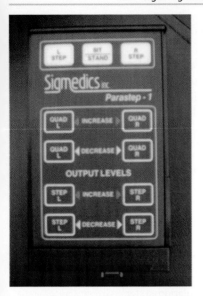

Fig. 12.8. The control panel of the commonly used FES system in the USA called "Parastep", produced by Sigmedics

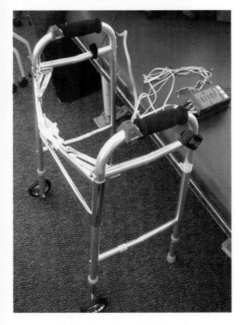

Fig. 12.9. The complete "Parastep" system comes with a walker equipped with control buttons on both sides

The microcomputer microchip handles all stimulation signal shaping, control, synchronisation and stimuli distribution to the various stimulation sites

The Parastep system generates trains of pulses to trigger action potentials of selected nerves at the quadriceps (for knee extension), the common peroneal nerve (for hip flexion withdrawal reflex), and paraspinals/gluteus maximus (for trunk stability)

Electrode Connection

Total of 12 electrodes or six pairs are used

Lower thoracic lesions (T9–T12) may only need four pairs of electrodes

Most patients use a walker (that comes with the set) for balancing and support

Stimulation current and charge densities are well within safety limits (Graupe and Kohn 1994)

Advantage of Parastep

Non-invasive

Personal stereo-sized external stimulation system

Comes with a walker to help balance and weight distribution

Don time 10 min, doff time 4 min

Reports from University of Miami showed effects of cardio-pulmonary conditioning

Others report decreased depression scores, decreased spasticity

Disadvantage of Parastep

Cost

Ambulance performance and results differ widely – depend on level of lesion, age, obesity and general condition (Graupe et al., Crit Rev Neurosurg 1998)

12.4.2.7.2   Hybrid FES/RGO Systems

Mechanism of the RGO Orthosis

Basic design is like a hip-knee-ankle-foot orthosis, with provision of stability and support. Those with some knee contracture can have the knees locked in extension

Equipped with a cable mechanism linking the two hip joints. This is to prevent bilateral hip flexion in standing and also provide a reciprocating motion of the two lower limbs when in motion

Mechanism of Reciprocating Motion

- When one leg is undergoing swing phase, the contralateral leg is forced by the cable mechanism to undergo push-off
- The mechanical braces allow antigravity support and stability

Calibration

- Orthosis of RGO is custom fitted and calibrated for individual use by orthotist
- Calibration involves adjustment of tension in the cable system and thoracic straps
- On-site orthotist support is needed

Electrode Placement

- The FES is built into the system, and used for the purpose of propulsion
- Surface electrodes are placed over hamstrings and quadriceps of each thigh
- It provides simultaneous hip flexion and contralateral hip extension while minimising the participation of upper extremities and trunk

Advantage of Hybrid Systems

- Can possibly provide more stability and support, even for those with partial knee and/or hip contracture
- Reports of decreased spasticity, decreased cholesterol level, increased cardiac output and vital capacity (Solomonow et al., Orthopedics 1997)

Disadvantage of Hybrid Systems

- Donning and doffing requires lot of time and effort
- Need frequent monitoring for pressure sores
- Malaligned orthosis can lead to negative ambulation habits (Crit Rev Neurosurg 1998)
- Requires on-site orthotist support and frequent calibration and adjustment of tension in cables
- Among 70 patients reported from Louisiana State University, only 6 finally used this RGO system in their daily activities

12.4.2.7.3   Other Systems

Percutaneous Systems

- These involve 8- or 16-channel stimulation of strategic muscles involved in posture and walking via percutaneous insertion of IM electrodes. The stimulation sequence being microprocessor-controlled and fine tuned for each patient, who were also given AFO (Kobetic et al., IEEE Trans Rehabil Eng 1997)
- The relevant motor points were predetermined for each muscle using surface stimulation prior to percutaneous electrode stimulation
- Some groups used ultra-fine percutaneous IM electrodes, as well as sensors to help detect knee buckling (Shimada et al., Arch Phys Med Rehabil 1996)
- The eight-channel stimulation frequently led to scissoring, and 16 channels seemed to perform better
- The muscles stimulated mostly include: erector spinae, hamstrings, posterior adductor magnus, tensor fascia lata, iliopsoas/sartorius, vastus lateralis/intermedius, and tibialis anterior/peroneus longus (Crit Rev Neurosurg 1998)
- However, complications like electrode wire breakage, infection, patient's reluctance limit the use of this mode of FES

Totally Implantable Systems

- This involves invasive implantation of electrodes directly onto motor nerves or roots, and with radiofrequency controls
- Most reports seem to discuss its use for standing rather than ambulation
- Number of channels varies a lot, and many systems also have knee sensors to detect knee buckling and this will trigger stimulation of quadriceps (Davies et al., Stereotact Funct Neurosurg 1994)

12.5   Tackling Urinary Problems in SCI

12.5.1   Introduction

- During the acute phase, most acute SCI patients will already have been given an in-dwelling urinary catheter
- As soon as the patient stabilises, and starts to sit out, techniques like intermittent bladder catheterisation can be tried

■ Most decision-making depends on combined clinical assessment + urodynamic studies done at approximately 3 months post-injury
■ But first let us recapitulate the normal physiology of micturition

12.5.2   Normal Neurophysiology

■ Levels of controls:
  - Cortical – communicates with pontine micturition centre, also helps maintain voluntary continence by effecting contraction of the external urethral sphincter via somatic efferents. Cortex can act to inhibit the sacral micturition centre and reflex bladder contraction
  - Pontine micturition centre – coordinate the synergistic interaction of detrusor muscle and urethral sphincter
  - Parasympathetic – distension of bladder → activates the stretch receptors in the detrusor → activates the S2–S4 sacral micturition centre
  - Sympathetic – sympathetic activation creates tendency towards storage as opposed to voiding via its T10–L2 efferents, which relaxes the fundus (by action on beta receptors) and contracts the bladder neck (by action on alpha receptors)

12.5.3   What Happens with Lesions at Different Levels

■ Suprapontine level (e.g. CVA)
■ Supraspinal level (e.g. SCI)
■ Sacral or peripheral nerve lesion

12.5.3.1   Suprapontine Lesion

■ This results in frequency and incontinence
■ However, unlike the next category of lesion, it does not lead to detrusor-sphincter dyssynergia
■ These patients mostly suffer from CVA and as such are outside the scope of this book

12.5.3.1.1   Management: Suprapontine Lesion

■ Condom catheter
■ Frequent timed voids
■ Anticholinergic drugs

12.5.3.2   Supraspinal Lesion

- Lesions of the cord above the sacral micturition centre carry the risk of causing detrusor sphincter dyssynergia (DSD)
- Presents usually as retention – since sphincter fails to relax during bladder contraction
- Can create complications like UTI and/or recurrent and reflux nephropathy from the elevated pressure

12.5.3.2.1   Supraspinal Lesion: General Treatment Options

- Anticholinergic drugs
- With/without alpha blockers
- Intermittent or long term catheterisation
- Sphincterotomy particularly if DSD
- Voiding at low pressures using neurostimulation
- Stents
- Sphincter injection (e.g. botulin)

12.5.3.3   Sacral or Peripheral Nerve Lesion

- The result is detrusor areflexia, with denervation of the detrusor
- Causes overflow incontinence

12.5.4   Key Principle

- Unlike cases of suprapontine lesions, SCI situations not infrequently produce detrusor-sphincter dyssynergia
- Recognition of which is important since these complications can cause renal damage
- Frequently treatment by voiding cystometrogram (see later discussion in Sect. 12.5.5)

12.5.4.1   Sacral or Peripheral Nerve Level: General Treatment Options

- Suprapubic pressure and/or with added valsalva
- Cholinergic drugs
- Long-term Foley
- Intermittent self-catheterisation

12.5.5 Use of Urodynamic Studies in Management Decision-Making

- Objective:
  - Assess filling pressures and abnormalities of compliance
  - Voiding cystometrogram will be able to detect DSD, an important complication since elevated pressures will cause renal damage

12.5.5.1 Protocol for UMN SCI Injury with Tetraplegia

- Most will have poor hand function making intermittent self-catheterisation (ISC) difficult; may try ISC if there was recovery of hand function
- For males, DSD if present may need sphincterotomy. If DSD absent, long-term catheter (can consider suprapubic) with anti-cholinergic agents
- Similar management for females, but DSD less common

12.5.5.2 Protocol for UMN SCI Injury with Paraplegia

- Most patients will try ISC since UL function intact
- In males, consider sphincterotomy if DSD present; otherwise ISC with anti-cholinergic agents
- In females, DSD uncommon, most will try ISC and/or consider suprapubic if encounter frequent catheter-related complications

12.5.5.3 Protocol for LMN SCI Injury with Cauda Equina Lesion (or Conus)

- DSD not exist in these cases
- Most patients will try ISC + self compression
- An occasional male patient may need bladder neck incision procedure

12.5.6 Role of Elective Surgery to Tackle Urinary-Related Problems in SCI

- Examples:
  - Endoscopic distal sphincterotomy especially in some cases of DSD
  - Suprapubic catheter insertion
  - Insertion of stents
  - Occasional use of more major procedures
  - Augmentation cystoplasty for refractory DSD (more in men) or refractory incontinence in women
  - Anterior sacral root stimulation (of S2–S4 roots) for patients with bladder paralysis and incomplete emptying

12.5.7 Role of Elective Surgery in Other Areas in SCI

■ Occasionally for spinal stabilisation (if not already performed at acute stage)
■ Elective surgery to improve UL function in selected cases: e.g.
   – C5/6 SCI: attempt restoring triceps function by posterior deltoid-triceps or biceps-triceps transfer
   – C6 SCI: attempt restoring lateral key pinch by modified Moberg procedure (attachment of BR to FPL with concomitant stabilisation of CMCJ and IPJ of the first ray)
■ Surgical intervention for neural complications, e.g. post-traumatic syringomyelia

12.6   Bowel Dysfunction in SCI

12.6.1 Introduction

■ It is the author's view that discussion of bowel dysfunction is equally as important as urinary-related problems
■ Improper training of bowel function can predispose to skin breakdown, cause sepsis to a nearby pressure ulcer, and can affect attempts at subsequent conception (see discussion in the section on reproductive dysfunction)

12.6.2 Normal Neurophysiology

■ Normal bowel function is under three sets of controls:
■ Intrinsic system of contraction
   – Governed by the intrinsic contractility of the intestinal smooth muscles, and the intrinsic system of the nervous system
■ Intrinsic nervous system:
   – Submucosal plexus: involved in control of GI secretion and blood flow
   – Myenteric plexus: aid coordination of gastrointestinal movement (peristalsis) and process sensory input from the submucosal plexus
   – Thus, peristalsis can still occur if the gut is deprived of sympathetic and parasympathetic inputs
   – The well-known gastrocolic reflex is also mediated by the intrinsic nervous system of the GI tract
■ The parasympathetic system:

- Originate from cranial and sacral outflows
- Cranial outflow innervates oesophagus to transverse colon
- S2–S4 outflow innervates distal portion of the GI tract from descending colon to rectum
- General action: increased peristalsis, decreased sphincter tone, increased secretion
- The sympathetic system:
  - From T8 to L2 of spinal cord
  - Tends to inhibit decreased peristalsis
  - Increases sphincter tone
  - Decreases secretion, vasoconstriction

12.6.3 Normal Defecation
- Defecation reflex initiated by rectal loading, and mediated by the intrinsic neural system, which induces internal sphincter relaxation and lower GI peristalsis. This reflex alone inadequate for defecation
- Parasympathetic system reflex needed to further increase peristalsis and decrease internal sphincter tone for defecation
- The external sphincter contracts as a reflex upon relaxation of the internal sphincter after rectal loading. Whether the external sphincter contraction persists depends on cerebral descending signals; thus, defecation can be deferred until a more convenient moment
- During convenient times, the brain will send facilitatory signals to relax both the external sphincter and pelvic floor muscles

12.6.4 Bowel Dysfunction After SCI
- Initial event: paralytic ileus stage, treatment is supportive during this period
- With time, ileus subsides, peristalsis resumes since the intrinsic neural system still functions
- But function is not normal since loss of higher centre control, and if the lesion involves the sacral cord, parasympathetic reflex is further affected

12.6.4.1 Scenario 1: S2–S4 Sacral Cord Intact
- Here, both parasympathetic and intrinsic defecation reflexes are still intact
- Rectal loading can produce reflex defecation

■ But:
- Lost voluntary control
- Faecal retention can sometimes occur from spasticity of external sphincter and puborectalis

12.6.4.2   Scenario 2: S2–S4 Sacral Cord Damaged

■ As discussed, normal defecation requires the parasympathetic defecation reflex as the intrinsic reflex not strong enough
■ Thus, in this scenario, faecal retention and impaction is the rule
■ The subset of patients with concomitant decreased tone of external sphincter and pelvic floor muscles (LMN lesions) can have faecal incontinence

12.6.4.2.1   Protocol for Patients with Intact S2–S4 Parasympathetic Reflex

■ We make use of the intact parasympathetic reflex + intrinsic system reflex + gastrocolic reflex (which is stronger with the first meal of the day)
■ We need also to relax the external sphincter by gentle digital stretch and use of suppositories, and clear any impacted faeces

12.6.4.2.2   Protocol for Patients with Damaged S2–S4 Reflex

■ Mainstay is rectal emptying by manual means with suppository
■ And/or helped by contraction of abdominal muscles

12.6.4.3   General Adjunctive Measures

■ Try to train bowel motion at the same day of the day
■ Early mobilisation and standing posture (some special WC allow a patient to stand) also helps, partly from gravity effects
■ Dietician advice is to aim at faeces that are neither too soft or too hard

12.7   Tackling Reproductive Dysfunction after SCI

12.7.1   Introduction

■ The key here is whether the patient is a male or a female; he or she has to relearn and rediscover everything about his/her own body including sensation both above and below (if partial) the lesion; positioning that eases spasticity, body image, sensuality, etc.

12.7.2   Key Concept

■ Notice that discussion of reproductive function comes after bladder and bowel functional restoration

■ This is because good restoration of initial stages (not to mention more advanced stages) of sexual arousal is seldom smooth if there is no proper retraining or tackling of bladder and bowel function

12.7.2.1   Reproductive Restoration in Males

12.7.2.1.1   Key Elements to Achieve Reproduction in Males

■ 1. General bodily arousal
■ 2. Local arousal response of genitals
■ 3. Copulation and ability to maintain local arousal of genitals
■ 4. Ejaculation and/or orgasmic response
■ 5. Sperm of normal quality and quantity
   (Prerequisite: normal local anatomy and neural control)

12.7.2.1.2   Normal Controls

■ 1. Arousal from various sensory inputs, tactile, visual or otherwise
■ 2. Erection requires intact parasympathetic system reflex at S2–S4, facilitated from descending cortical signals. There are two types of erections: psychogenic and reflexogenic
■ 3. Duration affected by factors like presence of continual sensory input, psychogenic factors, etc.
■ 4. Ejaculation: this stage will be discussed in the next subsection
■ 5. Nature of sperm depends on physiology and age of individual

12.7.2.1.3   Process of Ejaculation

■ Many texts mention that ejaculation is dependent on sympathetic nervous system
■ In fact, successful ejaculation depends on both sympathetic and parasympathetic systems:
   – Sympathetic: releases semen from testes to urethra (T10–L2 outflow)
   – Parasympathetic: propels semen out of urethra (S2–S4 outflow)

12.7.2.1.4   Question of Orgasm

■ Orgasm can sometimes occur in the absence of ejaculation (since the other major dimension of orgasm is at the level of the brain)

▪ An occasional SCI male patient can have orgasm-like sensation in the absence of ejaculation

12.7.2.1.5 Effect of Complete SCI

▪ Effect on the five key steps:
- 1. To be successful in this stage is not always easy, needs to know the feelings of the new body, areas with better sensation, psychological status important, e.g. difficult arousal if depressed
- 2. Erection sometimes does occur, e.g. psychogenic erection if there are still some connections between cortex and cord, but this connection may be lost in complete SCI; reflexogenic erection needs an intact S2–S4 reflex arc, thus erection may still be preserved
- 3. The determining factors same as in second step, but attention to positioning to prevent triggering undue spasticity and autonomic dysreflexia
- 4. Control of ejaculation mentioned, if lesion really complete, successful ejaculation rather rare. This is because the process normally also depends on a coordination centre in the brain that also receives input from visual, auditory besides sensual paths. If SCI really complete, the rather complex process of ejaculation will usually be much affected

12.7.2.1.6 Effect of SCI on Sperms and Fertility

▪ Decreased sperm motility and increased fragility very common, reason not certain
▪ Some experts feel this is the main reason for infertility in male SCI patients
▪ These observations, however, do not depend on the level of SCI
▪ Fertility frequently diminished due to sperm changes and retrograde ejaculation

12.7.2.1.7 Treatment Options in Complete SCI

▪ To tackle problems at the five key steps:
- 1. Re-discover the sensual body parts and treat any psychological disturbance, maintain morale
- 2. See options for erectile dysfunction
- 3. Same as (2), be sure to have good training of sphincter habits, and empty bladder and bowel prior to copulation

- 4. See options for obtaining sperms
- 5. Sperm banking, artificial insemination, in vitro fertilisation, etc. described, but pathogenesis of changes in nature of sperm in SCI not completely understood

12.7.2.1.8 Options of Treatment of Erectile Dysfunction
- Drugs, e.g. Sildenafil (Viagra)
- Injectable medication
- Others, e.g. tension rings and vacuum devices

12.7.2.1.9 Options of Treatment for Failure of Ejaculation
- Sperm can be obtained by:
  - Vibratory stimulation device (ventral penile shaft is stimulated), needs intact L2–S1
  - Electro-ejaculation via rectal probe, but retrograde ejaculation may occur
  - Needle aspiration

12.7.2.1.10 Effect of Partial SCI
- Effect on the five key steps:
  - 1. Patient must re-discover the sensitive part of the body, manoeuvres that trigger spasticity need be avoided
  - 2. Erectile dysfunction less common
  - 3. Erectile dysfunction rarer because both the sacral reflex arc and psychogenic mechanism may still be intact
  - 4. Ejaculation is less rare, but sometimes retrograde ejaculation may occur
  - 5. Problems with sperm just discussed

12.7.2.1.11 Treatment Options in Partial SCI
- Principle same, to tackle the five key steps
- If erectile dysfunction and failure of ejaculation occurs, treated along similar lines

12.7.2.1.12 General Adjunctive Measures
- Counselling by fertility specialist
- Good training of bowel and bladder habits
- Empty bowel and bladder before attempted copulation
- Patient taught about signs of autonomic dysreflexia, cease copulation behaviour if autonomic dysreflexia and consult physician
- Sperm banking

12.7.2.2   Reproductive Restoration in Females

12.7.2.2.1   Key Elements to Achieve Reproduction in Females

1. General bodily arousal
2. Local genital arousal and lubrication reflex
3. Copulation
4. With/without orgasm
5. Presence of ova ready for the process of fertilisation by sperm (prerequisite: normal local anatomy and neural control)

12.7.2.2.2   Normal Controls

1. Arousal commences with tactile or other stimuli like visual, and other senses
2. Lubrication in females can be by psychogenic or reflexogenic mechanisms
3. It is believed that both parasympathetic and sympathetic firing occur as arousal plateaus
4. Orgasm is manifested both locally and at brain level by endorphin secretion
5. Ovulation depends on controls of the hypothalamic–pituitary axis

12.7.2.2.3   Question of Orgasm

Not infrequently, females after SCI report ability to reach orgasm or sensations resembling orgasm

Overall, 50% of females with SCI can achieve orgasm (Ann Neurol 2001)

12.7.2.2.4   Effect of Complete SCI

Effect on the five key steps:
- 1. Amount of sensation left depends on level of injury, need to rediscover sensitive and sensual areas of the body
- 2. Lubrication frequently affected since central descending signals to thoracolumbar sympathetic outflow are affected; reflexogenic mediated lubrication may still be intact if S2–S4 reflex arc is still intact
- 3. Achieving plateau of emotions can be hindered by lack of lubrication, spasticity, autonomic dysreflexia. Need to discover positions of comfort and those less prone to triggering unwanted spasticity
- 4. Question of orgasm was discussed

– 5. Immediately post-SCI, menses stops, but in most cases recommences within 6 months. Ability to conceive usually maintained in most females with SCI

12.7.2.2.5 Treatment Options in Complete SCI
▨ To tackle the five key steps:
– 1. If depressed or with psychological disturbance, need psychologist. Otherwise need to re-discover sensual areas, and good training of bladder and bowel functions
– 2. Lubrication by gel done by self or spouse
– 3. Avoid positions that induce spasticity, empty bladder and bowel before attempted copulation
– 4. Question of orgasm discussed
– 5. May consult endocrinologist if menses does not return and/or fertility specialist

12.7.2.2.6 Effect of Partial SCI
▨ Effect on the five key steps:
– 1. Need to re-discover sensual and sensitive parts of the body
– 2. Lubrication probably less affected
– 3. Copulation may sometimes be hindered by spasticity and autonomic dysreflexia
– 4. Orgasm possible in 50% as mentioned
– 5. Ovulation usually not affected

12.7.2.2.7 Treatment Options in Partial SCI
▨ To tackle the five key steps:
– 1. Assess need for psychologist consultation, and re-discover sensual areas of own body
– 2. Assess need for lubrication
– 3. Avoid positions that induce spasticity, empty bladder and bowel before copulation
– 4. Question of orgasm discussed
– 5. Most can conceive, if endocrine disturbance suspected, consult endocrinologist or fertility experts

12.7.2.2.8 General Adjunctive Measures
▨ Counselling by fertility specialist
▨ Good training of bowel and bladder habits

- Empty bowel and bladder before attempted copulation
- Patient taught about signs of autonomic dysreflexia, cease copulation behaviour if autonomic dysreflexia occurs and consult physician
- Education on contraception, precautions of pregnancy and delivery

12.7.2.2.9 Precautions of Pregnancy
- Premature labour can occur
- Somewhat increased risk of autonomic dysreflexia and/or spasticity
- Increased UTI chance
- Increased difficulty with WC and transfer and weight shifts, additional carers needed
- Occasionally, respiratory embarrassment
- Increased chance of small for date babies
- If SCI level above T6, spinal anaesthesia recommended during delivery

12.7.2.2.10 Contraception Methods
- Contraceptive pills may increase deep vein thrombosis in face of LL paraparesis
- Barrier methods possible if good hand function
- IUCD: can be risky if loss of sensation, also may be late in detection of complications like pelvic inflammatory disease

12.8   Common Complications

12.8.1   Chronic Pain in SCI Patients
- This will be discussed in more detail in the chapter on pain management
- High incidence of pain is noted in a recent Swedish SCI study (Budh et al., Clin Rehabil 2003) constituting up to 64% among 456 SCI patients; other researchers like Boivie quote an incidence of 30%
- Pain was most common with incomplete spinal cord lesion, ASIA D
- Also, there were some correlation between pain and higher age at time of injury and the female gender

12.8.1.1   Key Message
- A proper knowledge of the pathomechanics and management of chronic neuropathic pain is most important
- Neuropathic pain will be discussed in Chap. 15

12.8.2   Autonomic Neuropathy (Autonomic Dysreflexia)

- Characterised by acute hypertensive episodes, often triggered by some sensory stimulation below the level of injury. The chemicals involved include dopamine, dopamine-beta-hydroxylase and norepinephrine. These agents are released due to the stimulation of the (still intact) sympathetic neural tissue at the inter-medio-lateral grey matter below the level of SCI triggered by the ascending volleys of activation below
- Pathogenesis in summary: after SCI, the supraspinal centres cannot act to decrease the sympathetic response. This syndrome is seen at cord lesions at/above T6 in the majority of cases (i.e. above the major T6–L2 sympathetic outflow). The hypertensive episodes cannot simply be controlled by the body's carotid or aortic receptors. High index of suspicion is required

12.8.2.1   Possible Triggers

- Any type of noxious stimulus, most commonly bladder or bowel
- Urinary: UTI, urinary retention, blocked Foley, renal colic, cystoscopy procedures
- Bowels: faecal impaction
- GI causes: appendicitis, cholecystitis, thrombosed haemorrhoids, even a rough per rectum examination or rough digital evacuation
- Ulcers: pressure ulcers
- Others: heterotrophic ossification (HO), deep vein thrombosis (DVT)/ phlebitis, ingrown toenails (IGTN), even intercourse, etc.

12.8.2.2   Symptomatology

- Above the level of SCI: can cause vasodilatation and sweating
- Below the level of SCI: vasoconstriction and pallor, patient usually become nervous and uneasy, with rising blood pressure and pounding headaches. Too high BP can cause cerebral haemorrhage and even death. Suspect the diagnosis if there is sudden increase in BP of 20–40 mmHg, or 15–20 mmHg in the adolescent. A systolic BP of 150 mmHg is regarded as a potentially dangerous level

12.8.2.3   Management

- Put patient upright to reduce cerebral hyperperfusion, loosen tight clothing, take off pressure stockings in the lower limb
- Continuous BP monitoring every 5 min

- Identify and treat aforementioned triggers, e.g. if bladder distended, decompress by Foley catheter (remember to use lignocaine gel to urethra before inserting Foley). If Foley blocked, either replace Foley and if one attempts to irrigate, do not use large amount of fluid to irrigate – bladder distension can cause further rise in BP. Use fluid at body temperature, not cold fluids
- If unresponsive to above measures, consider anti-hypertensive agents, e.g. nitroglycerine, nifedipine and/or prazosin, hydralazine
- Nifedipine can be administered by the bite and swallow method for prompt action, avoid the (erratic absorption) sublingual route
- Some situations where dysreflexia is frequently triggered by, say, bowel programme, may consider prophylactic medication such as captopril

12.8.3   Post-Traumatic Syringomyelia

- May occur from 2 months to 2 years post-SCI
- Estimated incidence 5–10%
- Suspect if: progressive weakness, ascending sensory loss, may cause bulbar weakness, diaphoresis, Horner's syndrome, or pain worsened by straining
- Diagnosis by MRI
- Management: symptomatic, decompress if progressing in size or deficit

12.8.4   Urinary-Related Complications

12.8.4.1 Catheter-Related Complications

- Pressure necrosis at external urethral meatus
- Urethral dilatation
- Blockade and encrustation
- Urethral erosion

12.8.4.2 Urinary System Complications

- Recurrent urinary tract infection
- Reflux nephropathy – especially if DSD+
- Renal stones
- Urethral stricture
- Cancer of the bladder (rarer)

12.8.5   Pressure Sores

■ Prevention is the best strategy
■ Cause of mortality in 4% of SCI cases
■ In particular, these patients should undergo pressure mapping to identify areas of high pressure, and the nature of seating material planned accordingly, sometimes need moulding; the same pressure mapping should be used to identify the effects of weight shifting in different directions
■ Frequent turning in bed, and avoidance of contractures is a must, and use of air cushions (Fig. 12.10)

12.8.5.1 Classification of Pressure Ulcers

■ Most follow National Pressure Ulcer Advisory Panel Guidelines:
  – Stage 1: intact epidermis with non-blanchable erythema
  – Stage 2: blisters or partial thickness skin loss present
  – Stage 3: full thickness involvement, with spared underlying fascia
  – Stage 4: full thickness involvement with deep structures involved; muscle, bone, or tendon

12.8.5.2 Management

■ Prevention: as mentioned
■ Treatment:
  – Patient and health staff education on the importance of pressure relief (pressure and shear are the most important factors, pressure

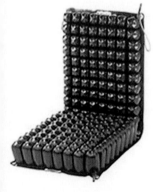

Fig. 12.10. The popular "ROHO" air-cushion system for pressure relief

of 70 mmHg for 2 h was shown by Kosiak to be adequate to cause histologic changes in animals)
- Identify and tackle other contributing factors (e.g. urinary or faecal incontinence, poor nutrition, anaemia)
- Treat infections if there are active signs of sepsis, but routine antibiotics treatment (of these usually colonised ulcers) is not encouraged
- Adjunct modalities to promote wound healing sometimes of use (see Chap. 2 on use of physical forces in rehabilitation)
- Non-response or significant sepsis requires surgical debridement and/or later flap coverage as required

12.8.6 Effect on Reproductive Function
▦ Discussed under Sect. 12.7

12.8.7 Respiratory Complications
▦ These complications mostly occur in acute stage
▦ Especially in patients with cervical cord injuries and ventilator-dependent patients
▦ As for thoracic cord injuries, recent studies indicate that high thoracic cord injuries are significantly more prone than low thoracic SCI (Cotton et al., J Trauma 2005)

12.8.8 Orthostatic Intolerance and Cardiovascular Deconditioning
▦ Recovery from acute spinal cord injury (SCI) is frequently complicated by orthostatic intolerance that is due to the combined effects of the disruption of the efferent sympathetic pathway and cardiovascular deconditioning occurring due to prolonged confinement to bed. Tilt table training in initial phases recommended (Fig. 12.11)
▦ The recent studies showing similar physiological changes of astronauts returning from space is worthy of further studies. Altered nitric oxide metabolism and its role in the pathogenesis of microgravity-induced cardiovascular deconditioning and the possible relevance of these new findings to orthostatic intolerance in patients with acute SCI and its potential therapeutic implications will be eagerly awaited (Vaziri, J Spinal Cord Med 2003)

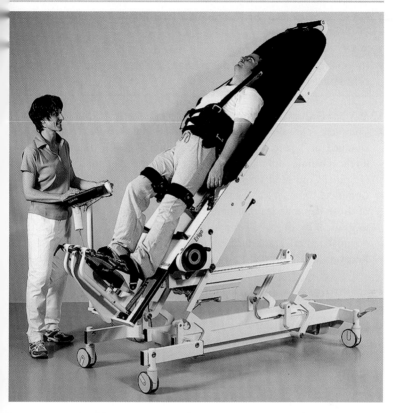

Fig. 12.11. The tilt-table is sometimes useful for slowly training SCI patients with ortho-static intolerance; the model here is also produced by the Swiss company, Hocoma

12.8.9 Psychological Disturbance
■ Examples include:
- Depression
- Loss of body image
- Sleep disorders, etc.

12.8.10 Miscellaneous Complications
■ These include: heterotropic ossification, deep vein thrombosis, osteo-porosis, etc., discussion of which is beyond the scope of this book

12.9   Prognosis of Recovery After SCI

12.9.1   General Comment
- In general, motor level is better than sensory or neurologic level in correlating function

12.9.2   Group with Complete SCI
- Complete paraplegics: 73% with neurologic level remaining unchanged at 1 year, 18% improve by one level, 9% improve by two levels. Overall, only 5% eventually become community ambulators (J Spinal Cord Med 1998)
- Complete tetraplegics: some recovery not unusual. At 1 month >90% of those key muscles that have recovered to grade 1 or 2 may recover to grade 3 by the 1 year mark (according to Kirshblum). Around 25% of most rostral grade 0 fibres may also recover to grade 3 at 1 year. Recovery of UL power, if any, mostly occurs in the first half year

12.9.3   Group with Partial SCI
- Prognosis of recovery much better
- Incomplete paraplegics: nearly half have enough useful motor recovery to ambulate at 1 year (according to Kirshblum)
- Incomplete tetraplegics: 80% regain useful power of hip flexion and knee extension by 1 year mark

12.9.4   Partial Cord Syndromes
- The prognosis varies between different entities, and was discussed in the earlier parts of this chapter

12.9.4.1   Expected Level of Function with Different Levels of Involvement

12.9.4.1.1   Lesion Above C4 Level
- In very high lesion survivors the phrenic nerve sometimes spared, or on phrenic nerve pacing
- Not all are ventilator-dependent
- Initial stage requires specially trained nursing staff and equipment
- Upon discharge, may mobilise with special wheelchair triggered by breathe/blowing (sip and puff) or mouth stick

- Environmental control unit tailored to individual and voice-assisted computer-mediated control of environment
- AT: environmental control units of assistance in this category of patients, exact equipment frequently needs to be individually tailored to the deficits present

12.9.4.1.2 C4 Complete Lesion

- Patients tend to be even more ventilator-dependent, especially in the initial stage
- Requires specially trained staff and equipment for care
- AT: environmental control units (ECU) of assistance in this category of patients, exact equipment frequently needs to be individually tailored to the deficits present. ECU can be made to be triggered by mouth-piece
- Upon discharge, may mobilise with special wheelchair triggered by breathe/blowing (sip and puff) or mouth stick

Examples of Components of Environmental Control Unit

- Usually based on assessing different devices by remote control from a special wheelchair unit
- Details of assistive technology (AT) were discussed previously (Sect. 12.3.4) and the underlying principles in Chap. 6 on assistive technology

12.9.4.1.3 C5 Complete Lesion

- Preserved motor control: deltoid and/or biceps
- Sensory level: lateral upper arm
- ADL possible:
  - AT that may help: balanced forearm orthosis to allow arm placement in ADL
  - Feeding, typing can be further helped by long opponent orthosis that affords element of wrist stability, or use dorsal wrist splint placed at dorsal surface of forearm to maintain the wrist in extension
- Powered wheelchairs with hand control are usually used

Balanced Forearm Orthosis

- Useful for those left with weak elbow flexors; the use of balanced forearm orthosis can be used for arm placement during usual ADL like feeding. Wrist stability is provided for equipment with utensil slots and pen holders

New Neuroprostheses for C5 Cord Lesion: NESS H200

- The NESS H200 system was developed to treat and prevent impairments and complications associated with disorders and injuries to the central nervous system. People with impaired upper-limb muscle control, loss of strength and reduced functional abilities (often associated with spasticity) may be candidates for this new technology
- The NESS H200 is an exoskeletal device worn on the hand and forearm (Fig. 12.12)
- The device includes five electrodes positioned above certain muscles responsible for different forms of movement. Once the NESS H200 is fitted, it controls the function of the hand by a coordinated stimulation of nerves and muscles. The comfortable positioning of the hand by the exoskeleton device, together with the functional microprocessor-controlled activation of otherwise paralysed muscles, is designed to improve hand function for those who have experienced a stroke or C5 spinal cord injury

12.9.4.1.4   C6 Complete Lesion

- Preserved motor control: patient is in addition capable of active wrist extension
- Sensory level: lateral forearm and lateral hand
- ADL possible: these patients use tenodesis to effect opposition of thumb and index finger for daily activities
- AT that may help: the above is helped by tenodesis orthosis

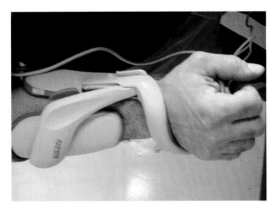

Fig. 12.12. NESS H200 system produced by Bioness

- Other possible aids: occasionally, slightly more demanding tasks that demand pinch strength via wrist-driven flexor hinge orthosis (see separate discussion below)
- Feeding is sometimes aided by short opponent orthosis equipped with utensil slots
- Patient at this level of injury may manipulate manual-type wheelchair on level surfaces helped by special gloves, with sliding board transfers. Although some still use powered wheelchair for negotiating longer distances

Wrist-Driven Flexor Hinge Splints

- Since the hand and wrist are a system of linked joints as mentioned in the companion volume of this book; this splint works via effecting grasp through a linked system where some hand joints are stabilised and others not
- Component parts include: tenodesis bar, forearm piece, palmer piece, and finger piece:
  - When patient effects wrist extension, the splint allows movement of some finger joints (mainly the index and middle fingers) to meet the thumb, which is held in position via the palmer piece to achieve grasp
  - If release is desired, patient allows gravity to plantar flex the wrist, to open up the fingers. Fine-tuning the amount of motion required done by adjusting the tenodesis bar

12.9.4.1.5   C7 Complete Lesion

- Preserved motor control: added triceps function and to some extent finger extension are a blessing
- Sensory level: up to middle finger
- ADL possible: most ADL can be independent with the help of tenodesis splintage
- AT that may help: manual wheelchair manipulation is much improved in the presence of triceps power, even with surfaces with slight slopes or mildly rough surfaces

12.9.4.1.6   C8 Complete Lesion

- Preserved motor control: all hand muscles are preserved except intrinsic ones

- Sensory level: medial hand
- ADL possible: WC use usually independent on level surface
- AT that may help: can drive specially designed cars using hand controls

12.9.4.1.7 T1 Complete Lesion
- Preserved motor control: essentially normal hand function
- Sensory level: up to medial forearm
- ADL possible: WC-independent
- AT: able to drive cars with adapted hand controls

12.9.4.1.8 Lower Levels
- The lower the thoracic level of the lesion, the more truncal control is maintained, and patients with low levels may have the potential capability for ambulation with the aid of special orthosis and/or electrical stimulation
- High cost of energy involved makes some patients prefer WC ambulation, with a much lower energy cost

General Bibliography

Nixon V (1985) Spinal Cord Injury – A guide to functional outcomes in physical therapy management (Rehabilitation Institute of Chicago Procedural Manual), Aspen, Maryland, USA

Consortium for spinal cord medicine, clinical practice guidelines. (website of paralysed veterans of America)

Selected Bibliography of Journal Articles

1. Bethea JR (2000) Spinal cord injury-induced inflammation: a dual edge sword. Prog Brain Res 128:33–42
2. Bracken MB, Holford TR (1993) Effects of timing of methyl-prednisolone or naloxone administration on recovery of segmental and long-tract neurological function in NASCIS 2. J Neurosurg 79(4):500–507
3. Geisler FH, Coleman WP et al. (2001) Measurements of recovery patterns in a multicenter study of acute spinal cord injury. Spine 26(24 Suppl):S68–S86
4. Rahimi-Movaghar V, Vaccaro AR et al. (2006) Efficacy of surgical decompression in regard to motor recovery in the setting of conus medullaris injury. J Spinal Cord Med 29(1):32–38

5. Vaccaro AR, Daugherty RJ et al. (1997) Neurologic outcome of early versus late surgery for cervical spinal cord injury. Spine 22(22):2609–2613

6. Vaziri ND (2003) Nitric oxide in micro-gravity induced orthostatic intolerance: relevance to spinal cord injury. J Spinal Cord Med 26(1):5–11

7. Hinckley CA, Ziskind-Conhaim et al. (2005) Locomotor-like rhythms in a genetically distinct cluster of interneurons in the mammalian spinal cord. J Neurophysiol 93(3):1439–1449

8. Santos-Benito FF, Ramon-Cueto A (2003) Olfactory ensheathing glia transplantation: a therapy to promote repair in the mammalian central nervous system. Anat Rec B New Anat 271(1):77–85

9. Johnston TE, Betz RR et al. (2005) Implantable FES system for upright mobility and bladder and bowel function for individuals with spinal cord injury. Spinal Cord 43(12):713–723

10. McCreery D, Pikov V et al. (2004) Arrays for chronic functional microstimulation of the lumbosacral spinal cord. IEEE Trans Neural Syst Rehabil Eng 12(2):195–207

11. Lu P, Yang H et al. (2004) Combinatorial therapy with neurotrophins and cAMP promotes axonal regeneration beyond sites of spinal cord injury. J Neurosci 24(28):6402–6409

12. Ashworth NL, Satkunam LE et al. (2006) Treatment for spasticity in amyotrophic lateral sclerosis. Cochrane Database Syst Rev CD 004156

13. Goldsmith MF (1985) Computerized biofeedback training aids in spinal injury rehabilitation. JAMA 253(8):1097–1099

14. Schonherr MC, Groothoff JW et al. (2005) Vocational perspectives after spinal cord injury. Clin Rehabil 19(2):200–208

15. McBride KE, Rines B (2000) Sexuality and spinal cord injury. A roadmap for nurses. SCI Nurs 17(1):8–13

16. Lovely RG, Gregor RJ et al. (1986) Effects of training on full weight-bearing stepping in the adult spinal cat. Exp Neurol 92(2):421–435

17. Conway BA, Hultborn H et al. (1987) Proprioceptive inputs resets central locomotor rhythm in the spinal cat. Exp Brain Res 68(3):643–656

18. Barbeau H, Rossignol S (1987) Recovery of locomotion after chronic spinalization in the adult cat. Brain Res 412(1):84–95

19. Behrman AL, Harkema SJ (2000) Locomotor training after human spinal cord injury: a series of case studies. Phys Ther 80(7):688–700

20. Edgerton VR, de Leon RD et al. (1997) Use-dependent plasticity in spinal stepping and standing. Adv Neurol 72:233–247

21. Hansen NL, Conway BA et al. (2005) Reduction of common synaptic drive to ankle dorsiflexor motoneurons during walking in patients with spinal cord lesion. J Neurophysiol 94(2):934–942

22. Graupe D, Davis R et al. (1998) Ambulation by traumatic T4–12 paraplegics using functional neuromuscular stimulation. Crit Rev Neurosurg 8(4):221–231

23. Solomonow M, Reisin E et al. (1997) Reciprocating gait orthosis powered with electrical muscle stimulation (RGO II): medical evaluation of 70 paraplegic patients. Orthopedics 20(5):411–418

24. Kobetic R, Triolo RJ et al. (1997) Muscle selection and walking performance of multi-channel FES systems for ambulation in paraplegia. IEEE Trans Rehabil Eng 5(1):23–29

25. Shimada Y, Konishi N et al. (1996) Clinical use of percutaneous intramuscular electrodes for FES. Arch Phys Med Rehabil 77(10):1014–1018

26. Sipski ML, Alexander CJ et al. (2001) Sexual arousal and orgasm in women: effects of spinal cord injury. Ann Neurol 49(1):35–44

27. Werhagen L, Buch CN et al. (2004) Neuropathic pain after traumatic spinal cord injury – relations to gender, spinal level, completeness, and age at the time of injury. Spinal Cord 42(12):665–673

28. Cotton BA, Pryor JP et al. (2005) Respiratory complication and mortality risk associated with thoracic spine injury. J Trauma 59(6):1400–1407

29. Waters RL, Adkins R et al. (1998) Functional and neurologic recovery after acute SCI. J Spinal Cord Med 21(3):195–199

30. Gittler MS, Kirshblum SC et al. (2002) Spinal cord injury medicine: rehabilitation outcome. Arch Phys Med Rehabil 83(3):S65–S71

31. Lee SU, Bang MS et al. (2002) Effect of cold air therapy in relieving spasticity, applied to spinalized rabbits. Spinal Cord 24(4):167–173

32. Dittuno PL, Dittuno Jr JF et al. (2001) Walking index for spinal cord injury (WISCI II): scale revision. Spinal Cord 39(12):654–656

33. Dittuno JF Jr, Dittuno PL et al. (2000) Walking index for spinal cord injury (WISCI): an international multi-center validity and reliability study. Spinal Cord 38(4):234–243

13 Burn Rehabilitation

Contents

13.1   Epidemiology

▦ Statistics in UK reveal a figure of 250 000 cases each year; 5% need hospitalisation
▦ The figure in US amounts to 750 000 emergency room visits, with 45 000 hospitalisations each year (J Burn Care Rehabil 1996)
▦ Mortality rate of burnt inpatients in UK is around 2%, but can be much higher in some developing countries
▦ Discussion in this chapter mainly centres on rehabilitation in subacute and chronic phases

13.2   The Acute Phase

13.2.1   Nature of Injury
▦ Flame burns and scalds are most common
▦ Other forms like chemical and electric burns rarer

13.2.2   Goal of Treatment
▦ Acute phase: removal from the burn scene, resuscitation, referral to burn centre if severe
▦ Subacute:
  – General[1] treatment: of acute complications – physical (e.g. inhalation injury, organ dysfunction) and psychological
  – Local treatment: e.g. prevention of deformity, aim at maintaining perfusion to zone of stasis
▦ Chronic: set functional goals, efforts towards reconstruction and resurfacing
▦ But rehabilitation should start immediately after hospitalisation, in all the three phases

---

[1] General body response in most cases with 30% burns

13.2.3 Prognostic Factors

■ Worse if:
- – Advanced age
- – High surface area involved
- – Inhalation injury
- – Presence of significant complications, like generalised sepsis

13.2.4 Increased Susceptibility in Major Burns to Sepsis and Shock Lung

■ Research in this area revealed that depletion of complement pathways (classic and alternate) was associated with sepsis, pneumonia and "shock lung"

■ Alternative pathway deficiency depletion was especially pronounced 1 week post-burn, and may contribute to the susceptibility of burn patients to bacterial sepsis (Gelfand et al., Ann Surg 1983)

13.2.5 Tackling the Hyper-Catabolic State

■ Many severe burn patients suffer rapid loss of muscle mass from the hypercatabolic state

■ This can further jeopardise the body's defence to infection

■ Recent literature on the use of anabolic steroids like oxandrolone appear promising (Burns 2003) via its role in decreasing nitrogen loss, increasing lean body mass and muscle protein synthesis

13.2.6 Shock Lung

■ Pathogenesis probably involved increased neutrophil aggregating activity in the plasma, neutrophil aggregates in the lungs, increased pulmonary vascular permeability, and increased lung oedema formation

■ The underlying mechanism is likely to be related to massive activation of the alternative complement pathway (J Clin Invest 1982)

13.2.7 Mortality

■ Animal research indicated that the severe activation of the alternative complement pathway not only predisposes to sepsis, or shock lung, but to increased mortality rate, but whether this can be extrapolated to humans is unsure (Gelfand et al., 1982). Possible role of strict glycaemic control in preventing mortality

▦ Recent studies point to the possible beneficial effects of better hyperglycaemic control in preventing infection and even mortality in adults and children (J Trauma 2005)

▦ Control of sepsis is important to prevent mortality and improve outcome, and will be discussed in the following section

13.3   Infection Control

13.3.1   Introduction

▦ Infection remains a leading cause of morbidity and mortality

▦ As such, proper strategies for prevention and management (particularly management of outbreaks) are important

13.3.2   Epidemiology

▦ Infection rate is higher in those with burns involving >30% of total body area

▦ In one big series involving 831 burn patients, the rate was 1.2% in those with <30% burn (755 patients), and 75% in those with >30% burn with regard to catheter-related blood stream infection (Carrougher, Burn Care Ther 1998)

13.3.3   Reasons for Predisposition to Infection

▦ Patients with significant burns have altered immunity, particularly excessive depletion of the alternate complement pathways that will predispose to sepsis

▦ Instrumentation and invasive monitoring by catheters sometimes act as route of entry for organisms

▦ Patients with extremes of age are also more infection-prone due to lowered defences

13.3.4   Organisms Involved

▦ Most prevalent gram-positives: *Staphylococcus aureus* (can be MRSA) and enterococci

▦ Most prevalent gram-negatives: *Pseudomonas*, *E. coli*, *Enterobacter*, *Acinetobacter* and *Klebsiella* spp.

- In many outbreaks, the importance of the colonised patient as a major reservoir for the epidemic strain was identified
- Overall, Gram-negative bacteria are more prone to causing invasive types of sepsis than Gram-positives

13.3.5 Situations in Which Occurrence of Multi-Bacterial Resistance Are More Likely

- Long hospital stay
- Critically ill patient with immunosuppression
- Routine use of prophylactic antibiotics
- Use of some antibiotics may predispose to certain strains (e.g. routine use of vancomycin may predispose to vancomycin-resistant *Staphylococcus aureus*)

13.3.6 General Management Strategies

- Strategies to prevent transferring exogenous organisms to patients:
    - Strict aseptic techniques in wound handling
    - Sterile gloves and dressings, and hand washing
    - Policies of isolation as required
    - Spatial separation between patients
- Strengthen the host: maintain proper nutrition and strengthen the intrinsic defences of the patient
- Strategies to control the transfer of endogenous organisms of the at-risk sites, and periodic surveillance culturing
- Stopping the breeding of bacteria resistance: avoid the routine use of prophylactic antibiotics

13.3.7 Policy of Antibiotics

- The burn wound (especially large ones) is frequently colonised by micro-organisms until wound is either closed or epithelialised
- Routine antibiotics will not eliminate colonisation, but invite bacterial resistance
- If antibiotics are needed, selection according to susceptibility pattern is needed, avoid broad coverage if possible and be on the look-out for other non-bacterial sepsis super-infection such as fungi
- Prophylactic antibiotics are mostly reserved to cover surgical procedures where indicated

13.3.8 Policy of Tackling an Outbreak

- Identify the organism and the type of bacterial resistance
- Trace the source of transmission, such as:
  - Hospital personnel (carrier)
  - Equipment (e.g. hydrotherapy units)
  - Items with potential to act as a source (e.g. pots of flowers)
  - Statistics from Boston burn centre indicated that in 85% of cases the source is endogenous flora
    (Mostly, the mode of transmission is contact, very occasionally droplets)

13.3.9 Extra Precautions in Two Patient Subgroups

- Those with major burns of >30% area
- Those patients colonised with multi-resistant bacteria
- (In children's burns unit, precautions against varicella and proper isolation as needed are required)

13.4 Rehabilitation in the Subacute and Chronic Phase

13.4.1 Introduction

- We will start by giving an overview of the process of assessment during the rehabilitation phase
- Then we will highlight the key problem areas and their management

13.4.2 Key Areas of Assessment: an Overview

- Checking patient's life history and priorities
- Assessing basic ADL
- Assessing instrumental ADL
- Motor testing
- Sensory testing
- Psychosocial and perceptual skills
- Pre-discharge preparation and post-discharge support

13.4.2.1 Checking Patient's Life History and Priorities

- COPM (Canadian Occupational Performance Measure) can be used to assess the patient's priorities

▩ COPM is usually used with Goal Attainment Scaling to help identify and agree upon goals of rehabilitation as the process of rehabilitation proceeds between the patient and the multidisciplinary team

13.4.2.2   Assessing Basic ADL
▩ Assessment by FIM (Functional Independence Measure) is recommended rather than simply using the Barthel Index
▩ Alternatives include: "Performance Assessment of Self-Care Skills", or "Klein-Bell Daily Living Scale"

13.4.2.3   Assessing Instrumental ADL and Community Integration
▩ Kohlman Evaluation of Living Skills is recommended
▩ Also, during later stage of rehabilitation assess community integration by "Community Integration Questionnaire"

13.4.2.4   Motor Testing
▩ Check:
 – ROM
 – Muscle tone and manual muscle testing
 – Document affected skin area and depth
 – Soft tissue status evaluation
 – If burns affecting arm/hand, serial charting of: nine-hole peg test of coordination (or use Purdue Pegboard) or Minnesota Rate of Manipulation Test. In addition, Jebsen Hand Function Testing was found to be very useful by many researchers in the literature on burns

13.4.2.5   Sensory Testing
▩ Somatosensory screening
▩ In later rehabilitation phase, assess need for more detailed testing, e.g. by monofilament testing

13.4.2.6   Psychosocial and Perceptual Skills
▩ Psychosocial problems if detected should be brought up in multidisciplinary team meetings and proper referral to psychiatrist and/or social service workers
▩ If brain function is altered, use mini-mental state testing and/or Lowenstein Occupational Therapy Cognitive Evaluation

13.4.2.7   If More Detailed Psychosocial Assessment Deemed Necessary

■ Consider further assessment by:
  - Allen Cognitive Level Test-90 (ACLS-90)
  - Occupational Case Analysis and Interview Rating Scale (OCAIRS)

13.4.2.8   Pre-Discharge Preparation and Post-Discharge Supports

■ Pre-discharge home visit
■ Meeting of the team with the family
■ Pre-discharge home leave during weekends to assess coping level
■ If return to work planned, assessment by the Worker's Role Interview
■ Home modification as required

13.4.3   Summary of Key Problem Areas in Rehabilitation Phase

■ Wound resurfacing
■ Hypertrophic scar management
■ Physiotherapy
■ Pain control
■ Control of infection (discussed already)
■ Psychological disturbance and support
■ Others: e.g. management of neuropathy, HO, pruritus
  (Occupational assessment was just mentioned)

13.4.3.1   Resurfacing of Burn Wounds

■ Split skin graft
■ Full thickness skin graft
■ Local flap
■ Free flap
■ Selective use of tissue expanders (mostly at scalp to help preserve hair-bearing skin areas)

13.4.3.1.1   New and Experimental Techniques

■ Hydrogel with adhesive semi-permeable film (Arch Surg 2006)
■ Tissue-engineered skin (Med Device Technol 2005)
■ Cryopreserved allodermis (J Burn Care Rehabil 1998)
■ Epidermal growth factor-impregnated collagen sponge in second degree burns (Arch Pharm Res 2005)

13.4.3.1.2 Use of Free Flaps in Reconstruction

▪ Free flaps may be indicated in severe and deep wounds
▪ The use of preoperative magnification angiography for both donor and recipient sites or transfer of free flaps or even digits is possibly a useful adjunct to increase the rate of success (May et al., Plast Reconstr Surg 1979)

13.4.3.2   Hypertrophic Scar

▪ Hypertrophic scarring is a major source of morbidity in patients with burns
▪ The physiologic characteristics are poorly understood, but increased neovascularity is typically seen in those wounds destined to become hypertrophic

13.4.3.2.1 Prevalence

▪ Studies indicate the prevalence of hypertrophic scarring of between 32 and 67% being commoner in non-white population (J Trauma 1983), correlation with age was inconclusive among different studies

13.4.3.2.2 Areas of the Body Less Prone to Scarring

▪ Palms of hand
▪ Soles of feet

13.4.3.2.3 Areas of the Body More Prone to Scarring

▪ Root of neck
▪ Sternal area
▪ Chest cage

13.4.3.2.4 Possible Pathogenesis of Hypertrophic Scarring

▪ Biochemical research from Harvard University indicated that burn wound healing abnormalities and scarring may be related to a change in the level of PGs or proteoglycan synthesis, and may be modified by IL-1 beta treatment (Garg et al., Biochem Mol Biol Int 1993)
▪ The same group of researchers also showed that the hypertrophic scar tissue after burns contained higher proportions of dermatan sulphate (DS), and chondroitin sulphate (CS) than normal skin fractions (Burns 1991)

13.4.3.2.5 Treatment Options for Hypertrophic Scarring

- Prevention: best strategy
- Pressure therapy/garment
- Proper patient positioning
- Use of splints and serial casting (with adjunctive physiotherapy)
- Tension-relieving surgery, e.g. Z plasty
- Excision and grafting (FTSG/PTSG) and/or flaps
- Use of newer coverage material like Integra (as dermal regeneration template) after contracture release (Plast Reconstr Surg 2004)
- Role of lasers

A Word About Pressure Treatment

- Pressure garments as prevention are worn 23 h a day for 9–12 months usually, and garments are replaced once every 3 months to ensure adequate pressure (J Trauma 1983)

Use of Lasers in Hypertrophic Scars

- Use of laser ablation of neovascularisation in sites of evolving hypertrophic scars, i.e. before the scar has matured (see Fig. 13.1), with the necessary eye precautions (Fig. 13.2)

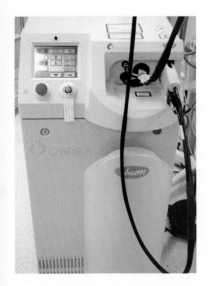

Fig. 13.1. This laser system is sometimes used to manage hypertrophic burns scars

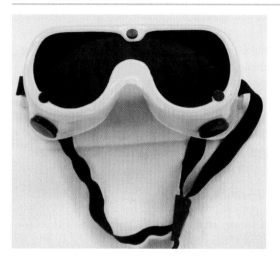

Fig. 13.2. Adequate eye protection is needed during laser treatment

Preliminary safety and feasibility studies are encouraging (J Burn Care Rehabil 1997)

Classification: the Vancouver Scar Scale
- Widely used in clinical practice and in documenting changes in scar appearance
- Good inter-rater reliability for research (Baryza et al., J Burn Care Rehabil 1995)

Further Classification of Highly Destructive Burn Wounds
- Based on a series of cadaver dissections, the Index of Deep Burn Injury (IDBI) was recently developed (Burns, 1997)
- The initial experience with the IDBI in a group of locally destructive "fourth degree" wounds was analysed with cadaveric dissections. This new index has the potential to improve our ability to describe very highly destructive burn wounds – the so-called fourth degree burn wounds

Key Concept
- Avoid tension in the scar

- Lasers may sometimes be useful in the management of *forming* hypertrophic scars, particularly those with persistent surrounding erythema that fails to go away, by ablation of neovascularisation
- Since scars cannot always be avoided, attempt to make them "more friendly" by taking tension off them (e.g. Z plasty) or sometimes using methods like lasers to avoid scars from getting out of hand

Skin Contractures and Scarring on the Growing Skeleton

- This can sometimes have a profound effect on the joint and the underlying soft tissue
- This effect of contracture has even more effect in the case of children who may be left with deformed, shortened and/or rotated bone and joints if not properly treated (see Fig. 13.3)

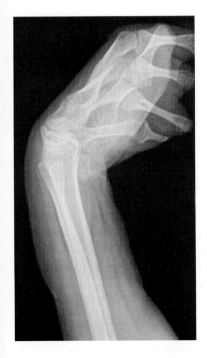

Fig. 13.3. The encasement induced by the hypertrophic integument caused abnormal bone growth in this growing child with upper extremity burns injury many years back

13.4.3.3   Key Physiotherapy Pearls

- Early ROM and weight-bearing
- Friction massage of scars is well described
- Early splinting throughout the hospital stay (protocol depends on different regions)
- Physiotherapy modalities to decrease pain
- Use of ultrasound to increase response to physical therapy is reported (Ward, J Burn Care Rehabil 1994)
- Selective use of: axial pin fixation and flaps
- Most papers report the use of early scar excision and sheet autograft wound closure
- But occasional use of other modalities in burn wounds such as LLLT lasers can be useful (Hawkins, Ann NY Acad Sci 2005)

13.4.3.4   Pain Control

- Pain is present in partial thickness, but not usually in full thickness burns, from damaged nerve endings
- Pharmacologic approaches work well for controlling tonic pain for many patients, but may be inadequate for controlling more severe phasic pain associated with burn treatment procedures, the latter may require additional short-acting opioid pain medications (Esselman et al., Phys Med Rehabil 2006)
- Nerve damage can produce neuropathic pain as well as sensorimotor disturbance from the associated neuropathy. Neuropathy is more commonly seen in electrical burns, alcohol abuse, or prolonged stays in intensive care units (J Burn Care Rehabil 2001)

13.4.3.4.1   Proper Pain Assessment

- McGill Pain Questionnaire – provides a subjective assessment of pain via the use of sensory, affective and evaluative word descriptors (Pain 1975)
- Visual analogue thermometer – adapted from Visual Analogue Scale and obviating the need for writing by means of plastic colour sliding strips (Burns 1994)
- Burn-Specific Pain Anxiety Scale (BSPAS) – used in assessing pain-related anxiety (Burns 1999)

13.4.3.4.2 Non-Pharmacological Interventions

- Virtual reality used as a distraction technique was recently reported to be useful in terms of pain control relative to controls (Hoffman et al., Pain 2000)
- Use of cognitive interventions, sensory focusing or music distraction was tried by Haythornthwaite, but not effective
- Other reported techniques include hypnosis (J Consult Clin Psychol 1997) and anxiety reduction techniques (Burns 2001)

13.4.3.5   Psychological Problems

- Common psychological problems include:
  - Sleep disorders
  - Post-traumatic stress reactions
  - Body-image dissatisfaction
  - Depression

13.4.3.6   Psychological Adjustment and Support

- Recent research has shown that even *slight* functional limitations were linked to *severe* depressions, similar to values found with patients with serious functional impairment. Interdisciplinary cooperation between plastic surgeons and psychosomatic specialists will optimise early intervention with patients exposed to social maladaptation (Pallua et al., Burns 2003)

13.4.3.7   Community Re-Integration

- The Community Integration Questionnaire was used by Esselman (J Burn Care Rehabil 2001) to assess areas like home integration, social integration and productivity (which measures school, work and volunteer activities)
- Productivity can be predicted by the patient's age, burn severity, and pre-injury job satisfaction (according to Esselman)
- Community re-integration is an important aspect of every burn-care rehabilitation program. There is evidence that a patient's ability to return to work is predicted by burn severity, and psychological problems. Also, the employment status at the time of the injury and co-morbid conditions such as substance abuse can limit the success of any vocational rehabilitation programme (Esselman et al., Phys Med Rehabil 2006)

13.5   Additional Management Pearls for Different Regions

13.5.1   Scalp
■ Tissue expanders sometimes of use here because of:
  - Inherent convex surface
  - Relatively unyielding deep surface
  - Rich vascular supply

13.5.2   Face
■ Klein and others propose decision-making at around day 10 to select areas that are not likely to heal within 3 weeks of injury to undergo excision and grafting (Fig. 13.4; J Burn Care Rehabil 2005)
■ Other commonly prescribed treatment like devices to prevent microstomia via stretching and wearing of facial masks, usually starting at 2 weeks postoperatively (Serghiou et al., J Burn Care Rehabil 2004)

13.5.3   Neck
■ The usual methods used in contracture prevention like pressure, stretching, splinting and surgery can be used to tackle troublesome scarring
■ Use of collars can be an adjunct in managing torticollis associated with neck burns (J Burn Care Rehabil 2003)
■ Position of the neck should either be in neutral or slight extension

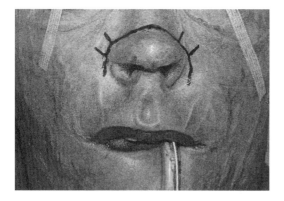

Fig. 13.4. Facial burns are not uncommonly associated with respiratory embarrassment as well as microstomia

13.5.4 Axilla

- Normal individuals have relatively thin skin in the axillary region
- Although reports of flap usage are sometimes reported in plastic surgery journals, try to avoid flaps in this area
- Whenever possible, use skin grafting, followed by postoperative splintage in abduction for adequate periods

13.5.5 Back

- The skin of the back of humans is very thick
- Seldom do we see really deep burns on the back
- In most cases skin grafting suffices
- An occasional patient may be considered for tissue expanders

13.5.6 Hand

- Burns involving the hand commonly cause deformity due to the superficial locations of the tendons. Examples include claw-hand, mallet finger and boutonnière deformities
- The principle of managing these burns includes early excision and grafting, ROM exercise, splinting, pressure garments and reconstruction (Burns 1998). In addition, adjunctive use of axial Kirschner wires to maintain functional joint positioning like 70–90° metacarpophalangeal joint flexion and proximal interphalangeal joint extension (J Trauma 1995)

13.5.6.1 Useful Tools for Assessing the Burnt Hand

- ROM: many researchers prefer to document the "total active motion", besides noting the motion of individual hand joints
- Jebsen Hand Function test: useful tool to predict hand function after burn injuries (Van Zuijlen et al., Burns 1999)
- Michigan Hand Outcome Questionnaire (Umraw et al., J Burn Care Rehabil 2004)

13.5.6.2 Challenging Scenario: Post-Burn Thumb Deformity with Loss of Prehension

- Reconstruction of thumbs so affected can be carried out by advancement and transferral of the second ray remnant onto the remaining metacarpal stump of the proximal thumb

▨ This technique combines the advantages of thumb lengthening and pollicisation procedures in a single operation and has been a useful method of restoration of single hand prehension in the severely burned hand (May et al., J Hand Surg 1984)

13.5.7 Lower Limb

▨ One of the major goals here is to aim at management options that allow the patient early weight-bearing, as recommended by workers like Burnsworth (J Burn Care Rehabil 1992) and Grube (J Trauma 1992)

13.6   Treatment Outcome and Prevention of Burns

13.6.1 Recent 10-Year Report of Outcome of Burns Care in Children

▨ Normal functional results were seen in 97% of second-degree and 85% of third-degree injuries; in children with burns involving underlying tendon and bone, 70% could perform ADL and 20% had normal function

▨ Reconstructive hand surgery was required in 4.4% of second-degree burns, 32% of third-degree burns and 65% of those with injuries involving underlying bone and tendon (Sheridan et al., Ann Surg 1999)

13.6.2 Prevention of Burns

▨ Most important since many cases are preventable

▨ Effected through law enforcement, survey of premises by fire services department, public education, adequate supervision of children by parents, proper insulation and safety measures in electrical appliances and stresses on work safety in workers dealing with chemicals and high voltage cables

General Bibliography

Carrougher GJ (1998) Burn Care and Therapy. Mosby, Missouri, USA

Selected Bibliography of Journal Articles

1. Brigham PA, McLoughlin E (1996) Burn incidence and medical care use in the United States: estimates, trends, and data sources. J Burn Care Rehabil 17(2):222–230

2. Gelfand JA, Donelan M et al. (1983) Preferential activation and depletion of the alternative complement pathway by burn injury. Ann Surg 198(1):58–62

3. Gelfand JA, Donelan M (1982) Alternative complement pathway increases mortality in a model of burn injury in mice. J Clin Invest 70(6):1170–1176

4. Pham TN, Warren AJ et al. (2005) Impact of tight glycaemic control in severely burnt children. J Trauma 59(5):1148–1154

5. Mason C (2005) Tissue engineering skin: a paradigm shift in wound care. Med Device Technol 16(10):32–33

6. Sheridan R, Choucair R et al. (1998) Acellular allodermis in burns injury: 1-year result of a pilot trial. J Burn Care Rehabil 19(6):528–530

7. Lee AR (2005) Enhancing dermal matrix regeneration and biomechanical properties of 2nd degree burn wounds by EGF impregnated collagen sponge dressing. Arch Pharm Res 28(11):1311–1316

8. May JW, Athanasoulis CA et al. (1979) Preoperative magnification angiography of donor and recipient sites for clinical free transfer of flaps or digits. Plastic Reconstr Surg 64(4):483–490

9. Engrav LH, Heimbach DM et al. (1983) Early excision and grafting vs non-operative treatment of burns of indeterminant depth: a randomized prospective study. J Trauma 23(10):895–898

10. Garg HG, Lippay EW et al. (1993) Comparison of the effects of interleukin-1 beta on proteoglycan synthesis by human skin and post-burn normal scar explant cultures. Biochem Mol Biol Int 31(3):583–591

11. Clayman MA, Clayman SM et al. (2006) The use of collagen-glycosaminoglycan (Integra) for the repair of hypertrophic scars and keloids. J Burn Care Res 27(3):404–409

12. Ward RS, Hayes-Lundy C et al. (1994) Evaluation of topical therapeutic ultrasound to improve response to physical therapy and lessen scar contracture after burn injury. J Burn Care Rehabil 15(1):74–79

14 Rehabilitation After Total Joint Replacement

Contents

14.1   Patient Selection and Expectations

14.1.1   Introduction

▨ Recent years have seen great enthusiasm and publicity as regards the use of MIS (minimal invasive surgery) and new surgical approaches (such as the two incisions surgical approach in THR) with hopes of quicker rehabilitation and shorter hospitalisation. Some units have reported performing MIS THR now as almost an outpatient procedure, while others report an impressive mean hospital stay of 1.5 days in TKR

▨ This chapter will help explore the latest evidence to see whether heated enthusiasm is warranted, besides touching on other aspects of rehabilitation

14.1.2   Pearls for a Successful TKR

▨ Patient selection
▨ Choice of implant
▨ Surgical technique:
  – Correct bone cuts and restoration of a favourable mechanical environment and alignment
  – Correct component placement
  – Correct ligament balancing
▨ Attention to PFJ and extensor mechanism preservation and restoration
  (Details of selection of implants, key surgical technique principles, common complications and their prevention have been discussed in the two companion texts of this book and will not be repeated in this chapter)

14.1.3   TKR: Patient Selection

▨ Realistic expectations
▨ Consideration should be given to other treatment options in younger adults. Examples: high tibial osteotomy (HTO) in the young adult high-demand labourer, uni-compartmental knee replacement in isolated medial compartment disease for selected patients around 60 years old

14.1.4 Pearls for a Successful THR

- Getting the right biomechanics – get the appropriate centre of rotation, the right offset, location of the greater trochanter, size of head, size of socket (larger area, less stress), and/or medialisation needed, but not excessive
- Getting better fixation (cemented/uncemented vs hybrids)
- Getting the optimal articulating couple for your patient
- Minimise wear (and friction)

14.1.5 THR: Patient Selection

- Realistic expectations
- Patient should be aware that there is no guarantee that any pre-operative leg length discrepancy will always be corrected postoperatively, although the surgeon will strive to equalise the leg length. Examples of the underlying reasons include: the balancing of soft tissue tension should not be sacrificed to equalise leg length or when, intraoperatively, the surgeon decides to go for a high hip centre
- The incidence of the different common complications should be told to the patient before signing the consent

14.2 Optimising Surgical Outcomes: Are Minimally Invasive THR and TKR the Answer?

14.2.1 Terminology: Less-Invasive vs Mini-Incision vs Minimally Invasive

- Since "minimal" literally means "barely sufficient", this term is not the best description
- Less invasive or mini-incision are likely to be better terms, but notice that there is a wide difference in the definition of "mini" in published papers by different authors both in THR and TKR

14.2.2 Is There Concrete Scientific Evidence for Minimally Invasive Surgery?

- If one prefers to have a scientific mind and insists that a randomised clinical trial (RCT) is necessary, only one RCT has been published recently, and the rest were mainly reports of different surgeons' experiences with different surgical approaches

■ Notice that in those papers there is a wide variety of definitions of "mini" incision, and many studies are in fact (strictly speaking) biased in that only patients with low BMI and good ROM are selected for the "mini" group. In such papers, it is perhaps unfair to compare a biased "mini" group with another "conventional" group and drawing conclusions stating that the "mini" biased group have better outcome

14.2.3 Patient Selection for MIS

■ Most published papers selected patients with low BMI, with relatively good ROM, an absence of significant deformity, and no prior hip or knee surgery

■ The reader should note this is a very biased group. To compare results of this group with "conventional" group is not without bias, and is rather like comparing oranges with apples

■ This is because many authors selected only patients with low BMI for the "mini" group undergoing minimally invasive THR, and concluded that there was good pain relief in the early postoperative period and increased patient satisfaction in the "mini" group. Much caution is needed when reading these articles

14.2.4 "Surgeon Selection" for Minimally Invasive Surgery

■ There are two sides of this coin
  – On the one hand, there are opinions expressed by some that minimally invasive surgery (MIS) is best reserved for surgeons who perform a large volume of total joint replacements a year (Orthop Clin North Am 2004)
  – On the other hand, some surgeons revealed they are starting to find patients who would rather select surgeons with less experience, but who do small incision surgery over more experienced surgeons who will not make promises about the size of incision or who perform standard incisions (Orthop Clin North Am 2004)

14.2.5 Are There Long Term Results of MIS THR or TKR?

■ There are no long-term studies or results available

14.2.6 One RCT on MIS Total Joint Replacement

■ Ogonda et al., J Bone Joint Surg Am 2005

■ Definition of "short" incision in this study < 10 cm, standard means > 16 cm
■ All surgeries by single experienced surgeon using the posterior approach to THR: no difference between the two groups with regard to blood transfusion, length of stay, early walking ability, or function scores at 6 weeks. No difference in accuracies of component placement

14.2.7 Minimally Invasive THR
■ The whole idea of MI THR should be looked upon as an "MI concept" rather than preoccupation with the exact length of the incision
■ It is unfortunate, as I have said, to note that some patients had started to prefer more inexperienced surgeons offering small incisions to more experienced surgeons (Goldstein, Orthop Clin North Am 2004)

14.2.7.1 Key Principles of MIS THR
■ This should at least include:
  - Aiming at minimising surgical trauma
  - With emphasis on decreased muscular trauma, e.g. sparing hip abductors, and mobile soft tissue window
  - Knowledgeable assistant
  - Proper training (whether by apprenticeship, surgical navigation, virtual reality or combined)
  - Proper equipment (eases exposure, decreased trauma)
  - Operative patient education
  - Pre-emptive analgesia and/or anti-emetics
  - Programmed and early postoperative rehabilitation

14.2.7.2 Key Concept
■ MIS THR is a concept or philosophy, the size of the incision is only one component, but definitely not the most important

14.2.7.3 Complications of MIS THR
■ In an article in Int Orthop 2006, despite the fact that the authors selected only low BMI patients for the "mini" group, they reported increased incidence of acetabular cup malpositioning

14.2.7.4 Approaches Used for MIS THR
- Posterior/posterolateral approach
- Anterolateral (abductor-sparing) approach
- Two-incision technique involving two approaches

14.2.7.5 Mini-Posterior Approach
- Essentially, using part of the traditional incision of the posterior approach
- One of the advocates (Dorr) thinks that computer-assisted orthopaedic surgery (CAOS) will be complementary to this approach (Iowa Orthop J 2005)
- Dorr found 90% of patients had normalised gait analysis by 10 weeks

14.2.7.6 Other Studies: Posterior Approach and/or Fluoroscopy
- Hartzband, Orthop Clin North Am: the author commented on the tendency towards vertical cup placement, eccentric acetabular reaming, and selecting a too posterior starting point for femoral canal broaching

14.2.7.7 Other Reports
- Goldstein et al., Orthop Clin North Am 2004: degree of bias since low BMI patients selected for "mini" group. This is the paper that commented that some patients now exercise their own bias by preferring surgeons who offer small incisions to more experienced surgeons

14.2.7.8 Anterolateral Approach
- Howell et al., Orthop Clin North Am 2004: degree of bias present since selected only "small" patients for "mini" group. Authors concluded the anterolateral technique was safe, there is no difference in blood loss, but in fact increased operating time
- Jerosch et al., Arch Orthop Trauma Surg 2006: definition of "mini" in this study 6–8 cm, both groups had early weight-bearing, no difference in complication rate, but commented that "mini" group seemed to have faster recovery

14.2.7.9 Two-Incision Approach with Fluoroscopy by Berger
- Essentially involves an anterior Smith Peterson, and a separate posterior incision for femoral broaching
- Requires the use of intraoperative fluoroscopy

■ Although excellent result (Clin Orthop Relat Res 2004) claimed by its proponents and now reported as an "outpatient" procedure, only 25% of patients for THR were subjected to this approach in the centre that proposed its use

14.2.7.10   Controversy Regarding the "Two-Incision" Technique

■ Although reported as having excellent results by its proponents, there are more and more reports of not uncommon complications (sometimes significant complications) by experienced surgeons in other centres

■ Common complications: femoral fracture (up to 5%) HO, lateral femoral cutaneous nerve palsy, etc. Dislocation rare

14.2.7.11   Other Seldom Mentioned Disadvantages of the Procedure

■ Possibility that the hip will intraoperatively become "too stable" after the two-incision technique: as Charnley has taught us that fine-tuning of soft tissue tensioning, and adjustment of offset is important intraoperatively in THR. New techniques like the two-incision techniques make intraoperatively attempted dislocation much too difficult since the THR is very stable once reduced

■ Repeated attempts at dislocation may in fact risk more soft tissue, nerve and bony trauma. Also, for those who have seen the two-incision technique performed before, the extent of manipulation of the LL if one wants to dislocate and reduce the hip 2–3 times, say, to fine tune the soft tissue tension, might increase the risk of DVT

■ For similar reasons, the same THR may be made more difficult to revise if subsequent revision is required

14.2.7.12   Author's View

■ The current marked discrepancy between the extremely good results reported from mainly one centre in the presence of significant complication rates in other centres by other total joint experts with vast experience reminds us of the analogy of the Sugioka's operation for hip with avascular necrosis. The apparent similarity is that in Sugioka's hands the operation was very successful. But the success was not easily repeatable in other centres since the operation was difficult

■ While it is too early to make any premature judgment and it takes a formal prospective randomised trial (preferably multicentre) to ascertain the result of the "two-incision" technique; there is an increasing amount of views from different experts that it is likely to be a difficult and demanding operation and not for the surgeon who only occasionally performs THR

14.2.8 Minimally Invasive TKR

- Repicci in the early 1990s had already introduced MIS for unicondylar replacement
- It is natural that the idea now involves tricompartmental total knee replacement

14.2.8.1 Key Concept of Minimally Invasive TKR

- The whole idea of MI TKR should be looked upon as a concept or philosophy
- The size of the incision is one component, but certainly not the most important
- The exact length of incision varies with the body build of the patient, among other factors

14.2.8.2 Components of the MIS Concept

- This should at least include:
  - Aiming at minimising surgical trauma
  - Emphasis on decreased muscular trauma, e.g. quadriceps sparing, and mobile soft tissue window
  - Knowledgeable assistant
  - Proper training (whether by apprenticeship, surgical navigation, virtual reality or combined)
  - Proper equipment (eases exposure, decreased trauma)
  - Good preoperative patient education
  - Pre-emptive analgesia and/or anti-emetics
  - Programmed and early postoperative rehabilitation
    (Tria is right: our main goal is to advance the science of medicine without compromising the ultimate result in the patient [Clin Orthop Relat Res 2003])

14.2.8.3 Complications

- Various groups have reported significant complications
- Four out of 30 tibial components showed signs of malalignment in the "mini" group (Dalury and Dennis, Clin Orthop Relat Res 2005)

14.2.8.4   Approaches Used for Minimally Invasive TKR

■ Using conventional approach except smaller medial arthrotomy
■ Subvastus approach
■ Midvastus approach
■ Lateral approach

14.2.8.4.1   Approach Same as Conventional, But Decreased Extent of Medial Capsulotomy

■ No difference in the two groups with regard to length of hospital stay, ambulatory ability, stair climbing, tourniquet time, radiologic alignment, or rate of complications (Tenholder et al., Clin Orthop Relat Res 2005)

14.2.8.4.2   Subvastus Approach

■ An old approach
■ Truly "quadriceps-sparing"

Increased Patella Clunk Syndrome Reported After Subvastus Technique

■ A recent paper reported that as there was increased ROM of TKR after MI subvastus approach, the authors (Schroer et al.) found a significant 6% of patients with patella clunk syndrome using posterior-stabilised (PS) prosthesis (Proc AAOS 2006)
  – This is very much predicted when it comes to the pathogenetic mechanism of "patella clunk" syndrome
  – Although the syndrome was coined by Hozack, it was the author who first highlighted the increased tendency and the mechanism for "patella clunk" to occur in TKR patients with increased ROM, reported in 2002 (Ip et al., Int Orthop), and later again in 2003 (Ip et al., Arch Orthop Trauma Surg)
■ (Another predisposing factor is patella baja or relative patella baja in situations where the joint line is elevated)
■ The fact that the same group was able to decrease after switching to a newer femoral component design again testifies the importance of femoral component design in the pathogenesis of the patella clunk syndrome as reported by the author previously (Ip et al., Int Orthop 2002)

14.2.8.4.3   Mini-Vastus Approach

- Proponents claim excellent results, e.g. increased flexion ROM, decreased pain medication, etc. (Clin Orthop Relat Res 2004)
- However, recent papers have reported complications like painful patella crepitus, retained cement, lateral peripatella soft tissue hypertrophy, less than optimal femoral component positioning, even open revision for uneven pressurisation while cementing componentry (Proc AAOS 2006)
- Another paper comparing mini midvastus and the conventional technique also reported significant complications like fracture of the lateral femoral condyle, and MCL injury in the mini midvastus approach group (Proc AAOS 2006)
- Common contraindications of mini midvastus approach include: significant valgus deformity, prior knee surgery, obesity, or very muscular individuals

14.3   Role of Surgical Navigation and Virtual Reality

14.3.1   Introduction

- Surgical navigation is, in the author's view, complementary to MIS total joint surgery
- Part of the reason is that with MIS, we expect some limitation in tactile sense and exposure, to which the surgeon is accustomed. This needs to be replaced by techniques like CAOS or fluoroscopy
- The complementary nature of CAOS is also reflected by others, e.g. Nogler (Surg Technol Int 2004), who says: "it seems inevitable that CAOS and MIS will converge"
- To add to this, there is also literature lending support to the theory that surgical navigation improves the accuracy of component placement (Wixson, Arthroplasty 2005; Nogler, Clin Orthop Relat Res 2004)
- How about soft tissue balancing? Newer CAOS systems that can now provide real-time feedback and soft-tissue tension devices that are compatible with the system have recently been made available for TKR
- But is CAOS completely without problems? One problem is that the current CAOS systems were mostly not originally designed with MIS in mind. But we will now discuss the larger problem

14.3.2 Problem of the Use of Surgical Navigation Becoming Generalised

- Proponents of surgical navigation on the one hand say it is potentially a very useful tool to teach the future generation of arthroplasty surgeons, but on the other hand mention that because of cost and other factors, these techniques will only be practised in a few centres!

- We all know that a technique or surgical procedure is only useful if it can be achieved by most surgeons; the above comments from the proponents alone cast doubt on its general applicability

- Besides, there are also problems associated with reimbursement (whether insurance companies are willing to pay extra for new techniques)

14.3.3 What is the "Second Best" Way or the "Best Alternative"?

- The answer of course is virtual reality

- Use of virtual reality (VR) as a teaching tool has already become reality and is no longer science fiction. Examples of the use of VR are given throughout this book

- If the software we use for VR training is basically similar to that of the surgical navigation, this will increase the compatibility of these two training platforms, allowing this useful latest technology to reach most hospitals and surgeons, instead of just a privileged few

14.3.4 A Word About Virtual Reality

- Virtual environment uses computerised images and sounds to represent reality

- Its use in training future generations of surgeons, which has already started both in general surgery and in orthopaedic surgery

- This has been made possible by previous projects like the "Virtual Human" project, which reproduces the human anatomy accurately on computer. Similar projects have been completed in the USA and also in China

- One such virtual reality platform under construction is the 'Virtual Interactive Musculoskeletal System' (VIMS) at the Orthopedic Biomechanics Laboratory at Johns Hopkins University, Baltimore, USA

14.4 Importance of Pain Control and Implications

14.4.1 General vs Spinal Anaesthesia

▨ Advantages of spinal (epidural) over general anaesthesia:
   - Less blood loss
   - Less DVT
   - Tend to have better analgesia postoperatively

14.4.2 Spinal vs Epidural

▨ Spinal: good pain relief with relatively low-dose morphine and pain relief lasts for 24–30 h. Site of injection below L2
▨ Epidural: usually delivered through catheter in the perioperative period; commonly used with local anaesthetic. Ideal site of epidural catheter placement in the middle of the involved surgical dermatome since epidural-related sensory blockade only occurs in the dermatomal zones near to the site of injection

14.4.3 Support for Epidural

▨ A randomised study from the Hospital for Special Surgery revealed that epidural anaesthesia was found to be associated with more rapid achievement of postoperative rehabilitation goals after TKR (Williams-Russo et al., Clin Orthop Relat Res 1996)

14.4.4 Patient-Controlled Epidural Anaesthesia

▨ Most patients who have epidurals will have an epidural catheter left in situ postoperatively to allow for patient-controlled supplemental dosing
▨ Beware of complications like epidural haematoma formation in the presence of concomitant anti-coagulation

14.4.5 Type of Opioid

▨ Morphine is more commonly used in total joint surgery since fentanyl has a much shorter action. Fentanyl is therefore more often used in day case surgery and lesser procedures that produce less pain (Rathmell et al., Anesth Analg 2005)
▨ This is especially the case in TKR where pain control usually tends to be more difficult than in THR (Anesth Analg 2003)

14.4.6   Minimising the Risk of Epidural Haematoma in the Setting of Concomitant Anticoagulation

- Epidural can only be considered if:
  - Prothrombin ratio/international normalised ratio (PT/INR) <1.5 if patient on warfarin
  - >10 h from last dose in the case of infusion of low molecular weight heparin
  - Subcutaneous intermittent heparin not common to produce epidural, still need to check prothrombin time (American Society of Regional Anesthesia)

14.4.7   New Option: Use of Epidural One-Shot Sustain-Release Morphine

- This method does not require the use of a catheter and is promising since this will not hinder the postoperative patient receiving physiotherapy and is safe with anti-coagulant regimen
- It works by slow sustained release of morphine from encapsulation in drug chambers located at the microscopic liposomes (Viscusi et al., 2003)
- Same caution and side effects as standard morphine administration, and cannot be given together with epidural local anaesthetics

14.4.8   Clinical Trial of One-Shot Sustain-Release Epidural Morphine in THR

- Proven to be better than placebo with the use of epidural sustain-release morphine (ESRM)

14.4.9   Use of Nerve Blocks in Total Joint Surgery

- Notice that owing to the nature of innervation of the hip; one needs in fact to block the lumbar plexus in order to be effective for THR, quite unlike the case of TKR
- To this end, the psoas compartment block may be used in the setting of THR (Mortin et al., Reg Anesth Pain Med 2005)
- Femoral nerve block may provide partial analgesia following TKR, but should not be used alone (Mortin, 2005)
- Some recent papers draw our attention to prevention of ulceration at pressure points such as heel ulcers after these nerve blocks by suitable protection (Todkar, Acta Orthop Belg 2005)

14.4.10 Use of COX-2 Inhibitors in TKR

■ In a multicentre RCT consisting of double-blind, single-dose parallel group (placebo vs. active comparator groups – parecoxib 20 mg i.v., parecoxib 40 mg i.v., ketorolac 30 mg i.v. vs morphine 4 mg i.v.); the group with parecoxib (40 mg) had the best patient satisfaction, and quicker onset of analgesia (Rasmussen et al., Am J Orthop 2002)

■ Other previous studies also revealed that parecoxib (40 mg i.v.) can lessen postoperative PCA use in THR (Malan et al., Anesthesiology 2003) and in TKR (Hubbard et al., Br J Anaesth 2003)

14.4.11 Multimodal Analgesia in the Setting of Total Joint Replacement

■ It has been shown previously that postoperative morphine usage was significantly decreased with administration of parecoxib or valdecoxib (Camu et al., Am J Ther 2002)

■ Common drug combinations in multimodal analgesia include: intravenous opioids and perioperative use of NSAIDs (just discussed), nerve blocks, or epidurals

■ In the subgroup of patients with OA knee or OA hip who have been on significant amounts of opioid-type medication prior to surgery, may need higher perioperative opioid doses and adjunctive nerve blocks and/or NSAIDs (according to Sinatra and Mitra)

14.4.12 Summary

■ From the rehabilitation point of view, use of multimodal analgesia can lessen pain, heighten patient satisfaction, and makes for earlier recovery

■ This is particularly the case because:
  – Many patients who have total joint replacements are elderly and pain can precipitate, say, cardiac events
  – Previous studies indicate that pain after TKR appears to be more than THR
  – Patients undergoing sequential procedures tend to have a lot more pain, which needs careful titration and prevention

14.5   Pearls in the Peri- and Postoperative Periods

14.5.1   Postoperative THR

14.5.1.1 Postoperative Weight-Bearing

- Most surgeons commence early full weight-bearing after cemented THR
- The immediate postoperative weight-bearing status after cementless THR depends on the degree of press-fit or primary stability obtained, but most surgeons prescribe a period of not less than 6 weeks of protected weight-bearing, theoretically to let the bone in-growth or on-growth get more stable footing

14.5.1.2 Minimising Joint Forces and Deforming Torques Postoperatively

- Common precautions to minimise joint force or torque in early postoperative THR patient:
    - Use of a cane on the contralateral side as walking aid
    - Avoid early straight leg-raising exercises, since these manoeuvres can produce high mechanical loads across the hip joint
    - Deforming torque is high on standing from a seated position, prescribe high chair and pushing off action by the upper limbs is recommended

14.5.1.3 Joint Protection Techniques

- These are mainly used to prevent dislocations in early postoperative period, particularly if a posterior approach was used
- Examples of common advice:
    - Use of abduction pillow while in bed
    - Avoid lying laterally in bed without a pillow between the legs
    - Avoid standing with feet turning inwards
    - Avoid low chair since will cause too much hip flexion, assess need for change of toilets or use raised toilet seats, bathroom equipped with proper hand rails
    - Avoid bending over to pick up objects, if really needed the operated leg should avoid excess hip flexion
    - Avoid excess hip flexion while arising from a chair, etc.
    - Suitable use of ADL aids (see Fig. 14.1) and home modification as necessary

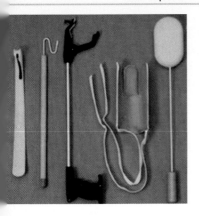

Fig. 14.1. Typical set of ADL aids useful for total hip and total knee arthroplasty patients

14.5.1.4 Muscle Strength Re-Training
▓ Preventing hip abduction weakness (initially isometric sets followed by muscle strengthening and resistance training) and hip flexion contractures (stretching useful) are important
▓ The above help avoid Trendelenburg lurch and gait anomalies
▓ Subsequent rehabilitation of the whole kinetic chain

14.5.1.5 Strength Training
▓ Adequate pain control important to prevent quadriceps shutdown
▓ For MI THR using two-incision techniques especially and surface replacements, since the hip is usually very stable, there is decreased need for the usual hip precautions

14.5.1.6 Ascending and Descending Stairs
▓ On descending stairs, place the two crutches one step lower, lower the operated leg followed by the sound leg
▓ On ascending stairs, put the sound leg one step higher, followed by the operated leg, then the two crutches

14.5.1.7 Prospects of Early Hospital Discharge with MIS
▓ Occasionally, patients can tolerate FWB with aids very early on, days 1–2 postoperatively after MIS procedures

- There are even claims that some patients have THR as outpatient procedure after the two-incision technique
- But as we can see from our discussion above, arthroplasty surgeons are highly selective on who gets MIS. Hence, for most patients (i.e. not the biased group) we aim at hospital discharge within 4–7 days depending on the type of procedure, and any postoperative complications

14.5.1.8 Resumption of Driving
- Decisions concerning the resumption of driving after THR depend on factors like the driving reaction time and the duration of post-surgical joint precautions
- A recent study showed that in general, patients managed to reach their preoperative driving reaction time at 4–6 weeks postoperatively (Ganz et al., Clin Orthop Relat Res 2003)

14.5.1.9 Resumption of Sexual Activity
- Previous studies reported that most patients were able to resume sexual activity within 1–2 months after surgery, and that males tend to resume the said function sooner than females. Most patients interviewed by questionnaires preferred the supine position (Stern et al., Clin Orthop Relat Res 1991)

14.5.2   Postoperative TKR

14.5.2.1 Role of Early Continuous Passive Motion
- Many centres performing MI TKR tend to use postoperative continuous passive motion (CPM) 0–100°, or sometimes with due regard to the ROM attained intraoperatively
- In the past, CPM has the track record of possibly increasing early ROM attained postoperatively, but the final outcome made no difference
- Whether the same holds if used with MI procedures remains to be seen:
  - Some units limit the ROM to as little as 40° while connecting the patient to CPM on the grounds that there is a theoretical danger of decreased transcutaneous oxygen tension (hence possible wound problems) with higher ROM. However, allowing ROM as low as this probably defeats the purpose of CPM (Fig. 14.2)

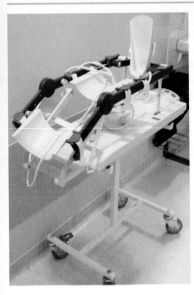

Fig. 14.2. Continuous passive motion (CPM) machine is not uncommonly prescribed for the postoperative total knee patient. See text for discussion of pros and cons of its use

- If CPM is used, it is recommended to disconnect for a few hours a day to allow full ipsilateral lower limb extension to prevent knee flexion contractures
- In addition, the results of the most recent prospective study do not support the addition of CPM to conventional physical therapy programmes after primary TKR, because CPM was shown to neither further reduce knee impairments or disability, nor reduce the length of the hospital stay (Denis et al., Phys Ther 2006)

14.5.2.2 Early Mobilisation and Weight-Bearing

- Most surgeons allow early and full weight-bearing after cemented TKR
- Cementless TKR is becoming less popular, but cementless femoral components have a better track record. Most of these latter hybrid constructs can be subjected to early postoperative full weight-bearing exercises

14.5.2.3 Dealing with Knee Stiffness

▦ The best predictor of postoperative knee ROM after TKR is preoperative knee ROM

▦ Proper restoration of ROM depends on proper bone cuts, posterior capsular release, and posterior osteophyte take-down. Given good surgical technique, the type of implant used may also have some bearing on ROM attained

▦ The possible role of CPM was mentioned. Attainment of at least 0–90° ROM is our goal upon hospital discharge, with a view to attaining a more functional range of 0–120° upon completion of physiotherapy training

▦ Manipulation under anaesthesia if used need to be undertaken early, i.e. within 2 weeks of operation to increase chance of success and prevent unwanted complications from late manipulations

14.5.2.4 Resumption of Golfing

▦ A previous study by Mallon in active golfers with TKR revealed that pain rates during and after play were significantly higher in golfers with left TKR than for those with right TKR, possibly due to increased torque on the left knee in right-handed golfers. It was recommended that TKR patients use a golf cart while playing, especially those who had left TKR who are right-handed (Mallon et al., Arthroplasty 1993)

▦ Contact sports should of course be avoided in both TKR and THR patients

14.6   Optimising Outcomes for Young Patients Who Have TKR and THR

14.6.1   Thought Process to Go Through Before Performing TKR in Young Patients

▦ Are there better options than TKR?

▦ Have we ascertained that our patient has realistic expectations and that there is a need for precautions such as avoidance of contact sports?

▦ Which compartment(s) of the knee is/are at fault, will a uni-compartmental arthroplasty suffice?

■ If TKR is decided upon, how can we optimise outcome for the patient?

14.6.2 Elements for Outcome Optimisation in the Young TKR Patient

■ Options other than TKR and uni-compartmental knee arthroplasty were discussed in detail in the companion volume to this book (*Orthopedic Principles – A Resident's Guide*) and will not be repeated here. Essential elements include:

– Preference is usually given to mobile-bearing knee replacement, which was discussed in detail in the companion volume to this text
– Use a knee design with good track record and good kinematic profile, e.g. with femoral rollback on knee flexion to optimise quadriceps moment arm, since these young patients tend to be more active and put more demand on their knees than older people
– Select a total knee design with a patella-friendly trochlea-articulating surface to minimise contact stresses of the patello-femoral joint (PFJ; Ip et al., J Orthop Surg 2003)
– Choose a femoral component with good surface finish
– The tendency nowadays is to use high X-linked polyethylene, although there is as yet no long-term report on the use of this newer plastic for TKR
– MIS technique (e.g. quadriceps-sparing approach) is an option that can be considered if the surgeon is experienced in the technique
– Adequate perioperative pain control with multimodal analgesia and prevent postoperative quadriceps weakness or shutdown from pain
– Aim at early FWB at days 1–2 after surgery

14.6.3 Thought Process to Go Through Before Performing THR in Young Patients

■ Seriously consider other options like a surface replacement (will be discussed shortly in Sect. 14.6.6) and detailed discussion of his or her expectations is important
■ If THR is somehow decided upon, then prior to performing surgery, the patient must understand:

– The expected restrictions and the need to avoid contact sports
– The incidence of common complications
– That sometimes revision is necessary for progressive worsening osteolysis, despite the fact that he or she may remain asymptomatic

14.6.4 Elements of Outcome Optimisation in the Young THR Patient

■ Preference is usually given to cementless fixation for both acetabular and femoral components. Although occasionally, cemented femoral fixation can be considered if the calcar:canal ratio of the proximal femur is deemed not best suited for cementless fixation

■ If cementless femoral component is chosen, then a tapered stem is preferred as it usually allows early or immediate weight-bearing

■ The option of MIS has been discussed previously and can be considered if the surgeon is experienced in the technique

■ Select a surgical approach that minimises violation of the abductor mechanism and a low dislocation rate for these younger, more active patients

■ Use an articulating couple with low friction so as to minimise the friction torque and wear rate, e.g. CoCr-Ceramic couple is an example

■ Adequate pain relief in the perioperative period with the use of multimodal analgesia

■ Active postoperative physiotherapy programme

■ Patients are usually encouraged to undergo a brief physiotherapy programme preoperatively, including teaching videos so that they will learn what to expect and the necessary precautions

14.6.5 The Option of Surface Replacement

■ Essentially consists of a metal–metal articulating couple that helps preserve bone stock as the femoral neck is retained

■ Popular in many countries outside US

■ Example: the Birmingham hip replacement

14.6.6 Advantage of "Surface Replacement"

■ Preserve bone stock

■ Preserve and maintain more normal hip biomechanics

■ Much better ROM because of the large (original-sized) femoral head

■ Can potentially allow quicker and better rehabilitation (see later discussion in Sect. 14.6.8) and participate in activities not usually expected or allowed after THR

14.6.7 Disadvantage of "Surface Replacement"

■ No long-term results to support the new technique as yet

- Femoral neck fracture estimated at 5%
- Compromised local vascularity to the femoral head/neck area
- Metal–metal wear debris can be carcinogenic/teratogenic. Thus, caution in young women awaiting pregnancy
- Contrary to popular belief, amount of wear particles can be even greater than with metal-poly couple, although the particles are much finer
- MIS is more difficult. But there is one recent report on MIS for Birmingham hip with apparently decreased pain, length of stay, and increased cosmesis (McMinn et al., Clin Orthop Relat Res 2005)
- As yet, there is no global standardisation or guidelines for the various companies manufacturing the componentry. For example, wear rates and other relevant data like wettability of the metals produced by the different companies are lacking

14.6.8 Relevance to Rehabilitation

- As the dislocation rate is much lower, hip mechanics and motion are more normal (retained original diameter of femoral head); this will have positive effects on rehabilitation in terms of:
  - Many of the normal hip precautions against dislocation are not required
  - Early return to activities that are not allowed after THR such as many sporting activities
  - Better ROM without many restrictions on ADL
- Long-term results of surface replacement for the hip are eagerly awaited

14.7   A Word on Outcome Measures

14.7.1 Recent Trends in the Use of Outcome Measures

- There is an increasing tendency to include more subjective measures from the point of view of the patient, e.g. in the form of questionnaires in studies of total joint replacement (and other fields of orthopaedics), besides including the traditional objective scores like the Knee Society Scoring System in TKR, or the Harris Scoring system in THR
- The following reveals two of the most commonly used subjective scores relevant to total joint replacement

14.7.2 Comparison of WOMAC and LEFS

- WOMAC = Western Ontario and McMaster Universities Osteoarthritis Index
- LEFS = Lower Extremity Functional Scale
- These are two popularly used functionally orientated health status measures, which involve the filling out of questionnaires by the patients
- As will be discussed in Chap. 18 on outcome measures, these questionnaires are not readily interchangeable and stress different aspects of similar pathology
- A recent comparison exists comparing these two questionnaires in patients awaiting or having undergone TKR (Jogi et al., Physiother Can 2005)
- The findings include:
  - Strong relationship between the WOMAC and LEFS, but individual scores are not highly predictive of one another or interchangeable
  - Therapists working with patients awaiting or having had TKR might find the WOMAC advantageous for facilitating communication with surgeons as well as comparison with data of similar patients in the literature
  - LEFS might on the other hand be preferable for facilitating comparison of patients awaiting and having undergone TKR with patients with other LL impairments

General Bibliography

Scuderi GR (2005) MIS Techniques in Orthopaedics. Springer, Berlin Heidelberg New York

Byrd JWT (2005) Operative Hip Arthroscopy. Springer, Berlin Heidelberg New York

Selected Bibliography of Journal Articles

1. Ogonda L, Wilson R et al. (2005) A minimal-incision technique in total hip arthroplasty does not improve early postoperative outcomes. A prospective, randomized, controlled trial. J Bone Joint Surg Am 87(4):701–710
2. Goldstein WM, Branson JJ et al. (2004) Posterior-lateral approach to minimal incision total hip arthroplasty. Orthop Clin North Am 35(2):131–136

3. Dorr LD, Hishiki Y et al. (2005) Development of imageless computer navigation for acetabular component position in total hip replacement. Iowa Orthop J 25:1–9

4. Hartzband MA (2004) Posterolateral minimal incision for total hip replacement: technique and early results. Orthop Clin North Am 35(2):119–129

5. Dalury DF, Dennis DA (2005) Minimal incision total knee arthroplasty can increase risk of component malalignment. Clin Orthop Relat Res 44:77–81

6. Nogler M (2004) Navigated minimal invasive total hip arthroplasty. Surg Technol Int 12:259–262

7. Ip D, Tsang WL et al. (2002) Comparison of two total knee prostheses on the incidence of patella clunk syndrome. Int Orthop 26(1):48–51

8. Ip D, Ko PS et al. (2004) Natural history and pathogenesis of the patella clunk syndrome. Arch Orthop Trauma Surg 124(9):597–602

9. Kim SJ, Wixson RL et al. (2005) Computer assisted navigation in total knee arthroplasty: improved coronal alignment. J Arthroplasty 20(7):123–131

10. Williams-Russo P, Sharrock NE et al. (1996) Randomized trial of epidural versus general anaesthesia: outcomes after primary total knee replacement. Clin Orthop Relat Res 331:199–208

11. Rathmell JP, Lair TR et al. (2005) The role of intrathecal drugs in the treatment of acute pain. Anesth Analg 101(5):S30–S43

12. Viscusi ER (2004) Emerging techniques in the treatment of postoperative pain. Am J Health Syst Pharm 61(1):S11–S14

13. Todkar M (2005) Sciatic nerve block causing heel ulcer after total knee arthroplasty. Acta Orthop Belg 71(6):724–725

14. Rasmussen GL, Steckner K et al. (2002) Intravenous parecoxin sodium for acute pain after orthopaedic knee surgery. Am J Orthop 31(6):336–343

15. Ganz SB, Levin AZ et al. (2003) Improvement in driving reaction time after total hip arthroplasty. Clin Orthop Relat Res 413:192–200

16. Stern SH, Fuchs MD et al. (1991) Sexual function after total hip arthroplasty. Clin Orthop Relat Res 269:228–235

17. Dennis M, Moffet H et al. (2006) Effectiveness of continuous passive motion and conventional physical therapy after total knee arthroplasty: a randomized clinical trial. Phys Ther 86(2):174–185

18. Mallon WJ, Liebelt RA et al. (1996) Total joint replacement and golf. Clin Sports Med 15(1):179–190

19. McMinn DJ, Daniel J et al. (2005) Mini-incision resurfacing arthroplasty of hip through the posterior approach. Clin Orthop Relat Res 441:91–98

20. Walker UA, Uhl M et al. (2006) Analgesic and disease modifying effects of interferential current in psoriatic arthritis. Rheumatol Int 26(10):904–907

Contents

15.1   General Introduction

15.1.1   Scope of the Problem

- Musculoskeletal pain, especially acute pain, is probably one of the most common presenting complaints seen not only by the orthopaedic surgeon, but also by the primary care physician
- It is estimated that the cost to US employers related to pain totals nearly $80 billion a year
- What is more important though is that there is evidence that orthopaedists tend to under-treat acute pain, according to recent studies, perhaps from the tradition of administering dosage of analgesics as needed

15.1.2   Introductory Comments

- Perhaps most individuals will consider pain as something "bad" because of the uncomfortable sensation it brings
- But one should look at pain from another viewpoint, which I termed: "the good, the bad and the ugly"

15.1.3   The Good, the Bad, and the Ugly

- Pain can be good sometimes because it helps to warn us against potential danger, such as when we step on sharp objects. An easy to understand example are those patients suffering from "congenital insensitivity to pain" – they tend to suffer multiple injuries including fractures and may have reduced longevity
- Pain can of course be bad, particularly if it turns chronic; there is increasing evidence that higher brain centres may take control and this can occur even if the initial insult or organic condition (if any) was settled, as we shall see in the discussion that follows
- Latter category will include a handful of patients that really do fake their symptoms in the quest for secondary gains or a few health professionals who underestimate the tremendous suffering of patients with chronic pain, which can lead to significant long-standing physiological as well as psychosocial effects

15.1.4   Pitfall in the Pattern of Emphasis of Pain Management

- It has been noted by the author that when experts talk about pain management in lectures, they talk about the reason being "the humanitarian need to cure pain". This sentence definitely has a very passive connotation – it gives the audience the idea that we treat pain as clinicians because it is only part of our obligation to our patient

■ Extremely few pain experts in fact stress the most important point and idea of pain management – which can be summarised in just four words: "to prevent chronic pain"

15.1.5 Key Concept

■ With advances in our knowledge of the nature of pain itself; the time is ripe for every clinician-scientist to stress the concept that the most important issue in pain management is to prevent chronic pain

■ This is because chronic pain is much more difficult to treat as the rest of this chapter will show. Once we achieve this end, other secondary gains will follow, i.e. fewer workers' compensation claims, less loss of revenue or work days. Prevention of chronic pain should be the main task of clinicians. If we can prevent acute pain (e.g. pre-emptive analgesia) so much the better. Certainly, our role is much more active than merely to "fulfil the humanitarian need to treat pain"

15.1.6 Other Reasons to Have Good Pain Management

■ Recent paper confirms a significant number of patients with postoperative pain (Apfelbaum et al., Anesth Analg 2003), and there is some suggestion that pain can sometimes be under-treated

■ It is common for patients receiving day surgery to be readmitted because of pain

■ Pain is one of the top health problems, costing employers in the USA nearly $80 billion a year (J Occup Environ Med 2003)

■ Proper pain treatment allows early mobilisation, preventing complications from associated immobility, and permits faster and earlier rehabilitation

■ Better patient satisfaction

15.2 Nature of Pain

15.2.1 Introduction

■ The reader will note there are many different definitions of pain

■ But the most popular definition is likely to be that of Merskey of the International Association for the Study of Pain

15.2.2 Definition of Pain

■ "Pain refers to an unpleasant sensory and emotional experience associated with actual or potential tissue damage, or described in terms of such damage"

15.2.3 Key Concept

■ Notice this definition of pain is good because:
  - It highlights that pain is very much a subjective experience
  - The definition puts equal weight on the sensory and emotional aspects
  - The definition implies that pain can potentially occur in the absence of actual tissue damage
  - The definition does not tie pain directly to an external stimulation of the nociceptors

15.2.4 Proposed Revised Definition

■ It is the author's opinion that the above definition can be bettered by adding a few qualifiers to make it more encompassing of the true state of affairs of what pain actually is

15.2.5 New Revised Definition

■ Pain refers to an unpleasant sensory and emotional experience (that may be associated with actual or feeling of potential tissue damage) and which is characterised frequently by special pain behaviour, the latter being determined by personal, physical and social context of the individual in question

15.2.6 Elaboration

■ Examples of personal factors: such as the patient's own beliefs and is affected by his mind and past learned experiences
■ Examples of physical factors: type and severity of the pathology
■ Examples of social factors: such as the behaviour and beliefs of his relatives and family

15.2.7 Examples of Importance of "Pain Behaviour" Especially in Chronic Pain

■ The well-known Waddell signs are in fact manifestations of "pain behaviour". It is perhaps unfair to immediately think of a non-organic cause of pain, even in the presence of some of these forms of pain behaviour

▪ Advanced CRPS (chronic regional pain syndrome) patients are known to have changes in the frontal lobe and bilateral limbic system with neuropsychiatric dysfunction, such as depressive and schizoaffective behaviours including even suicidal attempts if severe in some patients (Hooshmand, Chap. 9, in the book *Chronic Pain – Reflex Sympathetic Dystrophy*)

▪ Evidence from the fear-avoidance model of chronic pain (i.e. disability is largely determined by the erroneous belief that an increase in activity level is potentially harmful): recent research has found a relationship between self-reported disability and fear-avoidance beliefs, by demonstrating the relationship of fear of work to actual work-related behaviour (Vowles et al., Pain 2003)

15.2.8 Other Evidence in Support of and Practical Use of "Pain Behaviour" Assessment

▪ In a recent paper entitled: "Assessment of chronic pain behaviour: reliability of the method and its relationship with perceived disability, physical impairment and function", it was found that there was a strong correlation between pain behaviour (studied as a video-based assessment) and subjective pain report and disability. The author further concluded that pain and pain behaviour were the two most important determinants of self-reported disability (Koho et al., J Rehabil Med 2001)

▪ Certainly, further research on pain behaviour is very worthwhile

15.3 Pain Pathways

15.3.1 Summary

▪ Activation of peripheral nociceptors → activation of somatic pain sensory afferents in A-delta and C fibres → signal relayed to spinal cord → modulation at this level by "spinal gate" (see later discussion in Sect. 15.4.1) → signal relayed to higher brain centres (via various tracts to be discussed) → central processing and pain perception

▪ These processes have been termed "transduction, transmission, modulation, and perception" by previous workers like Ferrante. We will have further discussion on this simplistic model later when we discuss acute pain in detail

15.3.2   Nociceptors

- These pain-sensing peripheral receptors are present almost everywhere in the body (somatic and visceral) except the brain
- In the musculoskeletal system, they are present in skin, subcutaneous tissue, joints, bone, muscles and ligaments
- They can be depolarised by noxious stimuli, be it mechanical, thermal, or chemical

15.3.3   Spinal Grey Matter Cytoarchitectural Layout of Pain Fibres (According to Rexed)

- Afferents from muscles and deeper tissues end in Rexed laminae I, V, X
- Afferents from skin tend to terminate at Rexed laminae I, II and V at dorsal horn (J Contemp Neurol 1984)

15.3.4   Ascending Spinal Tracts Relaying Pain Information

- Spinothalamic tract
- Spinomesencephalic tract
- Spinoreticular tract
- Post-synaptic dorsal column fibres

15.3.4.1 Spinothalamic Tract

- The concept that pain is carried by anterolateral spinothalamic tract alone is rather over-simplified, since this is not the sole tract for the carriage of pain signal as taught in undergraduate medical school curriculum

15.3.4.2 Spinomesencephalic Tract

- This tract arises from the posterior horn and mainly ascends contralaterally
- Destination areas include tegmentum, periaqueductal grey matter, superior colliculus and cuneiform regions

15.3.4.3 Spinoreticular Tract

▧ This ascending tract has wide projections to areas of the brainstem (between medulla oblongata and the midbrain)

▧ Although the exact distribution still needs further research, there is evidence at least that points to the involvement of the reticular system of the brainstem in nociception (Physiol Rev 1987)

15.3.4.4 Post-Synaptic Dorsal Column Fibres

▧ The existence of this pathway, which was first described in 1968, was implicated by reports of pain abortion via commissural myelotomy (Exp Brain Res 1968)

▧ The destination of these fibres is unknown

15.4 Theories of Pain

15.4.1 Gate Theory of Pain (According to Melzack and Wall)

▧ The gate theory of pain was initially published in 1965 (with subsequent modification)

▧ Essentially, it states that pain is modulated at the level of the dorsal column of the spinal cord through a "gate" system, which can be "opened" or "closed" based on:
  - Peripheral (pattern of sensory afferent firing)
  - Supraspinal or central influences through the effect of the descending endogenous opiate system (DEOS; Melzack and Wall, Science 1965)

15.4.1.1 Modulation at the Spinal Level

▧ Normally, when peripheral nociceptors are stimulated, the evoked response travels through the smaller diameter C and A-delta afferents to the spinal cord, which are in turn relay to higher centres and perceived as pain via pain-transmitting cells (T-cells)

▧ Thus, it was observed that preferential activation of large diameter A-beta sensory afferents can activate inhibitory inter-neurones at substantia gelatinosa to close the spinal gate

15.4.1.2   Modulation from Cortex and Subcortical Areas

▪ This system originates from cortical and subcortical areas harbouring neurones capable of secreting opiate-like endorphins. These opiate-producing neurones are probably located at the periaqueductal grey matter and nucleus raphe magnus

▪ It is believed that firing of small-diameter sensory afferents can on the one hand depolarise T-cells, and on the other hand, activate a negative feedback loop that can cause inhibition of T-cells upon DEOS secretion of endorphins

15.4.1.3   Subsequent Modification of the "Gate Theory"

▪ Melzack and Wall subsequently published articles to include the modulating role of "cognition" in their gate theory of pain (Brain 1978)

15.4.1.4   What Exactly Have We Learned from the Gate Theory?

▪ According to Melzack's own words: "the gate theory's most important contribution to bio-medical science is to high-light the brain as the active system that filters, selects and modulates inputs. The dorsal horns, too, are not merely passive transmission stations but sites of dynamic action – inhibition, excitation, and modulation. The CNS is thus an essential component in the pain process (Melzack, Pain 1999)

15.4.1.4.1   Usefulness of Gate Theory to Explain Acute Pain

▪ The gate theory has been found to be a good model to explain many situations of acute pain

▪ It is, however, an overly simplistic model to explain chronic pain, which was the reason why Melzack came up with a subsequent neuromatrix theory

15.4.1.5   Examples of Evidence of Gate Theory Model to Assess Acute Pain

▪ Evidence of the existence of the DEOS pathways has been demonstrated in various studies via the use of the opiate antagonist naloxone (Clin J Pain 1985)

▪ An example will be abrupt cessation of pain relief from TENS application by the administration of naloxone

15.4.1.7   Other Examples

■ The well-known clinical phenomenon to most physicians or surgeons is the placebo response observed in some patients

■ This phenomenon may also be explained by the gate theory of pain, since the modified and updated model from Wall and Melzack brings to our attention the effect of cognition

15.4.1.8   Placebo Response

■ According to Wall, who is the neuro-anatomist who proposed the gate theory of pain together with Melzack, the placebo response may vary from 0–100%, and is likely to be stronger in those who have a deep desire to get well, i.e. the patient's own cognition or "expectancy". The placebo response will be described in detail shortly

15.4.2   New Model to Explain Chronic Pain: Neuromatrix Theory

■ Melzack theorises pain (especially chronic pain) as a multidimensional experience produced by patterns of nerve firing so-called "neurosignatures"

■ These originate from a widely distributed network called body-self neuromatrix

■ The activity of the neuromatrix is likely to be the prime mechanism for pain perpetuation (Melzack, Acta Anaesthesia Scand 1999; Melzack, Pain 1999)

15.4.2.1   Implication

■ Chronic pain arises from the output of a widely distributed neural network from the brain, as opposed to persistent peripheral sensory output evoked from sensory afferents

15.4.2.2   Modulating Factors of Neuromatrix

■ Melzack is of the opinion that the neuromatrix is modified by numerous factors:
  - Somatic sensory afferent firing
  - Individual's sensory experience
  - Possible genetic factors

15.4.2.3 But What Exactly is a "Neuromatrix"?

- Suggested reading is Melzack's view on phantom pain, to understand the concept of the new theory
- According to Melzack, the higher brain centres of our body perceive our body as a unity or "self". This comes about via a genetically built-in matrix of neurons for the whole body that can produce characteristic nerve-impulse patterns for the body and the myriad of somatosensory qualities we can feel
- Melzack termed the above network, whose synaptic links are initially determined genetically and sculpted by sensory input in later life, the "neuromatrix"

15.4.2.4 Possible Evidence in Support of the Neuromatrix Theory

- Recent reports from brain research units have found altered central sensorimotor processing in patients with chronic pain, such as in those with complex regional pain syndrome (Pain 2002)
- Decrease in psychomotor speed in chronic LBP patients vs. healthy controls (Percept Mot Skills 1998; Spine 1999), and diminished attention processing capacity was demonstrated again in chronic pain cases (Veldhuijzen, Pain 2006)

15.4.2.5 Altered Sensorimotor Processing and Cognition in Chronic LBP

- There are obviously two sides of the coin: it may be argued that these changes occur secondary to chronic pain affecting the patient (e.g. causing depression), rather than as possible evidence to support the neuromatrix theory
- However, if future research finds that these same brain changes occur in the majority of chronic pain (e.g. LBP) patients including those with adequate coping mechanisms and no depression, etc., then the evidence in such a circumstance will seem to be more in favour of the neuromatrix theory

15.4.3 Mechanisms and Importance of the "Placebo Effect" and "Nocebo Effects"

15.4.3.1 Introduction

- Despite the well-known fact that the placebo effect can have a profound effect on pain, it is not always discussed at length in every book chapter on musculoskeletal pain of orthopaedic texts
- However, study of the placebo effect can throw much light on pain treatment and is very important
- The placebo effect works on the phenomenon of "expectancy", i.e. the individual's brain expects there will be a response to treatment (Crow et al., Health Technol Assess 1999)

15.4.3.2 Terminology

- Concerning the subject of "expectancy" – just as the individual's brain can have positive expectation, i.e. possible placebo effect, sometimes the brain can have negative expectation, i.e. "nocebo effect", when the brain expects no effect from the treatment and/or with elements of uncertainties (Barsky et al., J Am Med Assoc 2002)
- Some therefore proposed a more encompassing term called "a meaning response" to include both these positive and negative effects that the individual's mind can have on the response to treatment (Brody et al., Adv Mind Body Med 2000)

15.4.3.3 Factors That Can Contribute to Producing Placebo vs Nocebo Effects

- What the patient expects the treatment will bring – preconceptions and beliefs, the effect of "meaning" or meaningfulness. An example will be prior exposure to a related medication that did or did not work for the patient
- Conditioning effect – e.g. if every time the patient had relief of pain after an electrical stimulation by application of an analgesic ointment, after some time, even giving an inert ointment can produce pain relief, this is an example of conditioned placebo response (Voudouris et al., Pain 1989)
- Expectancy effect – as a continuation of the conditioning effect, Kirsch et al. added another treatment arm to the experiment whereby individuals were told that the intensity of the electrical stimulation

would be lowered to assess the effect of the ointment. The result was a significant lowering of the placebo action; hence, it can be seen that even a conditioned effect can be altered by expectancy (Kirsch et al., Pain 1997)

15.4.3.4 What Research Has Been Done on the Mechanisms of the Placebo Effect?

■ Besides the above-mentioned studies on conditioning, other studies have revealed that:

- The brain's dopamine system is concerned with the stimulus associated with "expectancy" of a reward (Schultz, J Neurophysiol 1998), as does the associated "behaviour" of reward seeking (Philips et al., Nature 2003)
- The associated behavioural flexibility and attention is also linked to the brain's norepinephrine system (Aston-Jones et al., Biol Psychiatry 1999)
- The serotonin system has also been implicated in placebo analgesia, while the important component of the dopaminergic system – the anterior cingulate – becomes activated by placebo. In fact, Petrovic showed in the highly regarded journal *Science* that placebo and opioid analgesia have shared neuronal networking (Petrovic et al., Science 2002)
- The anterior cingulate is related to memory and cognition, as well as action/behaviour feedback (Botvinick et al., Nature 1999)
- In fact, the latest theory on the mechanism of placebo analgesia involves rACC (rostral anterior cingulated cortex) recruitment and enhanced functional connectivity of the rACC with subcortical brain structures crucial for conditioned learning, as well as descending inhibition of nociception (Bingel et al., Pain 2006)
- Patients with severe cancer pain for instance have recently been reported to benefit from stereotactic cingulotomy by turning the brain's attention and memory away from pain perception (according to Abdelaziz and Cosgrove 2002, in their chapter in *Surgical Management of Pain*)

15.4.3.5 Relevance of Studying the Placebo Effect in Orthopaedics

■ Understanding the placebo (or nocebo effects) potentially aids understanding of the effect of "centralisation" of chronic pain. The recent finding of sharing of neural networking between opioid and placebo analgesia reported in the journal *Science* is of particular interest

- We should remind ourselves that what the patient expects from our treatment (i.e. the personal context) has a large bearing on the outcome of our treatment. Realisation of the presence of nocebo effect is important in clinical practice
- The placebo effect should be taken into account in our design of study and be used as a treatment arm in many therapeutic interventions to avoid bias (e.g. use of sham needles in a study to investigate the effects of acupuncture)
- It is the author's view that this and related research on the subject lend further support to the mind–body interaction in medicine

15.4.3.6 Summarising the Light Shed by the Above Studies on Pain Mechanisms

- Widespread dopaminergic, serotoninergic, and norepinephrine circuits are confirmed with the placebo effect
- The important part of the dopamine system or anterior cingulate is not only activated by placebo effect, but modulates behaviour and memory, and attention
- There is evidence to suggest that opioid and placebo analgesia share common neuronal networking. The above circuitry may well be at least partly responsible in the process of centralisation in chronic pain pending further scientific research

15.4.3.7 Is This of Relevance to the Neuromatrix Theory We Just Discussed?

- The several brain systems that produce non-specific, rather generalised brain function modulation with links to the placebo effect listed below may well be involved to some extent by dint of its association with the limbic system, and with the current realisation that negative thinking like nocebo effect can also have influence on the brain, viz.:
  - Diffuse neurotransmitter projection systems and non-specific thalamocortical projection originating from basal forebrain to the rostral pons
  - Among these, the dopamine system of the brain (consisting mainly of the mesocorticolimbic, tuberoinfundibular and nigrostriatal pathways) is more related to presence of a reward

- Other systems include the serotonin system (whose cell bodies are located in a series of nuclei in upper pons and midbrain known as the raphe nuclei) as well as the norepinephrine system (located mainly at the locus ceruleus and tractus solitarius) linked to attention and behavioural flexibility (Aston-Jones et al., Biol Psychiatry 1999). It seems plausible, therefore, that the frequent finding of psychomotor and behavioural retardation in patients (see Chap. 16 on LBP) may well have some relationship with these systems
- The links to memory and emotional response of the placebo effect to the anterior cingulate (with its connection to the limbic system) help us understand that suffering from pain perception can be minimised by developing a lack of emotion and attention by the brain to the pain perception, thus adding a new dimension to our option of managing chronic pain by, for instance, stereotactic cingulotomy (according to Abdelaziz and Cosgrove 2002)

▦ (NB: to recapitulate a little on the topic of neuroanatomy – the hypothalamus is the centre of many endocrine and autonomic controls besides exerting influence on the behavioural outcome/aspects of one's emotion and affect, it is the "limbic lobe" (i.e. consisting of the para-hippocampal gyrus, cingulate gyrus, and lastly the subcallosal gyrus, which encircles the hypothalamus) that provides the circuitry through which emotional impulses from the hypothalamus could reach the cortex and vice versa via the Papez circuit; Kandel, Sci Am 1992)

15.4.3.8 Key Lesson to Learn

▦ When clinicians talk about "pain", what crosses their mind usually includes:
- Is it nociceptive or neuropathic?
- Is there centralisation?
- Is there associated psychosocial disturbance?

▦ However, the above and other basic science research studies reveal there is another a new dimension that is often not talked about, which is one that we may use in future to tackle chronic pain

▦ The new dimension to circumventing pain is to make the brain not pay attention to the pain, i.e. pain is still perceived, but there can be ways to tackle the brain pathways so that the brain itself ignores the perception. If this can be achieved, then not only will it relieve chronic suffering, it may even help to prevent the brain to "memorise" or effect further neuroplastic response expected of the centralisation process we talked about

▨ It is the view of the author that the recent finding of shared common neuronal networking between opioid and placebo analgesia reported in *Science* is important and warrants further research to elucidate the mechanism of "centralisation" in chronic pain patients

15.5   Classification of Pain

15.5.1 By Neurophysiologic Mechanism

▨ Nociceptive origin: somatic or visceral
▨ Non-nociceptive:
  – Neuropathic: peripheral or central (e.g. SCI)
  – Psychogenic
▨ To this, the author adds another group:
  – Unknown, e.g. many chronic LBP patients who have identified no source of nociceptive stimulus, with no nerve injury and no psychogenic factor can be grouped as having an "unknown" mechanism (further discussion on this point will be pursued in the Chap. 16 on LBP)

15.5.2 By Timing

▨ Acute
▨ Chronic
▨ P.S.: this classification is useful in many clinical situations, but in certain cases like LBP patients, the author suggests the addition of a third category: "acute-on-chronic". This is of use firstly to differentiate the really "acute" group from those who represent exacerbations of chronic LBP since the prognosis is very different, and secondly, it is good for research purposes since by mixing these two groups and labelling them "acute" we will have a heterogenous mix while studying the efficacy of different treatment modalities for "acute LBP" for instance

15.5.3   By IASP (International Association for the Study of Pain)

▥ In the revised version in 1994, this classification, which aims to standardise pain syndrome descriptions, consists of five axes, thus:
  – Axis I: anatomical region
  – Axis II: organ system
  – Axis III: temporal characteristics
  – Axis IV: patient's assessment of onset and intensity
  – Axis V: aetiology

15.5.4   Another Classification Suitable for Chronic Pain

▥ One useful classification particularly suited to patients with chronic pain is the "Emory Pain Estimate" model proposed by Brena in 1984

15.5.4.1   Emory Pain Estimate Model

▥ Essentially a 2-D strategy, with the following permutations:
  – Low pathology, high behavioural disturbance
  – Low pathology, low behavioural disturbance
  – High pathology, high behavioural disturbance
  – High pathology, low behavioural disturbance

15.5.4.1.1   Low Pathology, High Behavioural Disturbance

▥ These patients may have an element of symptom exaggeration
▥ High verbalisation
▥ Occasional drug or substance abuse

15.5.4.1.2   Low Pathology, Low Behavioural Disturbance

▥ These patients tend to have no/little identifiable pathology and rather ill-defined complaints

15.5.4.1.3   High Pathology, High Behavioural Disturbance

▥ These patients do have pathology
▥ But their adoption of sick role is at the same time quite dominant or significant

15.5.4.1.4   High Pathology, Low Behavioural Disturbance

▥ These individuals have organic pathology and know how to cope well with their condition

15.6   Further Analysis of Different Categories of Pain Causation

15.6.1   Nociceptive Pain

15.6.1.1 Importance of Nociceptive Pain
▓ Orthopaedic surgeons frequently manage patients with fractures and soft tissue damage, these are all usually mediated by peripheral nociceptors
▓ The same mechanism is also the cause of postoperative pain
▓ Pain management is very important as far as patient satisfaction goes, the following discussion will be looking at the body's response to this acute tissue damage

15.6.1.2 Nociceptor Activation
▓ Tissue damage will activate peripheral nociceptors
▓ The pain pathways after nociceptive firing have just been discussed
▓ But the acute cascade that follows tissue damage is far from that straight forward, as the following discussion will reveal

15.6.1.3 Concomitant Release of "Sensitising Soup" of Inflammatory Mediators
▓ After tissue damage or surgical trauma, a host of local inflammatory mediators will be released, e.g. histamine, prostaglandins, H^+ ions, bradykinins, cytokines, nitric oxide, leukotrienes, norepinephrine, etc.
▓ The admixture of mediators is collectively frequently called the "sensitising soup"
▓ The sensitising soup will generate inflammatory response that serves to amplify and prolong pain

15.6.1.4 Resultant Peripheral Sensitisation
▓ This refers to the local amplification of the inflammatory response effected by the sensitising soup
▓ In short, there is altered sensitivity of the nociceptors

15.6.1.5 Resultant Central Sensitisation
▓ This refers to amplification of the inflammatory response when mediators act on the CNS, causing thus "central sensitisation"
▓ This process is important and will be discussed in some detail

15.6.1.6   Mechanism of Central Sensitisation

Involves processes like:

- The primary processing of nociceptive information occurs in the dorsal horn of the spinal cord
- Nociceptive afferents trigger the release of glutamate (and other substances like substance P)
- Glutamate acts on N-methyl-D-aspartate receptors. Activation of these receptors plays a key role in neuronal sensitisation, a process that may underlie chronic painful states (Prog Neurobiol 1999)

15.6.1.7   Other Changes

Reduction of inhibitory inter-neuron tone in dorsal horn further enhances nociception

It is now realised that for transmission of nociceptive information to the brain, pathways other than the classic spinothalamic tract are involved. An example is the post-synaptic dorsal column pathway (see discussion of dorsal column stimulation under Sect. 15.6.2.14.11)

15.6.1.8   "Spinal Cord Wind-Up"

A term used by anaesthesiologists to describe the active central sensitisation process going on at the spinal cord. The spinal cord is now increasingly being recognised to be a very important pain-modulating organ in the body

Clinically, once central hyper-excitability ensues, the dose of analgesics like morphine to tackle pain will be higher. Whereas even giving a small dose of morphine was found by Woolf to be adequate to prevent central excitability

15.6.1.9   State of Hyperalgesia

Due to the release of multiple inflammatory mediators, there is amplification and a state of hypersensitivity to pain, described as "hyperalgesia"

15.6.1.10   "Primary" Hyperalgesia

Primary hyperalgesia refers to heightened pain sensitivity at the site of the tissue trauma or surgery, e.g. a smaller stimulus at the injured site is already adequate to generate pain perception

- One should avoid labelling the primary hyperalgesia effect as exaggeration on the part of the patient

15.6.1.11 "Secondary" Hyperalgesia

- Secondary hyperalgesia refers to a state of hypersensitivity in the nearby tissues, e.g. can sometimes produce allodynia
- Thus, in some cases, stimulation of nearby sites (not the original injury site) can have a lowered pain threshold, i.e. stimulus that usually will not produce pain can cause pain perception
- One should exercise caution not to label patients with allodynia as over-exaggerating. (The mechanism of the phenomenon of "hyperalgesia" has been described in Prog Neurobiol by Treede and is outside the scope of this book)

15.6.1.12 If Unchecked, Can Lead to Chronic Pain

- Chronic pain will be discussed later in this chapter
- Suffice it to say here that one of the difficulties in treating chronic pain is that the areas of the CNS affected or implicated are much wider. If left untreated or poorly treated, can even lead to structural changes in the CNS (a manifestation of neuroplasticity) and there is now evidence to suggest the newly altered circuitry might be "memorised" by our CNS

15.6.1.13 A Word About Neuronal Plasticity

- Neurons in our CNS have a capacity to change their connectivity, chemical profile, and hence function. This neuronal plasticity is believed to contribute to the altered sensitivity to pain just discussed
- Central sensitisation, if left untreated, can thus produce structural instead of functional changes

15.6.1.14 Strategies to Abort These Acute Changes

- These strategies will be discussed; they involve e.g. multimodal analgesia, pre-emptive analgesia

15.6.2   Neuropathic Pain

15.6.2.1   Introduction
▦ Included in this category are pains arising from damage to sensory fibres, or from the CNS itself and are frequently known as "neuropathic pain", examples are:
  – Spinal cord injury (SCI)
  – Injury to the peripheral nervous system (PNS), e.g. brachial plexus injury, or peripheral nerve damage

15.6.2.2   Features of Neuropathic Pain
▦ Described as a burning sensation
▦ Like electric-shock or lightning
▦ Pins and needles

15.6.2.3   Mechanism Causing Persistence of Neuropathic Pain
▦ Ectopic or aberrant activity
▦ Cross-excitation
▦ Neuronal hyper-excitability and other mechanisms

15.6.2.3.1   Ectopic Impulse Firing
▦ This ectopic firing occurs because proteins from cell body to distal axons are obstructed, or in other words, obstructed axoplasmic flow results in heightened excitability of these nerve injury sites
▦ Location of ectopic impulse need not always be the stump, can be at dorsal root ganglion, or sites of myelin injuries
▦ The origin of these ectopic impulses may involve partial axonal or perineural pathology that results in spontaneous firing
▦ Neuropathic pain can occur without peripheral lesions and can be produced by a variety of central lesions (e.g. spinal cord injury, sometimes in stroke)

15.6.2.3.2   Cross-Excitation
▦ Cross-excitation can occur in the presence of damaged myelin, owing to loss of insulation among the neurons

15.6.2.3.3   Neuronal Hyper-Excitability and Other Mechanisms

- Neuronal hyperexcitability is one of the hallmarks of neuropathic pain
- Other findings may include loss of inhibition at the level of CNS, and catecholamine hypersensitivity

15.6.2.4   Central Sensitisation Process

- This can occur when:
  - The heightened neural response to nociception input persists after the initial stimulus is gone
  - This phenomenon is more likely to occur when the intensity of the initial neural input to CNS was very high (Pain 1991)

15.6.2.5   Extent of the "Central" Sensitisation Changes

- Areas that can be affected are wide, e.g.:
  - Cerebral cortex
  - Thalamus
  - Brainstem
  - Dorsal horn of the spinal cord

15.6.2.6   Evidence That Higher Brain Centres Are Involved

- A good piece of evidence comes from the observation that sectioning the pain-carrying tracts of the spinal cord fails to relieve pain after the process of centralisation

15.6.2.7   Cellular-Molecular Reflection of the Central Sensitisation Process

- Manifestations at the cellular level:
  - Increased spontaneous firing of neurons
  - Increase after discharge to stimuli
  - Increased degree of response to stimuli
  - Increased receptive field (thus even nearby areas are sensitised)
- Manifestations at the molecular-receptor level:
  - Release of neuropeptides: acting via protein kinase to increase cellular activity
  - Release of glutamate: acts through gated ionic channels, e.g. NMDA receptors and G-protein receptors, with resultant elevated intracellular Ca^{++}

15.6.2.8   Neuroplasticity Phenomenon

▦ This refers to the observation that prolonged "centralisation" can cause structural and connectivity alterations

▦ Examples include altered connectivity, phenotypic changes in non-nociceptive neurons, and pattern of discharge

▦ Some even like the changes in connectivity to those reminiscent of the process of learning and memory

15.6.2.9   Key Concept 1

▦ Prolonged centralisation not only affects the physiology of CNS, but structure as well, e.g. new synapses, reconnect and growth of A-beta fibres to C-fibre territory, etc.

▦ The extent of CNS changes can be far greater than those parts of the central neuronal structures sub-serving the damaged neurological structure

15.6.2.10   Key Concept 2

▦ Please note that the phenomenon of centralisation can occur in the setting of either nociceptive or neuropathic type of pain

15.6.2.11   Key Concept 3: Management

▦ After "centralisation" has occurred, treatment is much more difficult

▦ Treatment should be aimed at both central and peripheral anomalies

15.6.2.12   Principles of a More Rational Pharmacological Approach

▦ Agents to tackle ectopic activity: anticonvulsants, sodium/calcium channel blockers

▦ Tackling loss of inhibition and/or descending facilitation: opioids, antidepressants, alpha-2 agonists, GABA agonists

▦ Agents to tackle centralisation: glutamate receptor antagonist, calcium channel modulators

15.6.2.12.1 Common Agents Used in Neuropathic Pain

▦ GABA-ergic agents

▦ NMDA antagonist

▦ Anticonvulsants

▦ Antidepressants

▦ Opioids

- Local anaesthetics
- Alpha-2 agonist
- NSAIDs
- Others

Antidepressants

- Include tertiary and secondary amines and can be used as first-line treatment in neuropathic pain
- Tertiary amines act to decrease reuptake of serotonin and NE at spinal cord brainstem and dorsal horn nuclei receptors. Secondary amines mostly decrease reuptake of NE
- Other possible mechanisms include: alpha blockade, anticholinergic and antihistamine action, reuptake inhibition of dopamine, effects on GABA-B and adenosine, Na-channel blockade, as well as NMDA-receptor antagonism (Jackson, Pain Practice 2006)
- Secondary amines (e.g. desipramine) appear to have fewer side effects than tertiary amines when used as analgesics in neuropathic pain (McQuay et al., Pain 1996)
- Previous reviews found antidepressants mainly useful in post-herpetic neuralgia and DM neuropathy. But it can be effective in CRPS (Harden, Am J Phys Med Rehabil 2005)

Newer Antidepressants

- These are the selective serotonin reuptake inhibitors (SSRI). These tend to be less effective in neuropathic pain, but have fewer side effects (Stacey, Am J Phys Med Rehabil 2005)
- An example of SSRI is duloxetine

Anticonvulsants

- Agents studied previously in papers include carbamazepine, gabapentin, phenytoin, lamotrigine and pregabalin
- Gabapentin is effective in DM neuropathy and post-herpetic neuralgia (JAMA 1998)
- Anticonvulsants in general like gabapentin and carbamazepine are useful also in CRPS (Am J Phys Med Rehabil 2005)
- Carbamazepine and phenytoin, if used, need serum level monitoring
- Gabapentin can have side effects of fatigue, drowsiness and the first dose administration should be at bedtime

Opioids

- Opioids are now regarded as one option in neuropathic pain, despite previous suggestions that they should be used for nociceptive pain (Rowbotham et al., N Engl J Med 2003)
- However, it remains a fact that their efficacy in nociceptive pain surpasses their effect on neuropathic pain
- The reason being that nerve injury induces downregulation of mu-opiate receptors in primary sensory neurons, their central terminals and post-synaptic spinal targets (Kohno et al., Pain 2005)
- Oxycodone, morphine and methadone have been used in phantom pain, post-herpetic neuralgia, and DM neuropathy
- Even tramadol has been used in neuropathic pain for its action on mu-opioid receptors and weak reuptake inhibition of norepinephrine and serotonin (Harati et al., Neurology 1998)

Local Anaesthetics

- Lidocaine as a 5% patch has literature support in neuropathic pain including CRPS (Backonja, Pain Med 2004) as it inhibits Na channels
- Other agents: clonidine (act on presynaptic alpha-2 receptors inhibiting NE release) or ketamine, which works by NMDA antagonism, and capsaicin, by depletion of substance P at unmyelinated C-fibres (Jackson, Pain Pract 2006)
- Systemic administration of these agents has also been recorded, e.g. systemic lidocaine and baclofen; the former via a decrease in C-fibre activity, while the latter via GABA-B agonist action

Steroids and NSAIDs

- There is some evidence to support steroid use in CRPS (Harden, Am J Phys Med Rehabil 2005)
- NSAIDs are mostly used in the literature for nociceptive pain. In fact, most neuropathic pain is resistant to NSAIDs

Combined Treatment

- Combination of different agents are sometimes needed in refractory cases and sometimes to avoid intolerable side effects

15.6.2.13   Phantom Limb Pain in Amputees

15.6.2.13.1 Introduction
- Phantom limb pain should be differentiated from phantom sensation; the latter is almost universal within 1 month of surgery (especially in UL above elbow amputee) and does not need treatment, the former occurs less frequently and is more common with proximal amputations

15.6.2.13.2 Phantom Sensation vs Phantom Limb Pain
- It should be noted that almost every amputee reports that they can feel sensation that seems to originate from the missing limb, a phenomenon known as "phantom limb sensation"
- But a much smaller proportion of amputees experience painful sensation from the phantom, which if present is called "phantom limb pain"

15.6.2.13.3 Nature of the Phantom Sensation
- Time course – most occur within 1 month of surgery
- Have feeling that the whole or part of the limb still exists (the latter condition called telescoping if the mid-portion sensation of the phantom is missing), there may be associated mild sensation of warmth or tingling, but not pain

15.6.2.13.4 Differential Diagnosis of Increasing Phantom Pain
- Can be part and parcel of the phantom limb pain condition getting worse
- CRPS
- Trigger areas etc. that may exacerbate pre-existing phantom limb pain
- Some are in fact stump wound complications
- Disease recurrence (e.g. if underlying disease is cancer)

15.6.2.13.5 Differential Diagnosis of Phantom Limb Pain from Stump Pain
- Phantom limb pain is believed to originate from neurons in the nociceptive pathways (supplying the affected limb) becoming overly active (or sometimes at higher centres)
- Usual causes of stump pain include:
  - Neuroma

- Bony prominence
- Poorly fitting prosthesis
- Nerve compression or neuropathy
- Wound complications, e.g. infection, breakdown

15.6.2.13.6 Management Options

▦ Pharmacological manipulation: just discussed (Sect. 15.6.2.12.1)

▦ Physiotherapy options discussed in Chap. 2

▦ Since patients with severe phantom limb pain frequently have cortical re-organisations (see ensuing discussion in Sect. 15.6.2.13.7), options like hypnosis, use of biofeedback (to be discussed in Sect. 15.6.2.13.9) and mirror (according to Lundborg from Sweden) have all been described. First we take a look at the changes in the cerebral cortex before talking about biofeedback

15.6.2.13.7 Changes in the Nervous System After Amputation

▦ After amputation, deafferentation occurs

▦ Those central neurons that receive information from the previously existent body part become unusually active

▦ Subsequent maladaptive changes in the thalamus and spinal cord may occur

▦ Severe cases of phantom limb pain are frequently associated with evidence of massive cortical reorganisation (Neurosci News 1998)

15.6.2.13.8 Melzack's View of Phantom Limb Pain (Pain 1999)

▦ The phantom can feel so real because the body that we normally feel is sub-served by the same neural processes in the brain. Although these processes can be modulated by peripheral inputs, they can act in its absence

▦ The origin of these topographical patterns probably lies in the brain; hence, suitable stimuli may trigger the patterns, but will not produce them

▦ The body is perceived by the brain as a unity or "self" and the perception occurs in higher brain centres as opposed to cord or peripheral nervous system

▦ The above brain processes are built-in by genetic specification, despite to some extent being modifiable by experience. The above concepts of

Melzack sow the seeds of his new "neuromatrix" theory, which is mentioned in Sect. 15.4.2

15.6.2.13.9 Use of Biofeedback
- Phantom limb pain (PLP) is a noxious, painful sensation that is perceived to occur in an amputated limb. It has been reported to occur in up to half of amputees
- A recent study provided some support for the use of biofeedback in the treatment of PLP and indicated the need for further definitive study (Harden et al., Appl Psychophysiol Biofeedback 2005)

15.6.2.14   Complex Regional Pain Syndrome

15.6.2.14.1 Terminology
- Previous terms of RSD and causalgia were replaced by CRPS Types I and II by IASP in 1994
- Type I CRPS: not associated with known nerve injury
- Type II CRPS: associated with known nerve injury

15.6.2.14.2 Aetiology
- As stated, Type II CRPS is associated with neural injury, e.g. chemical burns, post-herpetic neuralgia, SCI, etc.
- Type I can be associated with various aetiologies such as:
    - Trauma (e.g. Colles fracture)
    - Disturbed microcirculation (e.g. as in diabetes mellitus)
    - Associated with myocardial infarction (shoulder-hand syndrome)
    - Rarer: association with tumours, cervical spine pathology

15.6.2.14.3 Typical Symptomatology
- Allodynia
- Burning pain
- Temperature changes
- Colour changes
- Oedema
- Joint stiffness
- Trophic changes like hair loss

15.6.2.14.4 Key Concept
- Although IASP divided CRPS into Type I and Type II (previously called causalgia)
- The symptomatology of presentation are essentially the same for the two types

15.6.2.14.5 Main Stages
- Hyperaemic stage
- Dystrophic stage
- Atrophic stage

Hyperaemic Stage
- Also called acute stage, can occur anywhere within days or weeks post-injury, and lasts from weeks to months
- Refer to Sect. 15.6.2.14.3 for typical symptoms
- Can proceed to next stage if neglected

Dystrophic Stage
- Here, the extremity becomes stiff, cold, oedematous, may be associated muscle wasting and functional limitation, pain may worsen

Atrophic Stage
- Element of irreversibility is high at the atrophic stage
- Joint stiffness may become worse as may weakness

15.6.2.14.6 Differential Diagnosis
- Peripheral vascular disease (PVD)
- Thoracic outlet syndrome
- Raynaud's syndrome
- Carpal tunnel syndrome (CTS)
- Scleroderma

15.6.2.14.7 Diagnosis
- Clinical – only accurate if in Stage 2 or 3, need to look for orthostatic hypotension, and effect of Valsalva manoeuvre
- Thermography – can make diagnosis earlier
- Capillary blood cell velocity
- Bone scan

- Stellate ganglion block
- Laser Doppler fluxmetry
- Others: skin conductance response, quantitative sweat autonomic response test (MRI: sometimes used to rule out other conditions)

15.6.2.14.8 Key Concept
- The key to success in managing CRPS is early diagnosis and management
- While this may be true in many diseases, this is particularly relevant in conditions like CRPS
- Notice that in chronic end-stage disease, the patient may end up not only depressed, but may even have suicidal tendency

15.6.2.14.9 Role of Thermography
- Useful in early diagnosis of CRPS, and in some atypical presentations such as cervical CRPS
- Infrared telethermography can detect subtle temperature changes in different parts of the skin; it is a very sensitive test
- It is best to limit the diagnosis of CRPS in the presence of ≥ 1.5 to $2\,^{\circ}C$ difference (according to Hooshmand)

15.6.2.14.10 Thermography Compared with Bone Scan
- Bone scan is probably second best in diagnosis, but it is unreliable in very early disease, and tends to be very non-specific
- Most show an initial increase followed by decrease in activity on the scan for the body part affected by CRPS

15.6.2.14.11 Management
- Prevention: most important
- Treatment options:
  - Remove precipitating factors
  - Optimise drug treatment
  - Nerve blocks
  - Role of surgery, e.g. sympathectomy
  - Role of other procedures like SC stimulation

Prevention
   Index of suspicion
   Avoiding unnecessary surgery
   Avoiding some medications
   General advice

Things to Avoid

   Some drugs can potentially subject the patient to extra risk of CRPS: including alcohol (affects temperature regulation, significant intake destroys dopamine, serotonin and other neurotransmitters); narcotics like opioids; and abuse of substances like cocaine
   CRPS can be made worse sometimes by unnecessary surgery, well documented in the literature. Proceed only if absolutely essential
   Index of suspicion is needed in order to diagnose the condition early as the response to treatment is much affected by late (>6-month) diagnosis
   In our orthopaedic patients, the general encouragement of early use of the limb, early weight-bearing and active rehabilitation help prevent CRPS

Treatment Options

Drugs

   Examples of common agents used include:
   – Antidepressants (e.g. trazodone)
   – Alpha-2 blockers (e.g. yohimbine), alpha-1 blockers (e.g. terazosin), and beta-blockers (e.g. timolol)
   – Calcium channel blockers (counteract NE), e.g. nifedipine

Nerve Blocks

   Can be useful if administered early, e.g. stellate ganglion block (diagnostic and therapeutic)
   Need to prescribe active physiotherapy as an adjunctive treatment

Adjunctive Measures

   Active physiotherapy both at home and during training sessions
   Encourage the use of the affected body part
   Withdrawal of alcohol, and drugs like benzodiazepines, barbiturates, and graduated withdrawal of opioids

Surgery

- Sympathectomy, even if performed, does not always work, e.g. from persistent sympathetically maintained pain via the efferent sympathetic system coupled with associated supersensitive end organs to NE from alpha-1 receptor hypersensitivity (Drummond et al., Brain 1991) under which circumstance even alpha-2 blockers will not work
- Sympathectomy has the side effect of affecting the temperature regulation process
- Other invasive procedures like tractotomy, rhizotomy are usually not effective in CRPS (according to Hooshmand)

Other Reported Measures in Refractory Patients

- We will consider the option of dorsal column stimulation, which sometimes may work and is reserved for patients refractory to treatment
- Some patients noted diminished effect from dorsal column stimulation after an initial response, however

Drug Efficacy for Refractory CRPS

- At present, no analgesic drug totally relieves cases of chronic, resistant, neuropathic pain without producing significant unwanted side effects (Tulgar, Adv Ther 1992)
- This is one reason to consider options like electrical stimulation in refractory cases

Use of Intrathecal Bupivacaine in Refractory Pain from CRPS-I

- The subgroup of patients with refractory CRPS is difficult to treat
- A recent attempt by Lundborg to use intrathecal bupivacaine is reported to show efficacy in pain relief, but did not have any effect on allodynia, oedema and trophic changes (Acta Anaesthesiol Scand 1999)

Spinal Cord (Dorsal Column) Stimulation for Pain Relief

Introduction

- Dorsal column stimulation (DCS; sometimes just referred to as "spinal cord stimulation") has received considerable interest as an armamentarium in some patients suffering from chronic refractory pain including CRPS-I and failed back syndrome
- Although the mechanism is not entirely known, progress has been made in this interesting and important field

Terminology

In the past, it was commented on in one chapter of the famous text written by Wall and Melzack that: "…. It seems more appropriate to use the term 'spinal cord stimulation' rather than 'dorsal column stimulation'… that the actual neural tissue stimulated by the electrodes is unknown"

Argument for Retaining the Term Dorsal Column Stimulation
(Author's View)

Spinal cord stimulation as a method of pain relief can only be rendered effective when appropriate dorsal column fibres in the spinal cord are stimulated

Recent research indicates clearly that dorsal column nuclei can participate in persistent pain processes (Schwark et al., Brain Res 2001)

Mechanism of Action of Dorsal Column Spinal Cord Stimulation

The complete mechanism has not been elucidated

But the dorsal column nuclei were implicated in perpetuating the process of pain in recent research

In fact, based on the anatomical connections, the dorsal column nuclei may contribute to thalamic changes in persistent pain, as well as supraspinal centres that modulate pain transmission in the spinal cord (Brain Res 2001)

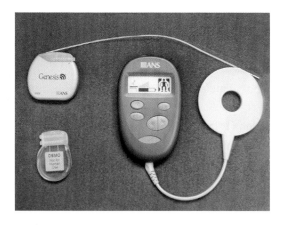

Fig. 15.1. A typical set-up of spinal cord stimulation with accessories

Comparison with Placebo

Experiments in human placebo controlled studies reveal that:
- DCS significantly alters pain transmission in humans, although the magnitude is sometimes not great
- The effect is not dependent on placebo
- DCS modulation of pain perception is not due to a general change in attention (Marchand et al., Pain 1991)

Administration

- Epidural electrode insertion performed under LA, with continuous verbal contact with the patient during surgery
- Select the final position of the electrode tip as determined by electrical stimulation. Carefully adjust electrode till the induced paresthesia corresponds to area of pain
- For painful UL conditions, the electrode tip is usually at low cervical or high thoracic position. The mid to high cervical levels are avoided to prevent changes in stimulation intensity during head motion
- The usual level of the electrode tip for LL conditions is usually in the low thoracic region
- The patient usually wears an external device for 1 week; if tolerated and effective, internalise the device

When to Abort the Procedure

- DCS fails to elicit paresthesia at the site of pain
- DCS causing intolerance and/or very unpleasant sensation in the patient
- Local conditions (e.g. sepsis) of the back contraindicating an epidural

Clinical Use

- Indications where the available evidence is stronger:
  - CRPS
  - Neuropathic pain
    (Anaesth Intensive Care 2004)
- Occasionally indicated (evidence less strong):
  - Failed back surgery syndrome (need careful patient selection)
- Other recent reported indications:
  - Cortical limb ischaemia
  - Vascular disorders, angina
  - Even movement disorders (Adv Ther 1992)

Drawbacks
- Invasive procedure
- A few patients have unpleasant sensation, sometimes more than their pain
- Limited paresthesia coverage (Holsheimer, Neurosurg 1997)

Elaboration on the Role of Paresthesia Coverage
- In DCS, it should be noted that the pain is only alleviated when the electrically induced paresthesia covers the painful area, meaning that the induced input to the fast-fibre system should be identical to the chronic pain input (Krainick, Surg Neurol 1975)

15.6.2.15   Newer Advances in Refractory Neuropathic Pain: Motor Cortex and Brain Stimulation

15.6.2.15.1 History
- Electrical stimulation of the human brain began in the 1950s and early 1960s by workers like Heath and Pool
- Previous targets of stimulation in an attempt to obtain pain relief have included: periaqueductal grey matter, periventricular grey matter, and sensory thalamic nuclei belonging to the neospinothalamic tract for treatment of mainly deafferentation pain

15.6.2.15.2 The Exciting Development of Motor Cortex Magnetic Stimulation
- It was Tsubokawa and coworkers who initially reported on the use of epidural motor cortex stimulation (MCS) in eight patients with central and neuropathic pain in 1991
- Since then, use and effectiveness of MCS has been reported by other groups

15.6.2.15.3 Role of Motor Cortex in Pain Modulation
- Motor cortical transcranial magnetic stimulation was found to modulate non-nociceptive sensory perception besides acutely provoked pain in healthy individuals (Lefaucheur, Neurophysiol Clin 2004)

15.6.2.15.4 Mode of Stimulation

- Effected by chronic high frequency sub-threshold repetitive motor cortex stimulation by surgically implanted epidural electrodes (after an initial procedure to ensure it works for the patient)

15.6.2.15.5 When Should This Procedure Be Contemplated?

- Pain refractory to all other forms of treatment
- Refractory neurogenic (especially of the upper extremity and face) and central pain
- A recent long-term (10-year) experience study reveals that it is mainly used for intractable neuropathic pain (Rasche et al., Pain 2006)

15.6.2.15.6 Clinical Use

- MCS is now regarded as an established therapy for the treatment of complex central and neuropathic pain syndromes (according to Brown)
- Examples of its use:
  - Limb stump pain
  - Pain after spinal cord injury
  - Post-herpetic neuralgia
  - Trigeminal neuropathy
  - Thalamic infarction

15.6.2.15.7 Proposed Mechanism of Motor Cortex Stimulation

- Increased regional cerebral blood flow in the ipsilateral ventrolateral thalamus – an area in which corticothalamic connections from the motor and premotor areas predominate (Brown, Neurosurg Focus 2001)
- Possible role in modulation of sensory perception mentioned

15.6.2.15.8 Difficulty to Be Surmounted

- Precise placement of the electrode over the motor cortex region that corresponds to the area of pain is essential for success (Mogilner et al., Neurosurg Focus 2001)

Recent Improvements in Correct Cortical Mapping

- In the past, localisation was by means of standard anatomical landmarks together with image guidance

Recently, methods that make for high accuracy of localisation include:
- Functional MRI imaging guidance – the data so obtained can be integrated to the frameless stereotactic database. Thus, the integration of functional and anatomical imaging data ensures increased location accuracy and aids surgical planning (Mogilner et al., Neurosurg Focus 2001)
- Intraoperative electrical cortical mapping (Am J Neuroradiol 2005)
- Combining functional MRI (with volumetric rendering of 3-D magnetic resonance data) and intraoperative electrical stimulation in the awake patient (Gharabaghi et al., Neurosurgery 2005)

15.6.2.15.9   Contraindication to Brain Stimulation
- Psychotic patient
- Pain not belonging to the common recorded indications
- Psychogenic pain

15.6.2.15.10 Other Areas of the Cortex Under Study
- Prefrontal cortex
- Other areas of parietal cortex

15.6.3   Psychogenic Pain

15.6.3.1   Key Concept
- It is probably incorrect to think that a considerable number of patients suffering from chronic pain such as chronic back pain are faking their pain or malingerers, as there is increasing evidence that once centralisation occurs, the pain is much more difficult to control

15.6.3.2   Note
- Discussion of psychogenic pain is outside the scope of this book
- However, some of the methods used by psychiatrists in managing chronic pain, such as cognitive-behavioural methods, will be discussed (refer to Sect. 16.5 on chronic LBP management in Chap. 16)

15.7   Discussion of Acute vs Chronic Pain

15.7.1   Acute Pain

15.7.1.1 Word of Caution

- As will also be highlighted in the Chap. 16 on LBP, it is the author's opinion that as far as this simple classification of acute vs. chronic pain, which most clinicians use, is concerned, it is highly advisable to add the category "acute-on-chronic"
- This is to remind the treating physician that the chances are that the prognosis in this subgroup of patients will be different from that of patients really suffering from acute pain

15.7.1.2 Key Concept 1

- Every attempt must be made to abort the pain at the acute stage, for it is now increasingly realised that many cases of chronic pain have more central modulation and are much more difficult to treat
- Another important finding is that pain may still somehow exist long after the initial (pathologic) process has come to an end

15.7.1.3 Key Concept 2

- If the pain or noxious stimulus is very marked and acute, there is increased likelihood of the pain becoming chronic and the time course of this transformation may be shorter than expected
- A recent study revealed that neuroplastic changes of central neurons (in a manner similar to that of chronic intractable pain) can occur as early as after 24 h of severe pain (Arnstein 1997)

15.7.1.4 Physiological Responses to Acute Pain

- Peripheral vasoconstriction
- Increased HR and cardiac workload, sometimes precipitate a cardiac event
- Increased sweating
- Increased respiratory rate
- Increased hospitalisation
- Acute nociceptive pain is sharp and intense (as opposed to visceral pain, which is dull and poorly localised)

15.7.1.5 Recapitulate Events Surrounding Acute Pain from Tissue Damage

▪ Tissue injury, nociceptor activation
▪ Concomitant release of "sensitising soup" of inflammatory mediators
▪ Causing peripheral sensitisation and later central sensitisation with pain amplification
▪ State of hyperalgesia (primary and secondary)
▪ If left unchecked, can lead to chronic pain

15.7.1.6 Recapitulating the Sites Where We Can Stop Pain in Its Tracks

▪ At the tissue level – sometimes called "transduction"
▪ Along the signalling path towards the spinal cord – sometimes called "transmission"
▪ At "central" level in the spinal cord – sometimes called "modulation"
▪ At higher and cortical brain centres – called "perception"
▪ These terms were used nicely in the book on postoperative pain management by Ferrante and VadeBoncouer
▪ But after reading this chapter, the reader can tell that transduction, transmission, modulation and perception are not the whole picture; they left out an emerging new strategy whereby our CNS can still perceive the pain, but does not pay attention to the pain – although more useful in chronic refractory pain

15.7.1.7 Groups of Analgesics at Our Disposal in Acute Pain

▪ Central action only: opioids, tramadol
▪ Central + anti-inflammatory action: NSAIDs, COX-2, steroids
▪ Central + alpha-2 agonist activity: clonidine
▪ Weak analgesic: acetaminophen
▪ Local anaesthetics
▪ Others: anticonvulsants, antidepressants

15.7.1.7.1 The Opioids

▪ Extremely effective as first-line drug for anticipated severe pain
▪ Morphine is more lipophilic and diffuses more widely if injected into the neuraxis than fentanyl
▪ Reduction in dosage can be achieved in multimodal analgesia (see discussion in Sect. 15.7.1.7.5)
▪ Long-term use may cause abuse (e.g. oxycodone) and addiction

15.7.1.7.2   Non-Selective Traditional NSAIDs

- Originally thought to cause pain relief by anti-inflammatory action
- Recent research indicated there is also a central action – since prostaglandin E_2 also implicated in the central sensitisation process of pain via protein kinase and dorsal horn neuron activation, and potentiates NMDA channel opening (Woolf et al., Science 2000)
- Peripheral as well as central inhibition of prostaglandin E_2 can be effected by COX-2 inhibitors like valdecoxib (Gierse et al., 2002) and celecoxib (Tegeder et al., J Neurochem 2001)

Side Effects of Non-Selective NSAIDs

- Predisposition to upper GI ulceration, sometimes GI bleeding (most common with aspirin), but can be occult with no symptoms (Singh, Arch Inn Med 1996)
- Affect platelet function
- Possible effect on the cardiovascular and renal system (especially in the elderly)

15.7.1.7.3   Selective COX-2 Inhibitors

- Less GI ulceration, in some studies incidence of GI ulcer approaches that of placebo, possibly less occult GI bleeds
- What about cardiovascular safety that has attracted so much attention in recent years?

Cardiovascular Adverse Events: Selective and Non-Selective NSAIDs

- Cardiovascular adverse events have been reported in major journals such as N Eng J Med by Nussmeier et al., 2005 for the COX-2 inhibitors

Current Status

- Many COX-2 inhibitors have been withdrawn from the market because of cardiovascular side effects, such as rofecoxib with its associated cardiovascular risk (especially thrombotic events like acute myocardial infarction), as demonstrated in the APPROVE trial in 2004
- Celecoxib is the only agent used in USA, but even celecoxib showed some degree of cardiovascular risk over placebo in the APC trial

Non-selective agents like naproxen also demonstrated increased cardiovascular and cerebrovascular risk over placebo, as demonstrated in the ADAPT trial

Current FDA Position on NSAIDs

The cardiovascular risk associated with celecoxib (the only COX-2 available in USA) is similar to that of non-selective NSAIDs

Further scientific studies are needed to ascertain the long-term cardiovascular risk of NSAIDs as a group. Box warnings on GI and cardiovascular risks will be issued to all marketed NSAIDs including celecoxib

Circumventing the Side Effects of COX-2 Inhibitors

Celecoxib is the only FDA-approved COX-2 inhibitor. It will be prudent for those patients with cardiac disease to take aspirin together with the drug to minimise side effects. For dosing and individual recommendation, a cardiologist needs be consulted

Effects of NSAIDs on Bone Healing

Another worrisome side effect of NSAID use is the possibility of hindering bone healing in patients with fractures and those patients receiving fusion, like a spinal fusion operation

To summarise the current knowledge concerning effects of NSAIDs on bone healing:

- Animal experiments revealed lesser inhibition of bone healing if given ketorolac (non-selective inhibitor) compared with valdecoxib (a COX-2 inhibitor)
- Fracture healing returned to normal on drug cessation and when PG levels are restored normal
  These, together with other basic science studies by Dr Einhorn, showed that:
- COX-2 (i.e. isoform 2 of the cyclo-oxygenase enzyme) is essential for bone healing
- Inhibition of COX-2 inhibits healing and bone healing is restored upon its withdrawal
- Furthermore, COX-2 inhibition seems to have more effect on indirect (endochondral type) bone healing as opposed to direct bone healing according to experiments on rats at University of Hong Kong (Cheung et al., 2006)

A recent RCT did not reveal a negative effect of celecoxib on spinal fusion in humans: no significant difference in spinal fusion rate between the celecoxib and placebo groups at the 1-year mark (Reuben and Ekman, J Bone Joint Surg 2005)

15.7.1.7.4   Other Drugs
Many of the other agents have already been discussed in Sect. 15.6.2 on neuropathic pain

15.7.1.7.5   Use of Multimodal Analgesia
Works by combining different analgesic agents and aborting the course of pain production at multiple sites

Frequently results in lower doses of individual agents, with lowered total dose of opioid usage and less pain increasing satisfaction (Kehlet et al., Anesth Analg 1993)

A common combination involves combined use of NSAIDs and opioids

Advantages of Combined Opioid and NSAID Usage
Opioid starting effect, lessen side effects of opioids, e.g. vomiting, respiratory depression, addiction, and decreased opioid consumption by 30%

On one hand opioids decrease rest pain, while NSAIDs decrease dynamic pain (e.g. when patient moves or during physiotherapy)

Shown by studies to be efficacious

15.7.1.7.6   Pre-Emptive Analgesia
Attempts to effect nociceptor blockade prior to the painful stimulus such as the surgeon's knife

Studies indicate this strategy helps prevent central sensitisation, which is a feat that cannot be accomplished by giving general anaesthetics

Previous studies confirmed the pre-emptive effects of COX-2 inhibitors like rofecoxib in arthroscopic knee surgery with decreased total opioid usage and prolonged postoperative analgesia (Reuben et al., Anesth Analg 2002)

Similar RCT evidence exists for combined pre- and postoperative use of celecoxib in knee arthroscopy (Ekman et al., 2004)

A common combination will be using preoperative i.v./oral analgesic with perioperative local anaesthetics (such as nerve blocks and/or intra-articular) and either spinal or epidural

■ Recent studies have reported the use of preoperative use of NSAIDs, which was shown to improve postoperative pain control

■ Postoperatively, the patient may be given a short course of COX-2 besides patient-controlled analgesia (PCA)

Advantages of PCA

Helps maintain the dose of opioids within therapeutic range, not so low as to cause pain, or so high as to cause sedation and may decrease total opioid usage

Care should be exercised to prevent pump errors and PCA is contraindicated if the patient is confused or delirious. Newer generations of pain pumps are preferred for better titration and accuracy of drug delivery if continuous analgesic drug infusion is prescribed (Fig. 15.2)

New Alternative: Iontophoretic Transdermal Fentanyl

Works by iontophoretic mechanism

Active drug fentanyl hydrochloride

Application to chest or upper arm

There are six 40-µg doses per hour

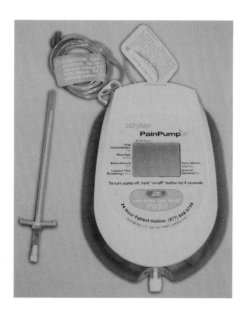

Fig. 15.2. Newer generation of analgesic drug infusion pumps may provide better titration and accuracy of drug delivery

- Efficacy comparable to PCA
- Some support for its use in recent clinical trials (Viscusi et al., JAMA 2004)
- But needs monitoring for respiratory depression, which needs naloxone infusion if it occurs

15.7.2   Chronic Pain

15.7.2.1 Introduction

- Most define chronic pain as pain of longer duration (> 3 months)
- Not infrequently, there is lack of evidence of pathology or tissue damage (although a handful with real pathology can now be detected with modern technology, see the Sect. 16.3.3 on upright MRI in chronic LBP in Chap. 16)
- Rather unpredictable prognosis
- Treatment is more difficult, and requires multidisciplinary approach

15.7.2.2 Physiological Responses to Chronic Pain

- Dull and persistent
- HR and respiratory rate normal
- Frequently depressed and apathetic
- Can occur even when the initial noxious stimulus is gone, and in these situations can be said to be serving no useful purpose

15.7.2.3 Mechanism of "Centralisation" in Chronic Pain

- Recent research indicates that:
  - Persistent pain can result in sensitisation of neurons in the spinal cord dorsal horn and produce physiological changes in sites such as the thalamus that receive projections from the dorsal horn
  - The dorsal horn nuclei receive both primary afferent input and projections from the dorsal horn, and recent research indicates that these nuclei may well be involved in participation of chronic pain processes (Schwark et al., Brain Res 2001)
- The process of centralisation in chronic pain frequently involves higher brain centres, as has been alluded to previously in this chapter (Sect. 15.6.2.6)

15.7.2.4 Other Players in the Process of Pain Modulation

▨ Other possible players (not yet mentioned so far) include:
- Role of neurotrophins
- Non-neuronal glial and immunocompetent cells can play a role in the process of modifying nociception (Millan, Prog Neurobiol 1999)

15.7.2.5 Models That Can Be Used to Explain Chronic Pain

▨ Examples include:
- Emory Pain Estimate model (discussed in this chapter and the next)
- International Classification of Functioning Disability and Health model (ICF; discussed in Chap. 1)

15.7.2.6 Conclusion

▨ It is hoped that the above discussion on pain management will allow the reader to gain a fresh look at the problem of pain next time he or she deals with an acute or chronic pain problem
▨ Further discussion of chronic pain and relevant issues like return to work are found in Chap. 16 on back pain

General Bibliography

Melzack R, Bonica JJ (1984) Textbook of Pain. Churchill Livingstone, New York, USA
Melzack R (2003) Handbook of Pain Management: a Clinical Companion to Textbook of Pain. Churchill Livingstone, USA

Selected Bibliography of Journal Articles

1. Melzack R (1999) From the gate to the neuromatrix. Pain 6(Suppl):121–126
2. Melzack R (1999) Pain – an overview. Acta Anaesth Scand 43:880–884
3. Melzack R, Wall PD (1965) Pain mechanisms: a new theory. Science 150:971–979
4. Wall PD (1978) The gate control theory of pain modulation. An examination and re-statement. Brain 101:1–18
5. Apfelbaum JL, Chen C et al. (2003) Postoperative pain experience: results from a national survey suggest postoperative pain continues to be under-managed. Anesth Analg 97(2):534–540
6. Vowles KE, Gross RT (2003) Work-related beliefs about injury and physical capacity for work in individuals with chronic pain. Pain 101(3):291–298

7. Koho P, Aho S et al. (2001) Assessment of chronic pain behaviour: reliability of the method and its relationship with perceived disability, physical impairment and function. J Rehabil Med 33(3):128–132

8. Veldhuijzen DS, Kenemans JL et al. (2006) Processing capacity in chronic pain patients: a visual event-related potentials study. Pain 121(1/2):60–68

9. Crow R, Gage H et al. (1999) The role of expectancies in the placebo effect and their use in the delivery of health care: a systematic review. Health Technol Assess 3(3):1–96

10. Barsky AJ, Saintfort R et al. (2002) Nonspecific medication side effects and the nocebo phenomenon. JAMA 287(5):622–627

11. Brody H (2000) Placebo and health: three perspectives on the placebo response: expectancy, conditioning, and meaning. Adv Mind Body Med 16(3):216–232

12. Voudouris NJ, Peck CL et al. (1989) Conditioned response model of placebo phenomenon: further support. Pain 38(1):109–116

13. Hollerman JR, Schultz W et al. (1998) Influence of reward expectation related neuronal activity during learning in primate striatum. J Neurophysiol 80(2):947–963

14. Aston-Jones G, Rajkowski J et al. (1999) Role of locus coeruleus in attention and behavioral flexibility. Biol Psychiatry 46(9):1309–1320

15. Petrovic P, Kalso E et al. (2002) Placebo and opioid analgesia – imaging a shared neuronal network. Science 295(5560):1737–1740

16. Millan MJ (1999) The induction of pain: an integrative review. Prog Neurobiol 57(1):1–164

17. Treede RD, Meyer RA et al. (1992) Peripheral and central mechanisms of cutaneous hyperalgesia. Prog Neurobiol 38(4):397–421

18. Harden RN (2005) Pharmacotherapy of complex regional pain syndrome. Arch Phys Med Rehabil 84(3):S17–S28

19. Stacey BR (2005) Management of peripheral neuropathic pain. Arch Phys Med Rehabil 84(3):S4–S16

20. Rowbotham MC, Twilling L et al. (2003) Oral opioid therapy for chronic peripheral and central neuropathic pain. N Eng J Med 348(13):1223–1232

21. Harati Y, Gooch C et al. (1998) Double blind randomized trial of tramadol for the treatment of pain of diabetic neuropathy. Neurology 50(6):1842–1846

22. Backonja MM, Serra J (2004) Pharmacologic management: lesser studied neuropathic pain disease. Pain Med 5(Suppl 1):S48–S59

23. Drummond PD, Finch PM et al. (1991) Reflex sympathetic dystrophy – the significance of differing plasma catecholamines concentrations in affected and unaffected limb. Brain 114:2025–2036

24. Tulgar M (1992) Advances in electrical nerve stimulation techniques to manage chronic pain: an overview. Adv Ther 9(6):366–372

25. Lundborg C, Dahm P et al. (1999) Clinical experience using intrathecal bupivacaine infusion in three patients with complex regional pain syndrome type-I. Acta Anaesthesiol Scand 43(6):667–678

26. Schwark HD, Ilyinsky OB (2001) Inflammatory pain reduces correlated activity in the dorsal column nuclei. Brain Res 889(1/2):295–302

27. Marchand S, Bushnell MC et al. (1999) The effects of dorsal column stimulation on measures of clinical and experimental pain in man. Pain 45(3):249–257

28. Carter ML (2004) Spinal cord stimulation in chronic pain: a review of the evidence. Anaesth Intensive Care 32(1):11–21

29. Holsheimer J, Wesselink WA (1997) Effect of anode-cathode configuration on paresthesia coverage in spinal cord stimulation. Neurosurgery 41(3):654–659

30. Krainick JU, Thoden U (1975) Spinal cord stimulation in post amputation pain. Surg Neurol 4(1):167–170

31. Lefaucheur JP, Drouot X et al. (2004) Neuropathic pain controlled for more than one year by monthly sessions of repetitive transcranial magnetic stimulation the motor cortex. Neurophysiol Clin 34(2):91–95

32. Rasche D, Ruppolt M et al. (2006) Motor cortex stimulation for long term relief of chronic neuropathic pain: a 10 year experience. Pain 121(1/2):43–52

33. Brown JA (2001) Motor cortex stimulation. Neurosurg Focus 11(3):E5

34. Pirotte B, Neugroschl C et al. (2005) Comparison of functional MR imaging guidance to electrical cortical mapping for targeting selective motor cortex areas in neuropathic pain: a study based on intra-operative stereotactic navigation. Am J Neuroradiol 26(9):2256–2266

35. Gharabaghi A, Hellwig D et al. (2005) Volumetric image guidance for motor cortex stimulation: integration of three dimensional cortical anatomy and functional imaging. Neurosurgery 57(Suppl 1):114–120

36. Arnstein PM (1997) The neuroplastic phenomenon: a physiologic link between chronic pain and learning. J Neurosci Nurs 29(3):179–186

37. Woolf CJ, Salter MW (2000) Neuronal plasticity: increasing the gain in pain. Science 288(5472):1765–1769

38. Tegeder I, Niederberger E et al. (2001) Effects of selective COX-1 and -2 inhibition on formalin evoked nociceptive behaviour and prostaglandin E2 release in the spinal cord. J Neurochem 79(4):777–786

39. Nussmeier NA, Whelton AA et al. (2005) Complications of the COX-2 inhibitors parecoxib and valdecoxib after cardiac surgery. N Engl J Med 352(11):1081–1091

40. Reuben SS, Ekman EF (2005) The effect of cyclo-oxygenase-2 inhibition on analgesia and spinal fusion. J Bone Joint Surg Am 87(3):536–542

41. Kehlet H, Dahl JB (1993) The value of multi-modal or balanced analgesia in postoperative pain management. Anesth Analg 77(5):1048–1056

42. Reuben SS, Sklar J (2002) Pre-emptive multi-modal analgesia for anterior cruciate ligament surgery. Reg Anesth Pain Med 27(2):225–226

43. Viscusi ER, Reynolds L et al. (2004) Patient-controlled transdermal fentanyl hydrochloride vs intravenous morphine pump for postoperative pain: a randomized clinical trial. JAMA 291(11):1333–1341

16 Back Pain

Contents

16.1   Introduction

- Seldom do we find a condition that involves the interest of so many different groups of people including healthcare professionals like orthopaedists and therapists, osteopaths, chiropractors, healthcare administrators, and even politicians
- This is complicated by the fact that 80% of chronic LBP sufferers have elusive aetiology
- We shall start by clarifying some myths surrounding the topic of back pain

16.1.1   Epidemiology of Back Pain

- It is well known that acute LBP affects 70–80% of adults at some point in their lives, with peak prevalence in the fifth decade
- The drastic increase in LBP in the past two to three decades, according to Gordon Waddell, was attributed to an increase in work loss, compensation or sick leave issues, and disability allowances with huge economic cost as its aftermath

16.1.2   Myths Surrounding LBP

16.1.2.1 Myths Concerning Acute LBP

- That prolonged bed rest is needed
- That patients with acute back pain do not need close follow-up since LBP is so common
  - That 80–90% of acute back pain completely resolves without treatment within 2–3 months

16.1.2.2 Clarification of Myths

- As will be discussed in the later part of this chapter (Sect. 16.3.5.3.1), prolonged bed rest is detrimental and should be discouraged in most cases of acute back pain
- Readers who have read the Chap. 15 on pain management will know that the most important aspect of pain management is to "prevent chronic pain". Thus, patients suffering from acute pain should be followed more closely in the first few clinic visits at least to ensure proper management of his pain

- McKenzie showed in 2006 that only about 40% of acute back pain completely resolves without treatment within around 2–3 months

16.1.2.3 Myths Concerning Chronic LBP

■ Myths that the presence of the Waddell signs necessarily mean the patient is faking pain or that the pain is unreal
■ The myth that what we can offer in such cases is nothing but symptomatic treatment as no organic cause can be found

16.1.2.4 Clarification of Myths

■ Presence of Waddell signs does not automatically imply non-organic pain, as discussed in the last chapter, but in fact are frequently a manifestation of pain behaviour. Gordon Waddell never said in his book that Waddell signs necessarily always imply non-organic cause of back pain
■ Chronic back pain is a challenging clinical problem. As has been stressed throughout this book, many challenging clinical rehabilitation problems need multidisciplinary team assessment, goal setting, and proper assessment and monitoring. Just giving the patient some medication for symptomatic relief is not going to work

16.1.3   Basic Pain Pathophysiology

■ Detailed discussion of pain pathways and theories of both acute and chronic pain were discussed in Chap. 15

16.1.4   Pain Innervation and Pain-Sensitive Structures in the Spine

■ It is convenient to think of the spine as having a dorsal and a ventral compartment (Spine 1983)
■ The dorsal compartment consists of facets, dorsal dura, back muscles and ligaments; while the ventral compartment contains anterior longitudinal ligament, posterior longitudinal ligament, intervertebral disc, the vertebral body, ventral dura, nerve root, and prevertebral muscles
■ The dorsal rami innervates the dorsal compartment, the medial branch of which goes to innervate the facets
■ The ventral compartment is innervated by the sympathetic chain anteriorly, while the sinuvertebral nerve innervates the PLL

16.2   Back Pain Classification

16.2.1   Clinical Classification
- Acute: <6 weeks duration
- Chronic: >6 weeks duration
  - (Some propose to add in the category called "subacute")

16.2.2   Author's Proposed Clinical Classification
- Acute
- Chronic
- Acute-on-chronic

  (Whether one should retain the category "subacute" is debatable; it is mentioned because many papers from Scandinavian countries report the result of subacute back pain management)

16.2.2.1 Rationale for Adding the Important Category of Acute-on-Chronic
- Helps to remind all treating physicians that the management of acute exacerbation of chronic back pain is very different in treatment approach and prognosis compared with a new patient that comes to your office for a first episode of back pain
- Probably allows one to draw clearer and more accurate conclusions from research in LBP. As will be pointed out, much research can be improved if we have these clear categories in mind, rather than lumping these all together as LBP and trying to draw conclusions

16.2.2.2 Supporting Evidence from Epidemiological Studies
- Epidemiological studies (e.g. BMJ 1998) have also found out that the majority of chronic LBP patients have recurrent episodes sometimes punctuated by acute pain; it therefore pays to add a subgroup called acute-on-chronic LBP since this group has a similar prognosis to that for chronic LBP

16.2.3   Subclassification for Chronic LBP Taking Account of Disability
- Grade 1 = low pain intensity, low disability
- Grade 2 = high pain intensity, but low disability

- Grade 3 = moderately limiting, high disability
- Grade 4 = severely limiting, high disability
  (Von Korff et al., Pain 1992)

16.2.3.1 Validation of Von Korff Chronic LBP Classification
- Validated and found to be useful in UK (Pain 1997)
- Useful also in population studies in Canada, presented by Cassidy in the International Society for the Study of Lumbar Spine, 1997

16.3   Work-up for Acute Back Pain

16.3.1   History and Physical
- It is interesting to note that with advent of advances in radiological imaging, some centres actually proposed "omitting routine clinical examination in patients with LBP and/or radiculopathy" in recent research from Hull Royal Infirmary. The study concluded that "history alone correlated well with MRI results, and clinical examination is only considered in those preoperative patients to document neurology"! (presented at the "Combined Orthopaedic Associations" meeting in Sydney in October 2004)

16.3.2   Author's View
- The above conclusion illustrates the modern tendency of many young surgeons to rely heavily on MRI while paying less attention to a good physical examination

16.3.3   Rationale for a Proper Physical Examination in LBP Patients
- MRI is too sensitive a tool and frequently picks up pathology that may well be a red herring
- We are not going to order MRI in most of our patients anyway
- Sometimes the real diagnosis is very obvious only on physical examination, e.g. careful physical examination will pick up more subtle diagnosis like early cauda equina syndrome (example: may present in queer ways like asymmetrical saddle sensory loss, with reduced anal tone only, see detailed discussion in the companion volume of this book)
- For medico-legal reasons, proper documentation of the physical examination findings is important, especially if, say, the patient sud-

denly or subacutely deteriorates after your clinic visit you need to have such documentation in a court of law

- Proper and gentle physical examination enhances trust and doctor–patient relationship with your patient

- Finally, routine MRI with the patient in supine position may still miss some pathology that can be picked up only by standing or upright MRI (see Fig. 16.1). This new open MRI technology is also good because it can be used in patients with claustrophobia (see Fig. 16.2). As Dr. Paul Pavlov, Director of the St. Maartenskliniek (Netherlands) puts it: "This new technology from FONAR is unique in enabling us to evaluate the spine anatomy in the fully weight-bearing state and in multiple positions"

(N.B. The presenting symptoms and signs of common spinal pathologies were discussed in the companion volume of the book, as were "red flag" signs)

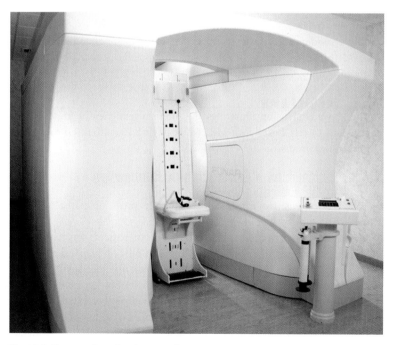

Fig. 16.1. The new "stand-up" or upright MRI, courtesy of FONAR, the MRI specialist

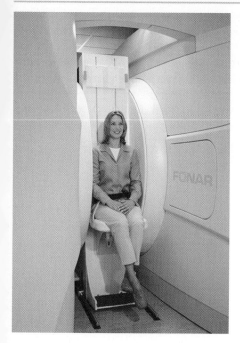

Fig. 16.2. The "open" MRI system is less frightening for some patients, and the upright posture feels more comfortable

16.3.4 Word of Caution

- Waddell's signs are more sensitive in chronic as opposed to acute back pain
- Details of Waddell's signs are listed, therefore, under Sect. 16.5 on chronic back pain

16.3.5 Management of Acute Back Pain

16.3.5.1 Key Concept

- There is every indication that the pathophysiology, management and prognosis inherent among patients with acute vs chronic back pain are very different
- This difference should be respected and separate discussions of acute vs chronic back pain are in order

16.3.5.2   Key Concept

▥ Every attempt must be made to prevent back pain in patients from becoming chronic

▥ This is because if chronicity sets in, the pain will be much more difficult to treat and the prognosis will be much more guarded

16.3.5.3   Interventions for Acute Back Pain

16.3.5.3.1 Bed Rest

▥ Waddell reviewed RCTs on this subject and found results showing that bed rest (especially if ≥4 days) was not an effective option for acute back pain (Br J Gen Pract 1997)

▥ A more recent paper in 1995 from N Eng J Med showed that bed rest resulted in significantly slower recovery compared with continuation of ordinary activities. Results of group with bed rest were worse in terms of sick leave, pain, Oswestry disability score, and lumbar flexion

16.3.5.3.2 Drugs

▥ Deyo reported in Spine 1996 evidence in support of the use of NSAIDs, and only fair evidence for muscle relaxants; other drugs were not favoured

▥ Koes subsequently conducted a study involving statistical analysis of pooled data of RCTs and the author suggested caution with regard to the initially keen support shown for NSAID (reported in Spine 1996)

▥ It thus appears that while NSAIDs seem to work, further studies are required to confirm their usefulness

16.3.5.3.3 Traction

▥ On reviewing 21 papers in 1995, only one paper was found to be of high quality, Van der Heijden concluded no inferences could be drawn (Phys Ther 1995)

▥ One paper was published in Spine 1997, but again did not differentiate patients into acute and chronic LBP. This study did not find traction to be an effective treatment

▥ Overall, further well-designed studies are needed to either support or refute traction as treatment for acute LBP

16.3.5.3.4   Spinal Manipulation

- Anderson reported positive effects of spinal manipulation in J Manipul Physiol Ther (1992), but like many other studies, did not differentiate between acute and chronic LBP
- A subsequent systematic review by Koes in Spine 1996 found that spinal manipulation was not always uniformly useful, but seemed effective in the subgroup with pain of 2–4 weeks' duration (Spine 1990), and those with limited straight leg raising (Physiother Pract 1988)
- A more recent trial by Cherkin (N Eng J Med 1998) compared three groups: chiropractic manipulation, McKenzie exercise, vs education leaflet. He did not find any difference among the three groups with regard to pain recurrence or days off work. The chiropractic group performed significantly better than the minimal intervention group at 4 weeks, but not at 3 months and the 1-year mark
- Thus, more recent studies on spinal manipulation seem to indicate some short-term effects, but there is doubt as to whether these effects will last in cases of acute LBP

16.3.5.3.5   Exercise

- A review in Spine 1995 by Faas reported that exercise was of no use in two trials with good study design, but some benefit was gained from McKenzie exercise in the other two trials with inadequate study design
- Dettori reported in Spine 1995 comparing flexion exercise vs extension exercise vs ice treatment. No difference was found between groups after 1 week, with regard to rate of recovery or rate of pain recurrence
- Trials subsequent to this mixed up acute and chronic LBP and it is therefore difficult to comment upon
- Thus, if anything, the evidence in support of exercise therapy was not strong. Further, better designed trials are needed for clarification

Word of Note

- Flexion exercises (like that of William's) are theoretically contraindicated in sciatica according to Nachemson's intradiscal pressure studies, as it will cause increased intradiscal pressure
- Although Nachemson's studies revealed increased intradiscal pressure with active extension, this does not contraindicate McKenzie's tech-

nique, which stresses passive extension (according to McKenzie's book on the lumbar spine published in 1981)
- Newer evolving strategies to tackle acute back pain by physiotherapists include postural strategies, positional release techniques, cranial-sacral therapy, etc. and are outside the scope of this book

16.3.5.3.6   Back Schools: What Are They?
- Back schools are popular in Scandinavian countries like Sweden
- They consist of educational programmes focusing on back care, mechanics and exercise (and more recently sometimes incorporate different types of practical exercise programmes like hydrotherapy)

Results of Back Schools
- A review in J Clin Epidemiol 1994 showed that two studies were in support of back schools, and two studies were not. However, the benefits arising from them appeared short-lived
- Di Fabio reviewed six RCTs in Phys Ther 1995 and found that back school alone improves knowledge and compliance; its efficacy in pain relief was positive only if combined with a comprehensive rehabilitation programme
- More recent studies have not found a positive effect of back school alone either (Leclaire, Arch Phys Med Rehabil 1996)

16.3.5.3.7   Effect of Acupuncture
- In a recent meta-analysis of 12 RCTs reported in Arch Intern Med (1998), acupuncture was found to be superior to many control interventions in the management of chronic LBP
- Other studies:
  - Another RCT reported in Clin J Pain in 2001 revealed a significant decrease in a group of chronic LBP patients at 1 and 3 months compared with placebo. Improvement occurred in the form of decreased pain-killer intake, better sleep and increased rate of return to work

16.3.5.3.8   Work Hardening and Vocational Conditioning
- Definition: work conditioning addresses the physical requirement for work (e.g. strength, flexibility, endurance) with an emphasis on functional outcomes, and usually performed by a single discipline specialist in the rehabilitation team

- Definition: work hardening refers to an interdisciplinary program addressing both the psychological and vocational needs of the patient
- Literature on this form of intervention in acute LBP is rare
- Lindstrom compared in Spine (1992) a treatment group with work conditioning vs a control treatment by the general practitioner. The result favoured the treatment group in terms of pain and time until return to work
- Mitchell also showed in Spine 1990 that a subgroup with work conditioning had earlier return to work, and resulted in fewer compensation claims
- Overall, there is some indication of the effect of work conditioning, even in more acute LBP patients

16.3.5.3.9   Multidisciplinary Programmes
- As for work hardening, there is more supporting evidence in the setting of chronic LBP
- Philips reported in Behav Res Ther 1991 on the positive effect of behavioural counselling within a problem-solving context to encourage exercise, socialisation and return to work. These results were better than psychotherapy alone in terms of pain resolution and return to daily activities

16.3.5.3.10 Important Role of Work-Site Visits
- The importance of work-site visits was highlighted by a recent Cochrane Library Review and deemed as an important element in multidisciplinary biopsychosocial rehabilitation for subacute LBP (Karjalainen et al., 2003)

16.3.5.4   Prognosis of Acute LBP
- Literature has it that 90% of patients with acute LBP episodes recover within 6 weeks, regardless of the type of therapy, and more than 50% can return to work within 1 week
- However, the rate of recurrence is high and is of the order of 50–80%
- But is there any method of predicting:
  - Who are likely to have LBP among healthy adults, and
  - Are there methods of predicting in which patients will acute LBP turn chronic?

16.3.5.5 Predicting Which Will Have Low Back Pain (Healthy Subjects)

▓ Static endurance testing is said to have a good predictive value; in one study the quoted odds ratio was 3.4 (Clin Biomech 1995)

16.3.5.6 Predicting in Which Patients Acute LBP Becomes Chronic LBP

▓ There is some evidence from the Scandinavian literature to indicate that lack of back extension power, as shown in bedside exercise testing, may be predictive of chronicity
▓ Burton also reported in Spine (1995) that disability at the 1 year mark may be predicted by psychological parameters far better than by using medical information

16.4 Common Spinal Interventional Procedures Performed by Physiatrists

16.4.1 Pain Originating from Facets

16.4.1.1 Facet Blocks

▓ Facet blocks are commonly performed, e.g. in the cervical or lumbar spine
▓ Of both diagnostic and therapeutic value. Can help locate the pain generator, and an occasional patient may find prolonged relief
▓ If positive response, but does not last, consider medial branch block

16.4.1.2 Medial Branch Block

▓ This procedure is usually advised before we do other interventional procedures like radiofrequency lesioning
▓ The site of injection is at the junction between the transverse process and the superior articular facet
▓ Figure 16.3 shows a patient with neck pain who underwent medial branch block

16.4.1.3 Use of Radiofrequency in Pain Arising from the Facet

▓ These patients mostly will have had facet block and medial branch blocks in the past

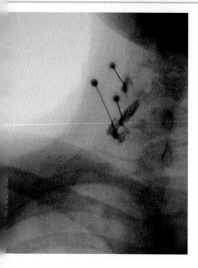

Fig. 16.3. Radiograph taken during "medial branch block", a type of spinal interventional procedure

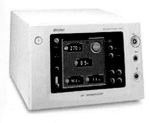

Fig. 16.4. Radiofrequency machine is currently used in many centres in spinal interventional procedures (Stryker)

- The illustration (Fig. 16.4) shows a radiofrequency (RF) machine at work
- The RF procedure sometimes needs to be repeated at the 1-year mark

16.4.1.3.1 Documentation During RF
- The following should be documented:
  - Initial positive sensory stimulation response (in Hz)
  - From no motor response to maximum stimulation (in Hz)
  - Temperature (in degrees)
  - Duration of RF (in seconds)
  - Impedance readings (in Ohms)

16.4.2   Discogenic Back Pain

16.4.2.1 Introduction

■ Role of discogram was discussed in the companion volume to this book

■ Recommended reading is a review article on discogenic back pain by Karppinen et al., Pain 2004

■ The new surgical option of disc replacement as an alternative option to spinal fusion will also be discussed

16.4.2.2 IDET Indication

■ The current indications for the use of intradiscal heating procedure include:
  – Annular tear
  – Internal disruption of the intravenous disc

■ Be sure the patient has had a positive injection response in previous discographic examination

■ The procedure involves threading an electrode tip around the annulus followed by heating

■ Different studies showed mixed results. Therapeutic mechanism not fully elucidated (Semin Musculoskelet Radiol 2006)

■ One possible reason why pain relief is not always obtained is that the innervations of the IV disc are complex, and say, for instance, if we can successfully coagulate the tissue near the annulus tear, we are not ablating all the pain fibres and pain can still persist

16.4.2.3 Radiofrequency for Dorsal Root Ganglion

■ This procedure has been tried by some, but not a widely popular technique yet for this diagnosis (Fig. 16.5)

■ If pain persists despite procedures like IDET, may consider fusion of the particular motion segment or disc replacement

16.4.2.4 Open Surgical Procedures

■ Spinal fusion – discussed in the companion volume to this book

■ Disc replacement (Fig. 16.6)

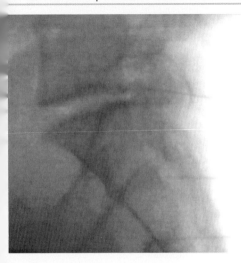

Fig. 16.5. Radiograph taken during radiofrequency procedure for dorsal root ganglion

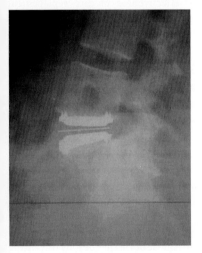

Fig. 16.6. Radiograph illustrating lumbar disc replacement

16.4.2.4.1   Current Status of Disc Replacement

- A typical possible candidate is single level disease, no nearby motion segment malalignment or degeneration
- FDA currently only approves one-level disease, although a recent paper from France in J Bone Joint Surg (2005) reported more than one

level in some of their patients when they reported their 7- to 10-year results

16.4.2.4.2   Pros and Cons of Disc Replacement

- Pros: theoretically avoid adjacent segment disease we expect from spinal fusion, maintains motion, removes pain generator
- Cons:
  - No long-term result (N.B. takes ≥10 years for a control group treatment arm (treated with fusion) to develop adjacent segment disease)
  - Revision can be difficult with local fibrotic reaction and abundant adhesions, but depends on model used

16.4.2.4.3   Word of Caution

- Although these procedures have attracted a lot of interest lately, longer term controlled clinical studies are needed
- Proponents have yet to prove cost-effectiveness of disc replacement over single-level fusion in the long term

16.4.3   Annular Tear

16.4.3.1   Role of Intradiscal Heating

- IDET may be indicated for annular tear
- But pain relief is not always assured for reasons just discussed

16.4.4   Sciatica

16.4.4.1   Epidural Injection

- Although an epidural injection can usually provide quick and significant pain relief in sciatica, the action usually is short lasting around 2–3 months and has to be repeated

16.4.4.2   Percutaneous Decompression

- Skryker has recently come up with the innovative idea by inventing the "percutaneous discectomy probe" (Fig. 16.7)
- This involves the percutaneous aspiration of disc material via a special probe that is threaded through an introducer cannula
- The most often stated goal of central nuclear decompression is to lower the pressure in the nucleus and to allow room for the herniated fragment to implode inwards (Pain Physician 2006)

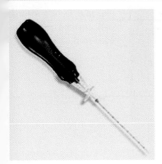

Fig. 16.7. Percutaneous disc decompressor, a new technology from the company Stryker

■ The procedure is done under LA. Contraindications include seque-strated disc, fractures, spinal stenosis, patients with pain from other causes, sepsis or severely degenerated disc

■ The clinical results of this interesting new procedure are eagerly awaited

16.4.4.3   Open Surgery

■ Emergency surgery is a must for spinal cord compression in the face of significant central herniation, or the cauda equina syndrome

■ Elective surgery usually needed for sequestrated discs and other diffi-cult scenarios, e.g. far lateral disc, failed previous interventional pro-cedures

16.4.5   Failed Back

16.4.5.1   Epidural Scope and Adhesiolysis

■ Despite initial enthusiasm, the use of epidural scope or related proce-dures is less common nowadays

■ This is partly due to rather unreliable pain relief, and the fact that ad-hesions, if present, tend to reform

16.4.5.2   Dorsal Column Stimulation

■ If causes like sepsis, recurrent disc, previous wrong diagnosis or wrong side surgery, significant spinal stenosis and causes like tu-mours were excluded, and the patient has refractory pain

■ If spinal cord stimulation of the dorsal column is considered, it will usually be given a trial run by keeping the stimulator external. If the method works for the patient, then internalise the device (Fig. 16.8)

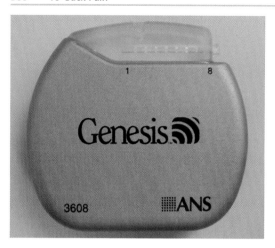

Fig. 16.8. Device for the performance of spinal cord stimulation

▓ A recent article quoted the rate of pain relief using DCS in failed back syndrome as 50–60%, but the author does caution that the strength of the current evidence of DCS in failed back is inadequate to advocate its use in all patients with this condition (Carter, Anaesth Intensive Care 2004)

16.4.6   Open Spinal Surgery

16.4.6.1   Introduction
▓ The indications for and contraindications of spinal surgery have been discussed in detail in the companion volume to this book: *Orthopedic Principles – A Resident's Guide*

16.4.6.2   Key Principle
▓ One must remember the teachings of well known figures like Nachemson:
  – The spine surgeon should avoid basing his decision to proceed to surgery solely on radiological images
  – The anomalies on imaging should correspond to the findings of history and physical signs (in many patients failed back or unsuccessful outcome stem from a hastily decided operation without taking into account the patient's symptoms and physical signs)

16.5   Chronic Back Pain

16.5.1   Work-up for Chronic LBP

■ It will be obvious after reading Chap. 15 that the following should be given due attention during the clinic visit of a patient with chronic LBP:
  - Pain behaviour – refer to Emory Pain Model and Waddell signs
  - The patient's perceptions and beliefs
  - The psychosocial context

16.5.2   Waddell's Signs

■ Signs are listed in the list below; if three or more of the 5 are positive, there is a *possibility* of non-organic basis
■ Waddell's signs
  - Non-anatomical regions of weakness or sensory loss
  - Non-anatomical or inconsistent tenderness
  - LBP on axial loading or sham rotation of the spine
  - Exaggerated pain response to non-painful stimulus
  - Inconsistent findings during distraction manoeuvres

16.5.3   Effects of Chronic LBP

■ It is well known that chronic LBP can have many systemic effects on the patient:
  - Effects on nervous system or neural control (see below)
  - Altered metabolism, e.g. fibrinolytic defect (Acta Orthop Scand 1991)
  - Psychosocial effects, e.g. depression, emotional distress

16.5.4   Effects on the Nervous System
or Neural Control in Chronic LBP

■ Altered sensory motor processing in the brain (Pain 2002)
■ Psychomotor retardation (Spine 1999)
■ Impaired postural control (Spine 1998)

16.5.5   Aetiology and Models to Use in Chronic LBP

16.5.5.1 Introduction

■ Most will agree that chronic back pain is difficult and challenging to manage
■ It will be useful to have some basic approach or models to work from in order to improve the results of treatment

- It is well known that in most patients chronic LBP is of unknown aetiology. Before considering models to tackle the problem of chronic LBP, let us first see why there has been little progress made in the past in eliciting the pathogenesis

16.5.5.2   Why Is It Difficult to Elicit the Aetiology of Chronic LBP?

- If we go back to the chapter on pain management, I have added the category "unknown" to include the majority of this category of patients
- Some difficulties related to the study of chronic LBP include: lack of a good animal model, does not fit easily into the nociceptive vs neuropathic model usually used, ethical issues involved in even thinking of inducing this syndrome in humans

16.5.5.3   Hypothesis on Pathogenesis of "Idiopathic" LBP

- Incidental intraoperative finding of epileptic-like activity in the thalamic nuclei among a group of patients with chronic LBP was reported in Acta Neurochir by Iwayama and Yamashiro in 1991
- Presence of reverberating circuits, i.e. groups of neurons stimulating themselves
- Abnormally low circulating endorphins

16.5.5.4   Models to Adopt in Managing Chronic LBP

- The International Classification of Functioning Disability and Health (ICF) model
- Emory Pain Estimate model
  (These have been discussed in detail in Chaps. 1 and 15)

16.5.5.4.1   Important Role of Social Context

- Recent evidence, such as studies on chronic back pain, that focuses on changing the social context can reduce disability as measured by sick leave or disability claims (Buchbinder et al., BMJ 2001)
- In this study, a concerted and prolonged advertising and education campaign in Victoria, Australia did change the knowledge and beliefs of both members of the general public and of general practitioners
- There was a significant decline in medical claims relative to a control state in the same country (New South Wales)

16.5.5.4.2 Emory Pain Estimate

- The Emory Pain Estimate model is one of the other useful models for tackling and categorising chronic LBP problems
- A careful study of the Emory Pain Estimate model led to one important point that was mentioned earlier; namely, that patients with positive Waddell signs have been repeatedly mentioned by some texts to be quite highly suggestive of non-organic pathology; this may have been over-emphasised
- If we look at category III of the Emory Pain Model, it is crystal clear that some patients can have "high" or genuine pathology and yet have "high" pain behaviour
- Learning point: the presence of Waddell's signs is essentially indicative of high pain behaviour, the presence of which does not and should not rule out an underlying organic disorder

16.5.6   Interventions in Chronic LBP

16.5.6.1 Exercise

- Has been shown to be an effective option in LBP with good results
- Examples: Manniche et al., Pain 1991; Hansen et al., Spine 1993

16.5.6.2 Work Hardening

- There is abundant support in the literature for this form of intervention in chronic LBP
- Examples: Hazard et al., Spine 1989; Mayer et al., JAMA 1987; Sachs et al., Spine 1990

16.5.6.3 Cognitive-Behavioural Approaches

- The reader will have come across these approaches frequently used by psychiatrists in managing back pain
- However, since many of these therapies are part of a fully comprehensive LBP programme in many hospitals, it is sometimes difficult to tell whether it is definitely useful or not
- It is the author's opinion that these therapies are sometimes useful in some individuals
- Let us not forget we mentioned the importance of personal context and beliefs in the new ICF model in Chap. 1
- The person's beliefs and cognition will definitely affect his illness behaviour and pain behaviour and relevant referral for assessment by clinical psychologists and psychiatrists should be initiated as necessary

16.5.6.3.1   What Does Cognitive-Behavioural Therapy Mean?

▓ These therapies are essentially based upon psychological principles for changing behaviour, and involve behaviour modifications. The term "cognitive" is frequently used because these therapies address factors like expectancies (remember we talked about placebo and no-cebo effects earlier), self-talk, the person's own beliefs and perceptions, interpretations, etc.

16.5.6.3.2   What Does Cognitive-Behavioural Therapy Involve?

▓ The therapy frequently involves several component procedures as a "package"

▓ The types of component procedures selected depends on the psychiatrists and which school of thoughts he follows, e.g. according to Ellis, Beck, or Meichenbaum

▓ Meichenbaum, for instance, believes that alteration of cognition will change the behaviour and emotions of the person (Meichenbaum, *Cognitive Behavior Modification*, 1977)

16.5.6.3.3   Examples of the Components of Cognitive-Behavioural Therapy

▓ Relaxation techniques
▓ Biofeedback
▓ Cognitive restructuring
▓ Coping skills or problem-solving training
▓ Stress management training
▓ Social skills training, etc.
   (The exact components selected depends on the individual patient and his illness)

16.5.6.4   Mind Body Interaction – Is There Any Scientific Basis for This Therapy?

▓ There is a growing enthusiasm in USA about the effects of "mind–body interaction strategies" in managing LBP, and whole books have been written on these subjects

▓ Although detailed discussion is outside the scope of this book, it is the author's belief that there is a scientific basis for a person's mind to affect the course of his or her illness, if only at least to affect the response to treatment, as can be seen in our detailed discussion on the placebo and nocebo effects and the basic science studies in support of these effects, in Chap. 15 on pain management

16.5.6.5   Multidisciplinary Approach

- Recent evidence suggests that a multidisciplinary approach that tries to alter several factors at once (multifocal intervention) may be beneficial
- In all 12 trials included in a recent systematic review, there was a psychological component that either generally focused on coping strategies or was in fact cognitive behavioural therapy
- Therefore, an approach that targets both impairment (through a functional restoration programme) and personal context (through cognitive behavioural therapy, etc.) seems to reduce pain more effectively than unifocal approaches (Guzman et al., BMJ 2001)

16.5.6.5.1   Further Evidence in Favour of Multidisciplinary Pain Programmes

- Further evidence in support of multidisciplinary pain programmes can be found in:
  - Nicholas et al., Pain 1992
  - Flor et al., Pain 1992

16.5.6.6   Importance of Work-Site Visit

- This has already been alluded to. This method has been proven to be useful, but has to be done early in the acute or subacute stage, and one should seldom wait until chronic LBP sets in
- For worker's compensation cases, the earlier the worker pays periodic visits to the work-site, the better. If clinically fit, light duties can be commenced early in the process of rehabilitation
- The longer a worker is off work, the less likely it is that he will eventually return to work

16.6   Commonly Used Assessment Measures

16.6.1   Subjective Assessment: Chronic LBP

- Roland Morris is the disability questionnaire used most (Roland and Fairbank, Spine 1983)
- Another popular score is the Oswestry low back pain disability questionnaire (Fairbank et al., Physiotherapy 1980)
- Others: Quebec Task Force

16.6.1.1   Roland Morris Score

16.6.1.1.1   Advantage of Roland Morris Score
- Used by most researchers and forms a good basis for comparative studies
- Good measure of early and acute disability and recovery
- Sensitive to change (Spine 2000)

16.6.1.1.2   Disadvantage of Roland Morris Score
- Not such a good measure for back pain patients with severe and chronic disability

16.6.1.2   Oswestry Score

16.6.1.2.1   Advantage of Oswestry Score
- Good tool to measure patients with severe disability

16.6.1.2.2   Disadvantage of Oswestry Score
- More complex to fill in
- Not so good for low levels of disability

16.6.2   Objective Assessment: Chronic LBP
- FCE: discussed in great detail in Chap. 17, but notice that doubts have been cast on the validity of FCE in recent papers
- Trunk Performance Test (Scand J Rehabil Med 1994)
- The Tampa scale for kinesiophobia: used to evaluate fear of movement and re-injury in workers (J Rehabil Med 2001) and a good tool for investigating pain behaviour
- Physical performance tests (Spine 1998)
- Shuttle walk test (Thorax 1992)

16.6.2.1   Advantage of FCE
- Reliability
- Reasonably objective
- Safe
- Print-outs have population norms for comparison
- Frequently used for vocational assessment, sometimes ordered by insurance companies, and useful for research and monitoring progress

16.6.2.2 Disadvantage of FCE

- It measures performance not capacity, still depends on patient's efforts
- Expense
- Needs a trained observer
- Time-consuming

16.6.2.3 Recent Doubts Cast on the Usefulness of FCE (in Workers with Chronic LBP)

- Better performance on evaluation was only weakly associated with faster recovery in workers with chronic LBP (Gross et al., Spine 2004)
- Contrary to functional capacity evaluation theory, better functional capacity evaluation performance, as indicated by a lower number of failed tasks, was in fact associated with higher risk of recurrence. The validity of functional capacity evaluation's purported ability to identify claimants who are "safe" to return to work is suspect (Gross et al., Spine 2004)

16.6.2.4 Possible Reason for the Observed Limitations of FCE in LBP

- It should be noted that functional capacity evaluations should be considered behavioural tests influenced by multiple factors, including physical ability, beliefs and perceptions (Phys Ther 2005)

16.7 Appendix: Myofascial Pain Syndrome and Fibromyalgia

16.7.1 Nature and Pathogenesis

- Myofascial pain is believed to result mostly from an original muscular injury that may release ionic calcium from breached sacroplasmic reticulum. The result is local ischaemia, depletion of ATP after local sustained contraction, with release of vasoactive substances like PG (prostaglandins) and serotonin that also sensitise the nociceptors

16.7.2 Location of Muscle Nociceptors

- The nociceptors in the muscles are believed to be specialised nerve endings that are at least partially ensheathed by Schwann cells; exposed areas have supply of vesicles and mitochondria (Mennell and Zohn 1976)

16.7.3 Result of Chronic Nociceptive Stimulation

▓ Chronic activation may trigger a self-sustaining cycle with enhanced local sympathetic activity and muscle tension, and possible later fibrotic changes (Bonica and Sola, 1990)

16.7.4 Classes of Myofascial Pain

▓ Primary – result from past trauma
▓ Secondary – no trauma

16.7.5 Characteristic Feature of Myofascial Pain Syndrome

▓ One main feature of this condition is the presence of trigger points. Pressure on these trigger points tends to reproduce the patient's pattern of pain

16.7.6 Microstructure of Trigger Points

▓ Studies under electron microscopy revealed evidence of hyaline changes and myofibrillar degeneration in the muscle fibres, as well as deposit of non-specific inflammatory residue in the interstices of the skeletal muscle (Mennell and Zohn)

16.7.7 Diagnosis of Myofascial Pain

▓ Diagnosis confirmed by inactivating the trigger point and methods include: stretching, injection of local anaesthetic (Travell et al., 1983)

16.7.8 Locating Trigger Points

▓ "Clinical" (by combination of spot tenderness, taut band, jump sign, pain recognition and local twitch responses)
▓ By algometer
▓ By thermography
▓ By electrical stimulation

16.7.9 Treatment

▓ Patient education, and stretching
▓ Cryotherapy: possibly acts via decreased temperature and stimulation of A-delta fibres, thereby suppressing C-fibres in the spinal gate
▓ Heat application
▓ Injection of local anaesthetic or use of iontophoresis
▓ TENS or related technique working according to the gate theory

■ Although some centres have started to use radiofrequency, this condition is not a common indication for radiofrequency

16.7.10   Fibromyalgia

■ This condition needs to be differentiated from myofascial pain syndrome
■ This condition occurs more frequently in females and is characterised by widespread chronic pain and systemic symptoms like sleep disturbance, depression and general fatigue

16.7.10.1   Diagnostic Criteria of Fibromyalgia

■ Guidelines from American College of Rheumatology:
  – Pain felt in ≥11 out of 18 predetermined points on physical examination
  – Pain and (usually bilateral) tenderness lasting ≥3 months involving both the axial region and above and below the waist

16.7.10.2   Pre-Determined Points in the Diagnosis of Fibromyalgia

■ Check on both sides:
  – Suboccipital muscle insertions
  – Low anterior cervical region
  – Second costochondral junction
  – Trapezius upper border
  – Supraspinatus
  – Lateral epicondyle
  – Superolateral gluteal area
  – Posterior aspect of greater trochanter
  – Medial knee

16.7.10.3   Treatment of Fibromyalgia

■ Education and exercise seem most important (Burckhardt et al., J Rheumatol 1994)
■ Other options:
  – Acupuncture, TENS, massage/relaxation therapy
  – Treat associated depression
  – Short course of analgesics, and/or tender point injections

General Bibliography

Newnham P (2002) Chronic Spinal Pain. Flivo Press, Meggen, Switzerland

Waddell G (2004) The Back Pain Revolution. Churchill Livingstone, Elsevier, UK

Cara E (2005) Psychosocial Occupational Therapy. Thompson Delmar Learning, New York

Selected Bibliography of Journal Articles

1. Waxman R, Tennant A et al. (1998) Community survey of factors associated with consultation for low back pain. BMJ 318(7199):1564–1567

2. Von Korff M, Le Resche L et al. (1992) Grading the severity of chronic pain. Pain 50(2):133–149

3. Waddell G, Feder G et al. (1997) Systematic reviews of bed rest and advice to stay active in acute low back pain. Br J Gen Pract 47(423):647–652

4. Harding L (1995) Treatment of acute low back pain. N Engl J Med 332(26):1787

5. Deyo RA (1996) Drug therapy for back pain: which drugs help which patient? Spine 21(24):2826–2832

6. Van Tulder MW, Scholten RJ et al. (2000) Non-steroidal anti-inflammatory drugs for low back pain: a systematic review within the framework of the Cochrane Collaboration Back Study Group. Spine 25(19):2501–2513

7. Van der Heijden GJ, Beurskens AJ et al. (1995) The efficacy of traction for back and neck pain: a systematic blinded review of randomized clinical trial methods. Phys Ther 75(2):93–104

8. Anderson R, Meeker WC et al. (1992) A meta-analysis of clinical trials of spinal manipulation. J Manipulative Physiol Ther 15(3):181–194

9. Koes BW, Assendelft WJ et al. (1996) Spinal manipulation for low back pain. An updated systematic review of randomized clinical trials. Spine 21(24):2860–2871

10. Cherkin DC, Deyo RA (1998) A comparison of physical therapy, chiropractic manipulation, and provision of an education booklet for the treatment of patients with low back pain. N Engl J Med 339(15):1021–1029

11. Faas A (1995) A randomized trial of exercise therapy in patients with acute low back pain: Efficacy on sick leave absence. Spine 20(8):941–947

12. Dettori JR, Bullock SH et al. (1995) The effects of spinal flexion and extension exercises and their associated postures in patients with acute low back pain. Spine 20(21):2303–2312

13. Koes BW, Van Tulder MW et al. (1994) The efficacy of back schools: a review of randomized clinical trials. J Clin Epidemiol 47(8):851–862

14. Di Fabio RP (1995) Efficacy of comprehensive rehabilitation programs and back school for patients with low back pain: a meta-analysis. Phys Ther 75(10):865–878

15. Leclaire R, Esdaile JM et al. (1996) Back school in a first episode of compensated acute low back pain: a clinical trial to assess efficacy and prevent relapse. Arch Phys Med Rehabil 77(7):673–679

16. Ernst E, White AR (1998) Acupuncture for back pain: a meta-analysis of randomized clinical trial. Arch Intern Med 158(20):2235–2241

17. Mitchell RI, Carmen GM (1990) Results of a multicenter trial using an intensive active exercise program for the treatment of acute soft tissue and back injuries. Spine 15(6):514–521

18. Philips HC, Grant L (1991) Acute back pain; a psychological analysis. Behav Res Ther 29(5):429–434

19. Karjalainen K, Malmivaara A et al. (2003) Mini-intervention for subacute low back pain: a randomized controlled trial. Spine 28(6):533–540

20. Karppinen J, Hurri H (2004) Discogenic pain. Pain 112(3):225–228

21. Pomerantz SR, Hirsch JA (2006) Intradiscal therapies for discogenic pain. Semin Musculoskelet Radiol 10(2):125–135

22. Singh V, Derby R (2006) Percutaneous lumbar disc decompression. Pain Physician 9(2):139–146

23. Tropiano P, Huang RC et al. (2005) Lumbar total disc replacement. Seven to eleven year follow up. J Bone Joint Surg Am 87(3):490–496

24. Carter ML (2004) Spinal cord stimulation in chronic pain: a review of the evidence. Anesth Intensive Care 32(1):11–21

25. Yamashiro K, Iwayama K et al. (1991) Neurones with epileptiform discharge in the central nervous system and chronic pain. Experimental and clinical investigations. Acta Neurochir 52:130–132

26. Buchbinder R, Jolley D et al. (2001) Population based intervention to change back pain beliefs and disability: three part evaluation. BMJ 322(7301):1516–1520

27. Manniche C, Lundberg E et al. (1991) Intensive dynamic back exercises for chronic low back pain: a clinical trial. Pain 47(1):53–63

28. Hansen FR, Bendix T et al. (1993) Intensive, dynamic, back-muscle exercises, conventional physiotherapy, or placebo-controlled treatment of low back pain. A randomized, observer-blind trial. Spine 18(1):98–108

29. Hazard RG, Fenwick JW et al. (1989) Functional restoration with behavioral support. A one-year prospective study of patients with chronic low back pain. Spine 14(2):157–1561

30. Mayer TG, Gatchel RJ et al. (1987) A prospective two-year study of functional restoration in industrial back injury. An objective assessment procedure. JAMA 258(13):1763–1767

31. Sachs BL, David JA et al. (1990) Spinal rehabilitation by work tolerance based on objective physical capacity assessment of dysfunction. A prospective study with control subjects and twelve month review. Spine 15(12):1325–1332

32. Guzman J, Esmail R et al. (2001) Multidisciplinary rehabilitation for chronic low back pain: systematic review. BMJ 322(7301):1511–1516

33. Flor H, Fydrich T et al. (1992) Efficacy of multi-disciplinary pain treatment centers: a meta-analytic review. Pain 49(2):221–230

34. Roland M, Morris R (1983) A study of the natural history of back pain. I. Development of a reliable and sensitive measure of disability in low back pain. Spine 8(2):141–144

17.1.2.2.1   Expanded Routine Task Inventory
■ Key elements include:
  - Able to follow directions
  - Able to maintain work place
  - Ability to perform simple to complex tasks
  - Ability to get along with co-workers
  - Ability to follow safety precautions
  - Ability to plan a work task for self and others

17.1.2.3   Work Traits
■ "General work traits" refer to abilities that are common to several jobs (Bryan, *Occupational Therapy and Practice*, 1990)
■ Most involve test batteries that assess several work traits, e.g. Valpar test
■ Tests of general work traits are better used to document gains before and after therapy

17.1.2.3.1   Drawbacks of General Work Traits
■ Drawbacks of test batteries like Valpar:
  - Cost
  - Over-simplification of work environment lacks content validity (Am J Occup Ther 1987)
  - Do not take into account other aspects like work place, cognitive or emotional factors or effects at work
  - Lacks predictive validity (according to Zila)

17.1.2.4   Work Conditioning
■ Work conditioning refers to the therapists emphasising aspects of general work conditioning as opposed to specific work tasks (according to Egan)

17.1.2.5   Work Hardening
■ In USA, work hardening needs accreditation by bodies like the Commission of Accreditation of Rehabilitation Facilities
■ The three major elements of work hardening:
  - Physical job demands
  - Cognitive job demands
  - Psychosocial job demands (Occupational Therapy Week, 1992)

17.1.3   Return to Work Issues for Patients with Physical Impairment

▪ In USA, the employer:
 – Cannot prescribe test that evaluates non-essential job functions
 – But can order assessment of essential job tasks for potential employees or prior to return to work of injured workers

17.1.4   Testing Specific Work Skills

▪ This may take the form of:
 – Standardised work samples (e.g. TOWER systems)
 – Simulated work samples
 – Using BTE (Baltimore Therapeutic Equipment) or other related systems like Lido-Workset (Fig. 17.1)
 – Or design special work sample after job analysis

17.1.4.1 Baltimore Therapeutic Equipment

▪ A machine providing work simulation with different handles and attachments simulating different jobs (according to Jacobs)

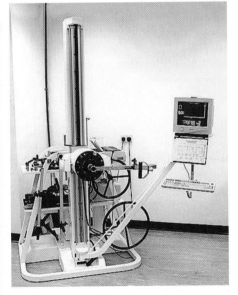

Fig. 17.1. The Lido Workset

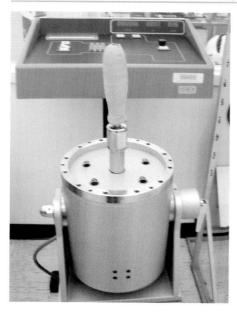

Fig. 17.2. Part of the BTE machine

- Can be adjusted to different heights and angles according to the exact nature of the patient's job (see Fig. 17.2)
- Validity of these and other work simulators have not been proven beyond doubt (according to Taylor)

17.1.4.2 Job Analysis
- Assess tools used by the job
- Assess the work-station
- Assess worker's capacity for job-specific force, position, or speed of bodily motions (according to Trombly)

(NB: to achieve the above frequently necessitates a work-place visit)

17.1.4.3 Criteria for Judging Worker's Compensation
- History of injury
- Injury from accident
- Injury that arose from employment
- Injury occurring in the course of employment

17.2   Functional Capacity Evaluation

17.2.1   Definition
- Functional capacity evaluation (FCE) is measurement of the patient's performance in a comprehensive series of standardised tests, resulting in data that can be interpreted according to the predictive validity of each test
- FCE helps answer the main concerns of employers: including functional progress of injured workers, and return to work issues; although it sometimes has other uses like pre-employment assessments

17.2.2   History
- Demands of functional assessment and evaluation began in the early 1980s with rise in disability claims
- In the past, research on FCE focuses mainly on specific sub-portion rather than the more important overall predictive validity of FCE. The latest research shows the various limitations of FCE

17.2.3   Advantages of FCE
- Identification of abilities helps determine what the patient can achieve
- Provides a comparison between functional capacity and PDC (physical demand classification) levels
- Objectivity – frequently used by claims managers, clinicians and attorneys

17.2.4   Indications for FCE
- Pre-employment
- Monitoring progress of functional rehabilitation
- Prior to return to work

17.2.5   Return to Work
- Identifying the point of maximal medical improvement – prevents prolonged costly, ineffective rehabilitation
- The employer can work with injured worker to set goals for return to work
- In addition, a guide to the extent that the worker can tolerate the physical demands of his job can be estimated in a report given in the language of the DOT (*Dictionary of Occupational Titles*, 1991, 4th Edition)

17.2.6   Role of Job Demand Analysis

■ Matching the person to the job
■ Ensures smooth and competent work performance
■ Decreases risk of injury
■ Better planning for return to work
■ Uniform criteria of hiring prevent administrative conflicts

17.2.7   Common Recommendations Given After Job Analysis

■ Job/task modification
■ Job reschedule
■ Ergonomics modifications
■ Environment modifications, e.g. work place layout, work aids

17.2.8   Main Types of Evaluation

■ For any type of occupation
■ For a specific occupation (Abdel-Moty, Clin J Pain 1993)
■ For a specific job
■ Readiness for return to work assessment
■ Solely to identify functional abilities of the worker

17.2.9   Issue of Reliability

■ If we obtain consistent data from FCE studies of our patients – can be referred to as reliable data
■ But "reliable data" do not necessarily mean that the effort is maximal
■ Thus, consistent data are necessary but not a sufficient condition to determine maximal effort. Inconsistent data, on the other hand, are invariably unreliable

17.2.10   What Is "Maximal Effort"

■ Maximal effort implies that the patient's data are not only consistent, but also represent the patient's best, yet safe, physiological effort

17.2.11   Tests to Assess Maximal Effort

■ Maximum voluntary grip strength
■ Rapid exchange grip
■ Other additional clues from:
  – Reasons for test termination, e.g. whether each test termination consistently reaches maximum heart rate

– Observations (by the therapist) of corresponding changes in motion patterns or physiology (e.g. HR/RR) during the report of symptoms (e.g. pain) by the patient

17.2.12　Can We Diagnose "Symptom Magnification"?

■ We do *not* use FCE to make comments on whether the patient is magnifying the symptoms
■ All we can do is to determine whether the patient's self-reported symptoms are consistent with observed behaviour

17.2.13　Assessing Functional Abilities

17.2.13.1　Ability to Reach Physical Demands
■ This aspect will be recorded according to the physical demand category (PDC) in the *Dictionary of Occupational Titles* (1991, 4th edition)

17.2.13.2　Assessment of Range of Motion
■ The respective ROM should be recorded and interpreted according to AMA guidelines

17.2.13.3　Cardiovascular Assessment
■ Fitness level can be determined via cardiovascular assessment using:
– Single-stage treadmill test and/or VO_2max
– Others

17.3　Overuse Work-Related Injuries

17.3.1　Terminology
■ Overuse musculoskeletal injuries
■ Repetitive stress injuries
■ Cumulative trauma disorders

17.3.2　Aetiologic Factors
■ Multifactorial and include:
– Physical factors
– Individual factors
– Psychosocial factors
– Ergonomic factors

17.3.3 Commonest Aetiology

■ Prolonged positioning away from the ideal posture will affect neural and other soft tissues in the upper extremity

■ Abnormal postures and positions may result in chronic nerve compression or may shorten muscles and, if the muscle crosses over a nerve, compression may occur. These postures may also contribute to muscle imbalance (Novak, J Orthop Sports Phys Ther 2004)

17.3.4 Pathomechanics

■ Tendinopathy affects millions of people in athletic and occupational settings and is a nemesis for patients and physicians

■ Mechanical loading is a major causative factor for tendinopathy; however, the exact mechanical loading conditions (magnitude, frequency, duration, loading history, or some combinations) that cause tendinopathy are poorly defined

■ Exercise animal model studies indicate that repetitive mechanical loading induces inflammatory and degenerative changes in tendons, but the cellular and molecular mechanisms responsible for such changes are not known

■ Injection animal model studies show that collagenase and inflammatory agents (inflammatory cytokines and prostaglandin E1 and E2) may be involved in tendon inflammation and degeneration; however, whether these molecules are involved in the development of tendinopathy because of mechanical loading remains to be verified

■ Finally, despite improved treatment modalities, the clinical outcome of treatment of tendinopathy is unpredictable, as it is not clear whether a specific modality treats the symptoms or the causes. Research is required to better understand the mechanisms of tendinopathy at the tissue, cellular, and molecular levels and to develop new scientifically based modalities to treat tendinopathy more effectively (Clin Orthop Relat Res 2006)

17.3.5 Predictors of Work-Related Repetitive Strain Injuries

■ The predictors positively associated with work-related repetitive strain injuries found in a recent population cohort study involving 2,800 workers include:
  - Female gender (odds ratio 1.98)
  - Some college or university education (odds ratio 1.98)

- Job insecurity (odds ratio 1.76)
- High physical exertion levels (odds ratio 2.00)
- High levels of psychological demands (odds ratio 1.61)

(Cole et al., Am J Public Health 2005)

17.3.6 Upper Limb Overuse Injuries

■ Many work-related overuse injuries involve the upper limb
■ Up until recently, criteria for classification of upper limb work-related overuse disorders had not been well described
■ In particular, many such injuries involve visual display units (see later discussion)

17.3.6.1 Criteria for Classification of Upper Limb Work-Related Disorders

■ Standardising terms and providing homogeneous criteria to achieve classification of upper limb damage due to biomechanical overload for increasing severity levels is absolutely essential
■ A recent attempt has been made by the consensus report by the Italian Working Group in 2005

17.3.6.2 Recommendations of the Working Group

■ The working group, which included the Italian Society of Physical Medicine and Rehabilitation and Italian Society of Clinical Neurophysiology, defined a general clinical procedure stressing objective examination and instrumental assessment (especially ultrasound and nerve conduction testing) regarding each portion of the upper limb concerned (shoulder, elbow and wrist/hand)

17.3.6.3 Risk Factors for Upper Limb Disorders
Due to Work-Related Visual Display Units

■ Physical risk factors include:
- Repetition
- Duration
- Working in awkward and static positions
- Forceful movements of the upper extremity and neck (J Occup Rehab 2005)
■ Attention to proper ergonomic principles in the design of visual display units such as computer work-stations is important (Delisle et al., Ergonomics 2006)

17.3.6.4   Treatment Principles

▨ Since frequently multifactorial, all factors need to be tackled:
- Job analysis and work place visit
- Patient education
- Postural correction
- Specific physical therapy programme to address the multiple levels of nerve compression and cervicoscapular muscle imbalance
- Behavioural modification at home and at work may be necessary (J Orthop Sports Phys Ther 2004)

17.3.6.5   FCE for Work-Related Upper Limb Disorders

▨ Work-related upper limb disorders in patients are commonly associated with reduction in functional capacity

▨ A validated instrument to test functional capacity in this patient group is unavailable

▨ But a recent paper does describe the functional capacity evaluation for work-related upper limb disorder patients working with visual display units and provides evidence of content validity (Reneman et al., J Occup Rehabil 2005)

▨ Eight tests were selected to cover all risk factors:
- The overhead lift
- Overhead work
- Repetitive reaching
- Handgrip strength
- Finger strength
- Wrist extension strength
- Fingertip dexterity
- A hand and forearm dexterity test

17.3.6.6   Preventing Future Injuries

▨ Prevention of further injuries needs attention to paid to:
- Ergonomic factors by the employer
- Attention to posture by the patient

17.3.6.6.1   Importance of Ergonomics

▨ Attention to ergonomics by employers has the following potential benefits:
- Increased work site safety

- Decrease in injuries hence decreased cost
- Manifestations of concern to workers
- Increased job satisfaction and productivity

17.3.6.6.2 Principle of Proper Positioning (after Church and Glennen)

- Proper positioning of body segments and posture in handling heavy items is important in prevention of back injury and lighter duties are usually prescribed for back-injured workers initially returning to work
- In computer workers, proper arm and wrist supports are particularly important to prevent overuse injuries like elbow lateral epicondylitis
- For patients with physical impairment, proper positioning and support are needed, especially for those with poor neuromuscular control and truncal weakness. Proper function positioning of the body part involved in handling equipment is essential

17.3.6.6.3 Principle of the Anatomical Control Site (after Galvin and Scherer)

- The control display and command panels of machinery need to be placed in the most comfortable position with due regard to the biomechanics and kinesiology of the human body
- In patients with physical impairment, the control buttons or control arm of the machinery should be within easy reach of the most functional body part of the patient
- For more impaired patients, the control panel should be made as simplistic as possible, such as the use of a single switch as opposed to rows of switches
- Even if the returning worker has fully recovered, work places that have awkward layout of machines or storage units may make it difficult to use the knowledge of "good body mechanics" taught to the patient by the therapist (Carlton, Am J Occup Ther 1987)

17.3.6.6.4 Principle of Simplicity and Intuitive Operation (after Saunders and McCormick)

- Design of the controls of machinery should be compatible with the intuition of most humans as far as possible just like closing a valve is by clockwise motion as opposed to a counter-clockwise manoeuvre
- These design considerations also serve to minimise errors
- For patients with physical impairments, these designs will make it easier and quicker to master

17.3.6.6.5   Principle of Notice Suitability (after Saunders and McCormick)

- Notices like warnings or precautions to take should be placed in easily visible parts of the machinery, preferably right next to the control arm or control button to prevent undue hazards
- For patients with physical impairment such as visual impairment, conveying a warning notice may need use another of the body's senses like use of a siren or sharp warning sound, assuming the hearing of the patient is not impaired

17.3.6.6.6   Principle of Allowance of Recovery from Errors (after Szeto A)

- Strategies in this respect are many, such as colour coding of wires, making the machinery or socket connection so that it fits in only one orientation, and prevention of harm to the operator by fusing the electrical appliances
- For physically impaired patients, with, say, decreased dexterity, then addition of a second set of safety measures like voice commands (e.g. undo connection) will be of help especially if there is concomitant visual impairment. This will also help prevent undue injury to our patient

17.3.6.6.7   Principle of Adaptability and Flexibility (after Szeto A)

- Machinery should be made user friendly and easy to handle. This will not only quicken the process of learning, but lessen the chance of error during busy handling of the machinery. Thus, the importance of a friendly human–machine interface
- For patients with physical impairments, the device and controls should be made to fit the person, and not the other way round. This is also the principle used in the design of assistive devices discussed in Chap. 6 on AT

17.3.6.6.8   Principle of Mental and Chronological Age Appropriateness (after Szeto A)

- Design of equipment should suit the age of the target group, for instance, rehabilitation equipment for children should preferably have adjustable heights as the child grows
- For patients with physical impairments, for instance CP and neurodegenerative brain disorders, sometimes they may have a mental age different from chronological age and corresponding adaptations need be made in either the machinery or rehabilitative devices

17.4 Towards Earlier Return to Work in Workers in Chronic LBP

17.4.1 Introduction
■ Many of the key strategies in rehabilitation previously discussed in this text are useful in planning work rehabilitation and earlier return to work in workers with chronic LBP

17.4.2 Goal Setting
■ Goal setting should commence once the multidisciplinary team have collected data from vocational, psychological and functional assessment

17.4.3 Function of Goal Setting
■ Clarify for the team and patient the goals with regard to vocation, function and psychological aspects
■ This process frequently helps in overcoming the not infrequent conflicts between different parties, i.e. patient's family, insurance companies, and the employers

17.4.4 Keys to Make the Goal Setting Process a Success
■ Goals should be tailor-made for the individual with due consideration of his occupational requirements
■ Throughout the process, the importance of active participation by the patient being needed for success is stressed

17.4.5 Functional Evaluation
■ Functional testing can reveal the patient's capacities and limitations
■ Functional capacity is compared to norms, and serial assessments are made to monitor progress
■ Slow or no progress may necessitate more frequent multidisciplinary meetings for evaluation

17.4.6 Programme of Functional Restoration
■ Most functional restoration programmes have the following elements:
  - Start with low demand aerobic, flexibility and toning exercises
  - Second part of the session will involve bicycling, and specific muscle group exercise

– This is followed by progressive lifting drills or other work simulation activities (Figs. 17.3, 17.4)

17.4.7 Psychological Programme

◼ Typically may consist of:
   – Emotional therapy, e.g. to create more realistic concepts of pain
   – Coping techniques and stress management, e.g. fear of re-injury
   – Inculcate more positive thinking and shy away from passive feelings of pessimism
   – Special psychotherapy for specific problems, e.g. depression

17.4.8 Social Issues

◼ In many cases, the multidisciplinary team may need to enlist the help of social workers to tackle problems such as finance, familial discord, etc.

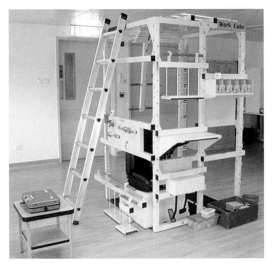

Fig. 17.3. The "Work-Cube" used by therapists for work simulation and work hardening

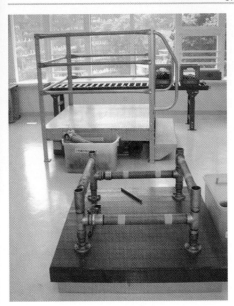

Fig. 17.4. Another example of a simulated work environment for the training of workers prior to resumption of work

17.5   New Strategy for Early Return to Work

17.5.1   Introduction

▪ The following describes a viable programme run by the government labour department of the author's home country

▪ It is known as the "Voluntary Rehabilitation Programme" and is sponsored by the insurers, since early return to work decreases the period of disability payment and forms a win-win situation for all parties involved: employer, employee and insurance companies

17.5.2   Voluntary Rehabilitation Programme

▪ Aim:
   – Inculcate the worker with a positive attitude towards work and sense of belonging
   – Quicker recovery
   – Earliest possible return to work or at least to the work environment
   – Rebuild confidence on resumption of duties
   – Rebuild self-esteem

17.5.3 Procedure
- Insurer identifies suitable injured workers
- Insurer provides rehabilitation service free of charge
- Work trial starting with light duties that can be tolerated by the patient (with prior job analysis)

17.5.4 Work Trial
- Prior job analysis and assessment of fitness for work trial by professionals
- The professional team will make recommendations concerning:
  - Type of work
  - Duration of work per day
  - Total period of work trial (most last between 1 and 3 months)

17.5.5 Obstacles to be Surmounted
- Small scale industries may have difficulty in arranging "light duties"
- Worries about new injury
- Employers or workers sometimes lack confidence

General Bibliography

Putz-Anderson V (1988) Cumulative Trauma Disorders – A Manual for Musculoskeletal Diseases of the Upper Limb. Taylor and Francis, Philadelphia

Enderle J, Blanchard SM, Bronzino J (2005) Introduction to Biomedical Engineering, Academic Press

Selected Bibliography of Journal Articles

1. Da Silva Cardoso E, Allen CA et al. (2004) Life skills and subjective well-being of people with disabilities: a canonical correlation analysis. Int J Rehabil Res 27(4): 331–334
2. Abdel-Moty E, Fishbain DA et al. (1993) Functional capacity and residual functional capacity and their utility in measuring work capacity. Clin J Pain 9(3):168–173
3. Novak CB (2004) Upper extremity work-related musculoskeletal disorders: a treatment perspective. J Orthop Sports Phys Ther 34(10):628–637
4. Cole DC, Ibrahim S et al. (2005) Predictors of work-related repetitive strain injuries in a population cohort. Am J Public Health 95(7):1233–1237

5. Colombini D, Menoni O et al. (2005) Criteria for classification of upper limb work-related musculoskeletal disorders due to biomechanical overload in occupational health. Consensus document by Italian Working Group. Med Lav 96(Suppl 2):5–26
6. Delisle A, Imbeau D et al. (2006) Comparison of three computer office work-stations offering forearm support: impact on upper limb posture and muscle activation. Ergonomics 49(2):139–160
7. Reneman MF, Soer R et al. (2005) Basis for an FCE methodology for patients with work-related upper limb disorders. J Occup Rehabil 15(3):353–363

Contents

18.1   Putting Outcome Measures into the Correct Perspective

18.1.1   Introduction

■ The reader will notice that there are more and more books on the market on the topic of outcome measures; we will consider the reason for the boom in interest in the coming discussion

■ But the most important thing to point out is that seldom, if ever, do books on outcome measures highlight the fact that the design of our research is much more important than which of the dozens of outcome measures for a given pathology we will pick for our research study

■ As the recommended outcome measures for the orthopaedic conditions discussed in this book were given in their respective chapters, this chapter will be short and will mainly concentrate on some basic principles

18.1.2   Definition

■ "Outcome" is defined as a change in a state or situation that arises as a result of some process of intervention

■ "Measure" refers to the quantification of data in some way, either in absolute or relative terms

18.1.3   Putting the Role of Outcome Measures into the Correct Perspective

■ The discussion that follows will hopefully put the role of the different outcome measures (the numbers of which are increasing by the minute) into the correct perspective

18.1.4   Key Concept 1

■ Although knowledge of what constitutes a good outcome measure is important, it is even more essential that the fundamental design of the research study or audit we are going to embark on is properly designed

18.1.5   Key Concept 2

■ Outcome measures can be likened to surgical tools that the surgeon uses

■ No matter how good the surgical tools we have, they cannot substitute for poor surgical technique

■ Similarly, no matter how good an outcome measure the researcher picks, it cannot overcome the deficiency of a poorly designed study
■ On the other hand, reasonably reliable study results that may be worthy of publication can sometimes be obtained by a very well-designed study even in the face of outcome measures of slightly poorer quality

18.1.6 Recapitulating Elements of a Good Study Design
■ Clear statement of the research goal
■ Elimination of bias, e.g. use of controls, single or double blind studies preferred
■ Clear statement of the level of evidence
■ Proper power studies before research begins to ensure the magnitude of sample size required
■ Selection of proper assessment and outcome tools appropriate to the pathology at hand, as well as with due regard to the goal of the study
■ Proper presentation and analysis of data
■ Proper selection and use of statistical analyses
■ Appropriate discussion and conclusion based on the findings of the study

18.1.7 Reason for the Recent Surge in Interest in Outcome Measures
■ The main reason comes from aspects of clinical governance and clinical audit, which will be discussed separately. Often, health authorities are reluctant to pay for services rendered unless supported by "good outcome"; an example is seen in "seating clinics" discussed in Chap. 6
■ Moreover, when it comes to rehabilitation, many health administrators still have the misconception that a subspeciality like rehabilitation can be easily assessed by the use of outcome measures

18.1.8 Limitations in the Use of Outcome Measures in Rehabilitation
■ The outcome of the rehabilitation service as a whole may differ from the outcome arising from any single component of the service, remembering that the rehabilitation process is a multidisciplinary process with multiple interventions

- Often, the final outcome can be influenced by factors the team does not have control over, e.g. community resources, level of unemployment (Clin Rehabil 2001)
- As pointed out by ICF of WHO, besides the above-mentioned social context factors and physical factors of the patient (such as the number of impairments), there are factors pertaining to "personal context", e.g. attitudes of family, patient's beliefs and expectations

18.1.9 Why the Recent Surge in Interest in Quality of Life Outcome Measures?

- Increased realisation that functional status rating tools that measure consumers' performance in activities that are meaningful to them allows service providers to detect changes in functional status based on perceived quality of life

18.2 Selecting the Appropriate Outcome Measure for Your Research

18.2.1 Key Elements of Any Outcome Measure

- The numerous textbooks on outcome measures are usually rather dogmatic: they just tell you what the key elements are without explaining why. Then follows a list of validated and non-validated outcome measures for common clinical conditions
- In view of the above, we will use an example of a clinician selecting an investigation into a clinical problem as illustration. In this way, it will be much easier to understand and demystify aspects of outcome measures

18.2.2 Using Selection of Clinical Investigations to Ease Understanding

- I believe the readers are mostly clinicians, and we order clinical investigations every day
- What, then, makes us choose a particular clinical investigation of a patient?

18.2.2.1   The First Question

- We first ask ourselves what is the aim of ordering an investigation. In this context, we will use a 4-week postoperative TKR patient with recurrence of knee pain as our example
- In this example, suppose the surgeon wants to rule out subacute sepsis after examining the patient, and this is the chief aim in mind

18.2.2.1.1   Corollary

- Similarly, in the case of outcome measures we must first have the aim of our clinical research before proceeding to choosing an outcome measure

18.2.2.2   The Second Question

- The second question we ask ourselves is what determines our choice if there is more than one possible investigation to choose from
- In this case, our options include: ESR, C-reactive protein, diagnostic knee tapping, bone scan, open biopsy, frozen section, etc. The list is endless

18.2.2.2.1   Corollary

- This scenario is rather like the situation in which there are many outcome measures for the same orthopaedic condition we want to study

18.2.2.3   The Third Question

- Given the options, what determines our choices?
    - Depends on the test sensitivity, specificity and reliability
    - We will remind ourselves exactly what we are looking for in each test, i.e. the content
    - We need to interpret the test results
    - We need to decide whether to do one or more such investigations in our patient
    - If all tests are negative, but we still suspect infection, is there a test that is sensitive to changes in the patient's condition?

18.2.2.3.1   Corollary

- Similarly, in choosing outcome measures for our study:
    - We need to reveal the content or in other words, what exactly is a given outcome measure looking at
    - We will also come across cases in which more than one outcome study is needed, e.g. including both subjective and objective types

- We need to know how to interpret the meaning of the scoring used in different outcome measures
- We need to know how sensitive our test is – in the field of outcome measures we choose to call this "validity"
- We need to know the reliability or inter- and intra-observer reliability
- We need to know how responsive the test(s) we selected is/are well enough to pick up subsequent changes in the patient's condition (for better or for worse)

18.2.2.4   The Fourth Question

- Finally, we need to sign the consent and the patient invariably will ask questions like: "Is the procedure going to be very painful? Will I be incapacitated for days?" – in short, patient's acceptability
- On the other hand, we know at the back of our minds how simple or how complex the procedure is – in short, whether it is a technically demanding procedure

18.2.2.4.1   Corollary

- Similarly, in the case of outcome measures, whether it is user-friendly on the part of the patient and surgeon needs to be considered

18.2.3   Summary of Key Considerations in Choosing Outcome Measures

- Review the aim of our study and nature of the pathology and study population
- Reliability
- Content validity and content interpretation
- Responsiveness to change
- Whether user-friendly to both the patient and the surgeon

18.2.4   Other Myths Concerning Outcome Measures

- Misconception that better outcome measure will automatically equate with better function
- In fact, it is interesting to note that the yardstick of what constitutes a good outcome measure differs widely in the eyes of different people: some prefer simple measures, others prefer more disease-specific, yet others prefer more generic ones

18.2.5 Caution in the Use of Outcome Measures

▪ The measure chosen should only focus on the intended area of interest, not on extraneous factors, i.e. do not get side-tracked

▪ The measure chosen should preferably have been validated previously for the measurement of the item we are studying. Example: use of GMFM-66 as a monitor of muscle strength in CP children throughout his/her rehabilitation process

18.2.6 General Conclusion

▪ Outcome measures are only tools, not solutions

▪ All parties must remember that the validity of conclusions of any study depends mainly on the study design and logic of the study

▪ Using good and appropriate outcome measures increases the chance of success of the study, but cannot compensate for bad study design

18.3 Use of Outcome Measures in the Field of Rehabilitation

18.3.1 Pitfall of Using Outcome Measures in the Field of Rehabilitation

▪ Rehabilitation involves a multidisciplinary team process, and the patient receives multiple interventions going through the process

▪ The desired outcome of the service is affected and constrained by many factors outside the team's control; hence, application of clinical governance in rehabilitation is not straight forward

▪ Since monitoring outcome may be an ineffective way of assessing (Mant et al., BMJ 1995), especially when it comes to rehabilitation, an alternative way is to monitor "adverse outcomes" such as falls leading to fractures, pressure sores, etc.

18.3.2 Point of Note

▪ The field of rehabilitation itself involves periodic re-evaluation of its process. Re-evaluation is a main component of rehabilitation besides the three other components; namely, assessment, goal setting and intervention

▪ Most will agree a most convenient and appropriate means of monitoring is to review patient documentation

Occasionally, use of a standard outcome measure is appropriate in a rehabilitation service dedicated mainly to the treatment of a major clinical condition, e.g. geriatric hip fractures

18.4   Recent Trends

18.4.1   What Are Some Recent Trends in the Use of Outcome Measures?

Many orthopaedic surgeons are accustomed to using more objective outcome measures, e.g. Knee Society scores in patients undergoing TKR

There is recently a trend towards an increase in the use of subjective outcome measures, not only in orthopaedics, but also in other fields of medicine

18.4.2   Use of Patient-Based Subjective Outcome Measures

These are definitely increasing in popularity

The reader will note that more and more peer reviewed papers have now included patient-based subjective outcome measures

18.4.3   Chief Argument for Using Subjective Patient-Based Measures

Particularly after operation, e.g. spinal fusion, while the X-ray may look perfect and the attending surgeon contented, the patient may still be dissatisfied, say, because of persistent pain

Patient satisfaction is becoming a very important subjectively based outcome measure, particularly after surgical procedure

Subjective measures like the use of questionnaires frequently correlate well with the results of clinical assessment of health status and work ability (Eskelinen et al., Scand J Work Environ Health 1991)

18.4.4   Author's View

In most cases, the use of subjective and use of objective outcome measures compliment each other

It is the author's view that many research studies require the concomitant use of both objective *and* subjective outcome measures

18.5   Other Areas of Interest

18.5.1   The Question of "Validation"

■ To better illustrate the concept of validation, we will use "Validation of Questionnaires" as an example

18.5.2   Elaborating the Concept of "Validation"

■ Validation of a questionnaire involves testing its test-retest reliability (reproducibility), responsiveness (ability to detect clinically important change), and validity

■ Face validity is the concept that questions are relevant. Content validity is determined by the consensus of experts. Construct validity is determined by correlating participants' answers to the questions with objective measurements

■ However, some experts feel that there is no accepted standard of what constitutes validation. Validation is self-proclaimed, usually after a study has been published in a medical journal (according to Sarins)

18.5.3   Question of "Specificity"

■ Use of outcome measures that are specifically useful for the condition at hand should be borne in mind

■ For example, if we intend to assess the subjective outcome of ACL-injured patients, we should use measures like ACL-QOL (quality of life) questionnaire, rather than, say, the WOMAC or SF-36

■ The Short Form-36 (SF-36) is a generic measure that includes questions about general health, activities performed, problems at work, emotional issues, physical activities, pain and personal feelings. One of the 36 questions (specifically, a question regarding the level of vigorous activities) could relate to knee instability. The SF-36 has been validated for quality of life, but not for knee problems

■ The Western Ontario and McMaster Universities (WOMAC) Osteoarthritis Index was developed to assess patients who have osteoarthritis of the hip and/or knee. The index consists of 24 questions related to pain (5), stiffness (2) and physical function (17). The response to each question is scored from 0 to 4. The maximum score is 96. None of the questions are about instability or sports participation

  – A patient who has a tear of the ACL, causing the knee to give way with pivoting motions and resulting in positive Lachman and pivot-shift tests, can still receive a score of 96. The WOMAC scale has been validated for osteoarthritis of the knee, but not for knee instability

- The ACL-QOL questionnaire was developed, pretested and validated for patients who have a torn ACL

18.5.4   Learning Points Concerning the Use of Questionnaires

- The more specific a questionnaire, the more sensitive it will be for discriminating outcomes between patients who have the disorder
- A one-time use of a questionnaire on the status of a condition is not a "measure of outcome". The answers to the questions are merely descriptions of subjective symptoms at a single point in time. Comparing responses to the same questions asked before and after intervention are subjective measures of outcome

18.6   Clinical Governance

18.6.1   Concept of "Clinical Governance"

- The modern definition of clinical governance in the eyes of health authorities should involve the process of monitoring and improving the quality of clinical services. Also, since the healthcare organisation needs to take responsibility for its own affairs, it tries to locate "power and responsibility" at a point within the system (usually by nominated individuals) to take full responsibility for the delivery of a quality service

18.6.2   Key Elements of Clinical Governance

- Reach an agreed definition of the quality aimed at
- Agree on who is responsible for achieving and maintaining the agreed standards
- Agree on how quality is to be measured

18.6.3   Concluding Remarks: Is There an Ideal Outcome Measure?

- There is no one measure that is ideal
- It is the author's view that many studies require the concomitant use of both objective *and* subjective outcome measures

- Outcome measures that are validated to the disorder we are studying are concise and easy to administer by team members and evaluated serial functional changes will be given priority
- As far as rehabilitation is concerned, since a multidisciplinary team is involved; one should understand that the outcome of the rehabilitation service as a whole may differ from the outcome arising from any single component of the service
- Only proper understanding of the principles and uses of outcome measures will pave the way to satisfying the basic elements of clinical governance

General Bibliography

Pynsent P (2004) Outcome measures in Orthopaedics and Orthopaedic Trauma. Oxford University Press, UK

Selected Bibliography of Journal Articles

1. Mant J, Hicks N (1995) Detecting differences in quality of care: the sensitivity of measures of process and outcome in treating myocardial infarction. BMJ 311:793–796
2. Tuomi K, Eskelinen L et al. (1991) Effect of retirement on health and work ability among municipal employees. Scand J Work Environ Health, 17(Suppl 1):75–81

New Evidence-Based Programme for Preventing and Rehabilitating Hip Fractures (Thesis Submitted to the Rehabilitation Board of HKCOS)

Contents

19.1   General Introduction: Importance of Hip Fracture Prevention and Rehabilitation

19.1.1   Introduction

■ This thesis discusses a new comprehensive programme for tackling both the rehabilitation and prevention of geriatric hip fractures patients based on the latest evidence and studies of the author as well as those of numerous researchers in different disciplines. In the author's opinion, any hip fracture programme that does not incorporate secondary prevention of falls and management of osteoporosis is doomed to fail in the long run

■ In addition, analyses of fall mechanisms as well as postural and gait changes in the elderly represent fundamental data if a rational rehabilitation programme for hip fractures and fallers is to be designed rather than going for a cook-book approach

■ Despite marked advances in surgical techniques, technology and anaesthesia, which all serve to improve the rates of survival and successful outcome for elderly people with hip fractures, it is common knowledge that not less than 50% of these hip fracture patients fail to achieve physical, emotional or social recovery back to baseline, with a significant number becoming unable to return home or function independently, even after operation (Magaziner et al., J Gerontol Med Sci 1990). Moreover, many hip fracture patients scored poorly during follow-up in the Physical Role and Emotional Role Subsets of SF-36 (Petersen et al., Osteoporosis Int 2002). The reason for the poor outcome observed, as well as the underlying cause of poor results of hip fracture rehabilitation, was seldom highlighted enough in the literature. As pointed out in previous texts by the author, the effect of a hip fracture on the elderly is not unlike the effect of a high-energy trauma on younger individuals. In the past and I should sadly say even in some hospitals in this day and age, despite the fact that due respect has always been given to high-energy trauma in younger patients, the attitudes of many healthcare workers towards geriatric hip fractures are exemplified by common expressions like "just another hip fracture". The impact of hip fracture goes well beyond its morbidity as reported in standard texts, for it carries with it the well-known one-year mortality rate of 15–30%, depending on different series, and often has a profound influence on the social and psychological aspects of these individuals

19.1.2 Hip Fracture Epidemiology

■ In the proceedings of the 4th International Symposium on Osteoporosis and Consensus Development Conference, data from the Chinese University of Hong Kong indicated that there is a definite rising trend of hip fracture in Hong Kong. The figure rose from 321 per 100,000 of the population in 1966 to an astounding 1,916 per 100,000 in 1991. This has turned into tremendous cost implications for the local health authorities, both in Hong Kong and in many countries around the world with an aging population

■ Rising trends of hip fractures in other parts of Asia were highlighted in Chap. 1 of the author's companion text *Orthopedic Principles – A Resident's Guide*, and similar trends have also been observed particularly in countries with an aging population such as in Sweden

19.1.3 Importance of the Study of Fall Prevention

■ Different definitions of falls are found in the literature. The definition derived from the work of the Kellogg International Workgroup is often quoted, which describes a fall as an event that results in a person coming to rest inadvertently on the ground or other lower level other than as a consequence of the following: sustaining a violent blow; loss of consciousness (LOC); sudden onset of paralysis, as in a stroke; or epileptic seizure (Sattin). Perhaps a simpler definition is that a fall means a sudden and unintentional coming to rest at a lower level or on the floor (Patterson)

■ Orthopaedic surgeons as well as healthcare providers are very eager to reduce the number of falls in the elderly

■ The chief aim is to reduce the number of hip fragility fractures, which have been extrapolated in the past to rise exponentially as the population ages. Besides, it is a well-known fact that hip fracture in the elderly carries significant mortality and morbidity, not to mention the use of many human and hospital resources as mentioned

■ Devising effective fall prevention and an evidence-based fractured hip rehabilitation programme is a far from easy job. Although the world literature contains abundant books and articles by various authors reporting their own hip fracture rehabilitation protocol, they seldom report their long-term results and often fail to tell the reader the rationale behind their approach Sadly it was noted that few protocols involve a more comprehensive secondary and not to mention primary hip fracture and fall prevention programme. Devising such a programme is far from simple, for it requires knowledge of many disciplines: neurophysiology, theoretical physics, biomechanics, bioengineering, orthopaedics, etc. to name but a few disciplines, as well as good surgical techniques and proper selection of fracture implants on the part of the attending surgeon

■ The major part of the programme discussed here has already been put into practice in the author's regional hospital and sister hospitals. It is the firm belief of the author that a thorough understanding of postural control and gait changes in the elderly is fundamental and forms the cornerstone of a good evidence-based programme

19.1.4   Why Do the Elderly Fall?

■ The main categories of fall are usually divided into intrinsic versus extrinsic causes. The next section will detail the author's finding that the relative importance of intrinsic causes climbs sharply as one ages, particularly when someone reaches their 80s

19.1.4.1 Examples of Extrinsic Causes

■ Slippery floor, and/or obstacles
■ Slippery bathroom
■ Lack of night lights
■ Improper shoe wear, etc.

19.1.4.2 Examples of Intrinsic Causes

■ Musculoskeletal problems, e.g. pain and deformity of LL, cervical myelopathy
■ Problems of vision, vestibular function, etc.
■ Neurological, cardiovascular causes and psychiatric disturbance
■ Acute illness
■ Urinary-related problems
■ Malnutrition
■ Medication-related

19.2 Evidence Accumulated from the Study of the "Double Hip Fragility Fracture Study" Conducted by the Author

19.2.1 Importance of Studying the Patient Subgroup with Double Hip Fragility Fractures

■ This is important for various reasons. First, the literature on double hip fragility fractures is sparse. Yet, this is an important group of patients to study since it offers a golden opportunity for us to reveal the categories of causes of falls among the elderly, as patients with double sequential hip fractures are almost always frequent fallers and very few of us will dispute this point. This is also a challenging group as far as rehabilitation efforts go, just as it is much more challenging to rehabilitate a bilateral amputee as opposed to within a unilateral scenario, but the good point in such a research project when, for instance, we want to compare the efficacy of different protocols, is that the patient can then act as his or her own control and the confounding complex medical co-morbidity factors are essentially the same. In addition, this group is also unique in as far as patient demographics and fracture patterns are concerned, as the ensuing discussion will show

■ The following details this latest research project on double geriatric hip fractures and the important lessons learned from it. The important findings will pave the way for a more rational and practical approach to hip fractures as a whole. This paper, which is entitled: "Do elderly with double hip fragility fractures form a unique subgroup among geriatric hip fracture patients?" will soon be published by the *Journal of Orthopaedic Surgery (Hong Kong)* (December 2006 issue)

19.2.2 Materials and Methods

■ The study population consisted of an unselected series of consecutive admissions of geriatric hip fracture patients with a history of one documented episode of hip fracture of the contralateral hip. There were 50 patients with double hip fractures noted during the study period of 18 months, and we only excluded patients who were too medically unfit to have any surgery. The method of assessment of our hip fracture patients will be discussed separately later in this chapter (Sect. 19.7.2). Attention was paid particularly to the following parameters:

- The cause of the fall – this piece of information was obtained from the patient himself/herself, the carer, any nearby eyewitness, etc. Not uncommonly, the patient only manages to remember this bit of history upon return to the friendly atmosphere of the home environment and it is documented by our community nurse or occupational therapist during home visits, or during subsequent outpatient follow-up
- Fracture pattern, type of surgery, any initiation of osteoporosis treatment after the first fracture, presence of other fragility fractures other than the hip in the past, and period of rehabilitation and outcome of each episode of hip fracture

19.2.3 Results

■ The demographics of the 50 patients under study are shown in Table 19.1
■ Table 19.1 illustrates clearly that:
- The vast majority of the patients with double hip fragility fractures are of advanced age with a mean age of around 80
- Subgroup analysis (by age) reveals that the vast majority of the elderly with advanced age suffered from trochanteric fractures – the implication is that if we believe that our population is aging, then chances are we will be seeing many more trochanteric hip fractures as opposed to fractured necks of femurs – and this will further guide our future endeavour to improve our surgical results of trochanteric hip fractures (Fig. 19.1)
- As for the causes of the fall, in this study, 50% of cases were due to intrinsic causes, 25% to extrinsic causes, 16% were truly multifactorial, and the remainder were from unknown causes. Furthermore, subgroup analyses of the causes of the fall reveal that extrinsic causes mainly accounted for the cause in the younger age group (aged 65–75), while the older one gets, the more likely the cause of the fall will be due to intrinsic causes (Fig. 19.2). And, as the reader is probably aware, it is easier to correct extrinsic causes (e.g. slippery floor, improper shoe wear, improper use of walking aids, etc.) than intrinsic causes. For this reason, our discussion in the ensuing sections will concentrate more on intrinsic causes, with great emphasis on recent advances in our knowledge on postural and gait anomalies with aging, as well as those changes detected in frequent fallers or those with high-level gait disorders

Table 19.1. Demographics of 50 patients studied

Patient	Age/sex	Interval of fracture (years)	Factor causing fall	Factor causing previous fall	Type of hip fracture (this episode)	Type of hip fracture last episode
1	F/83	2.5	Kicked obstacle	Slippery floor	Trochanteric	Femoral neck
2	F/91	3.0	LL weakness	LL weakness	Trochanteric	Trochanteric
3	F/85	3.5	Incoordination	LL weakness	Trochanteric	Trochanteric
4	F/84	4.0	Slippery floor	Kicked obstacle	Trochanteric	Trochanteric
5	F/94	1.25	Multifactorial	Multifactorial	Trochanteric	Trochanteric
6	F/87	0.75	Multifactorial	Multifactorial	Trochanteric	Trochanteric
7	F/83	2.0	LL weakness	LL weakness	Femoral neck	Femoral neck
8	F/84	2.5	Unknown	Unknown	Trochanteric	Trochanteric
9	F/91	1.25	Incoordination	LL weakness	Trochanteric	Trochanteric
10	F/75	3.5	Kicked obstacle	Kicked obstacle	Femoral neck	Trochanteric
11	F/65	2.75	Slippery floor	Improper shoes	Femoral neck	Femoral neck
12	M/94	1.25	Urinary urgency	Confusion	Trochanteric	Trochanteric
13	F/94	0.75	Poor vision	Poor vision	Trochanteric	Trochanteric
14	F/82	1.25	Incoordination	LL weakness	Trochanteric	Trochanteric
15	F/96	2.25	LL weakness	LL weakness	Trochanteric	Trochanteric
16	F/79	1.75	Improper shoes	Slippery floor	Trochanteric	Femoral neck
17	M/94	2.5	LL weakness	Incoordination	Trochanteric	Trochanteric
18	F/83	2.0	LL weakness	LL weakness	Trochanteric	Trochanteric
19	M/82	1.25	Confusion	Urinary urgency	Trochanteric	Trochanteric
20	F/89	0.75	Multifactorial	Multifactorial	Trochanteric	Trochanteric
21	F/93	2.0	LL weakness	LL weakness	Trochanteric	Trochanteric
22	F/75	2.0	Kicked obstacle	Slippery floor	Trochanteric	Trochanteric
23	F/85	1.75	LL weakness	Incoordination	Trochanteric	Trochanteric

24	F/87	0.75	Multifactorial	Multifactorial	Trochanteric	Trochanteric
25	F/93	1.5	Poor vision	Poor vision	Trochanteric	Trochanteric
26	F/87	1.75	Incoordination	LL weakness	Trochanteric	Trochanteric
27	F/65	3.0	Slippery floor	Improper shoes	Femoral neck	Femoral neck
28	F/90	2.0	LL weakness	LL weakness	Trochanteric	Trochanteric
29	M/93	1.25	Multifactorial	Multifactorial	Trochanteric	Trochanteric
30	F/75	2.5	Kicked obstacle	Slippery floor	Trochanteric	Femoral neck
31	F/80	2.0	Slippery floor	Kicked obstacle	Trochanteric	Trochanteric
32	F/89	1.25	Multifactorial	Multifactorial	Trochanteric	Trochanteric
33	F/84	2.0	LL weakness	LL weakness	Trochanteric	Trochanteric
34	F/83	1.5	Poor vision	Dizziness	Femoral neck	Femoral neck
35	F/85	4.0	Improper shoes	Slippery floor	Trochanteric	Trochanteric
36	F/84	2.5	Incoordination	LL weakness	Femoral neck	Femoral neck
37	F/83	2.0	Kicked obstacle	Slippery floor	Trochanteric	Trochanteric
38	F/75	2.5	Slippery floor	Improper shoes	Femoral neck	Femoral neck
39	M/90	1.25	Urinary urgency	Poor vision	Trochanteric	Trochanteric
40	F/75	1.5	Kicked obstacle	Kicked obstacle	Femoral neck	Femoral neck
41	M/77	0.5	Unknown	Unknown	Femoral neck	Trochanteric
42	F/81	2.5	LL weakness	LL weakness	Trochanteric	Trochanteric
43	F/85	1.5	Dizziness	Unknown	Trochanteric	Trochanteric
44	M/82	3.0	Confusion	Urinary urgency	Femoral neck	Femoral neck
45	F/90	1.5	Multifactorial	Multifactorial	Trochanteric	Trochanteric
46	F/94	1.5	LL weakness	LL weakness	Trochanteric	Trochanteric
47	F/84	2.5	Kicked obstacle	Slippery floor	Femoral neck	Femoral neck
48	F/89	1.2	Unknown	Unknown	Trochanteric	Trochanteric
49	F/82	3.5	Incoordination	LL weakness	Femoral neck	Femoral neck
50	M/85	2.0	Multifactorial	Multifactorial	Trochanteric	Trochanteric

- The major implications of the current research include:
  - We have to try to find out the real cause of the fall causing the current hip fracture, as the cause tends to repeat itself in the second episode of falling
  - Trying all our efforts to correct the cause identified. All of us know that 90% of the literature on hip fractures will mention that the cause of hip fracture is multifactorial. While this is often true, since the current study showed clearly that the immediate cause of fall is truly multifactorial in only 16% of cases, and that the causes tend to repeat themselves (or in other words, history tends to repeat itself, even when it comes to the question of a fall), the immediate concern of the care team should be to concentrate all their efforts on correcting the immediate cause as soon and as far as possible
  - Patients whose fall really does have multifactorial causes are more complex and require detailed assessment by a multidisciplinary team and frequent assessment in a fall prevention clinic – a topic to be discussed at the end of this chapter (Sect. 19.12). This is because it is quite impossible and not really cost effective to refer each and every patient to fall prevention clinics (Ip et al., J Orthop Surg, Hong Kong)
- Another very important finding that needs to be highlighted in this study is the statistically significant increase in the time needed for rehabilitation of these patients. In the current study, the rehabilitation protocol given after surgery for both episodes of hip fracture were the same, and it was shown that the time required for rehabilitation of a second episode of hip fracture is statistically significantly longer than for the primary or first episode, with a p value of <0.01
- To the author's knowledge, this is also the first study to confirm that statistically significantly more time is needed for rehabilitation of patients suffering a second episode of fragility hip fracture, given the same rehabilitation protocol and given the same type of fracture and surgery. Based on all the aforementioned, it is the belief of the author that patients with bilateral geriatric hip fracture form a definite subgroup of patients with hip fracture that merits more of our investigative and research efforts. Also, the study of this group of patients will throw light on the future planning of our rehabilitation and preventive efforts for geriatric hip fractures

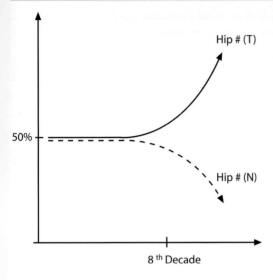

Fig. 19.1. Graph showing that as one ages (especially when someone reaches their 80 s), the proportion of trochanteric (*T*) hip fractures rises, while the proportion of fractured necks (*N*) of femur falls

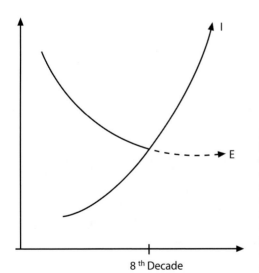

Fig. 19.2. Graph showing that as one ages (especially when someone reaches their 80 s) the proportion of falls due to intrinsic (*I*) causes rises significantly, while the proportion of falls due to extrinsic (*E*) factors does not

19.3   Science Behind Altered Postural Control in the Elderly: Basic Concepts

▓ Before we talk about strategies to prevent falls or of devising a rational hip fracture rehabilitation programme, we need to know the basic control mechanisms of human posture and walking. Studies of gait and postural deviations in the elderly are especially important, particularly the latter, since most falls in the elderly occur during walking

▓ But before we talk about these controls, we need to clarify two basic myths

19.3.1   Myth 1: "Human Gait Itself is Nothing More Than a Simple Automated Task"

▓ The above has recently been shown to be incorrect

▓ In fact, the act of human walking is a much more complicated task than simple automated processes like tapping our fingers on the table

▓ Human walking represents a complex cognitive task, especially involving executive function (according to Hausdorff). Much more discussion will be forthcoming in the pages that follow

19.3.2   Myth 2: "The Elderly Tend to Fall Since it is Part of the Aging Process"

▓ This was again shown to be incorrect

▓ In fact, as early as 1989, Woollacott showed in his book *Development of Posture and Gait Across the Lifespan* that normal aging and its subclinical signs and symptoms do not necessarily affect the functional status of elderly persons as long as the central nervous system can compensate for the cumulative sensorimotor degradation in adapting movements. Only when the central nervous system can no longer compensate will functional disabilities emerge

▓ Woollacott's findings were recently confirmed by careful research (Gait Posture 2005)

19.3.3 Control of Posture and Physiological Changes of Aging

19.3.3.1 Basic Components of Postural Control

▨ In humans, these include:
 – Sensory and proprioceptive input
 – Other senses located in the head: vision and vestibular systems
 – Motor output (as synergies)
 – Reflexes (their importance in quiet posture is doubted by some)
 – Central processing and integration of sensorimotor signals, possible cerebellar contribution
 – Higher cognitive functioning (does not refer to consciousness in this context, refers to adaptive movement strategies and anticipatory motions), activated in the presence of posture or gait perturbations

19.3.3.2 Role of Continuous Feedback

▨ Proper execution of balance and posture involves a feedback loop with:
 – Sensory input from vision, proprioception and vestibular apparatus of the inner ear
 – Central processing – involving the cerebrum, cerebellum, basal ganglia and brain stem
 – Muscular contractions to adjust balance

19.3.3.3 A Word on Sensory Inputs

▨ Vision – important sensory information and can normally compensate for the absence or unreliability of other sensory input
▨ Vestibular input is usually regarded as less crucial
▨ Proprioceptive input – located in the peripheral joints, especially at the soles of the feet, the lower limb muscle spindles and joints and cervical spine mechanoreceptors

19.3.3.4 Levels of Balance Control

▨ At the lowest level – involves sensory and musculoskeletal systems
▨ At a middle level – involves central processing areas – e.g. cerebellum, brain stem, motor and sensory cortices
▨ At the highest level – motor planning area involving the frontal lobes

19.3.3.5   The Normal Physiological Changes with Aging

▓ This involves:
  – Small increase in onset latency of long-latency postural reflexes
  – Reversal of the distal-to-proximal pattern of muscular activation in response to movement of the supporting surface, we will discuss more on this point later
  – In general, aging is associated with reduced mobility and often, gait velocity, step length and range of motion of lower limb joints are all decreased. This reduced performance capacity is often accompanied by reduced gait stability and increased risk of falling

19.3.3.5.1   Concomitant Lowered Strength in the Normal Healthy Elderly

▓ Recent research using isometric strength testing on a KinCom dynamometer (Rehab World, Hixson, TN, USA) confirmed a significant age-related reduction in strength (normalised to individual body weight) reaching statistical significance (Hahn et al., Gait Posture 2005)

19.3.3.5.2   Walking Speed May Be Decreased, But Not Always

▓ The fact that the gait velocities in healthy elderly volunteers need not be significantly lower than those in younger adults may indicate that they represent a more able-bodied section of the broader elderly population. It has been argued that it is quite possible for a sample of less active elderly individuals to demonstrate significantly slower walking speeds (Gait Posture 2005)

19.3.3.5.3   Possible Cause of Reduced Gait Speed in (Some) Elderly

▓ Recent studies cited kinematic alterations at the hip as being a cause of reduced gait speed in the elderly. As far as kinematic factors are concerned, a reduction in maximum hip extension in particular does not uncommonly act to limit gait speed early in the aging process (Riley, Gait Posture 2001)

19.3.4   Normal Controls in the Setting of Quiet Posture

19.3.4.1   Basic Physiology

▓ The relationship between the centre of pressure and centre of gravity is a valuable indicator of how the central nervous system sets ankle joint stiffness for the control of postural sway in the sagittal plane (Winter, J Neurophysiol 1998)

▪ During quiet standing for example, ankle dorsiflexors and plantar flexors act as springs to cause the centre of pressure to move in phase with the centre of the mass, making the body sway like an "inverted pendulum" about the ankles. Similarly, in dynamic conditions, such as gait initiation or one leg raising, any voluntary segmental movement is preceded by an early centre of pressure and centre of gravity displacement towards the supporting leg controlled by the ankle muscles

▪ With aging, however, there is often difficulty in controlling the anterior-posterior centre of gravity displacement during gait and particularly in decelerating its forward motion to regain a stable posture

▪ Studies revealed that the weaker coupling between the centre of pressure and centre of gravity motions with aging could be attributed to the inability of the ankle muscles to generate the levels of muscle torque required to maintain the foot fixed to the ground during performance of dynamic limb oscillations

▪ In fact, it has been proposed that a combination of slow activation and reduced high speed force generation of the ankle muscles may be one of the predisposing factors that increase the incidence of falls among the elderly. Moreover, the greatest decrease noted in tibialis anterior activation levels could be linked to recent works of Whipple's et al. showing the strength of ankle dorsiflexors to often be reduced significantly among all muscles in elderly fallers. This insufficient ankle muscle activity results in a highly unstable postural base, which in turn, restrains knee and hip motions of the stance limb

▪ Younger persons, on the other hand, generate sufficient levels of ankle muscle activity to create a stable postural base, which allows the "release" of extra degrees of freedom in the upper body. This is reflected in the "inverted pendulum" operation of the stance limb depicted by the progressively increasing joint range of motion from distal (ankle) to more proximal (hip) joints and greater trunk movement

19.3.4.2 Postural Control Changes in the Elderly

▪ In summary, insufficient ankle muscle activity, central integration deficits and increased anxiety to postural threat are important factors implicated in the weaker postural synergies and freezing of degrees of freedom seen in the elderly during performance of single limb oscillations (Hatzitaki, Gait Posture 2005)

19.3.4.3 Other Changes in Balance Controls in the Elderly

- Several studies have associated balance control limitations with a possibly less efficient information processing system responsible for the central integration of multiple sensory inputs (Perrin, Gerontology 1997; Hay, Exp Brain Res 1996)
- There are speculations from recent studies that the stabilising hip behaviour or strategy (which will be discussed in Sect. 19.3.5.2) results in an "en bloc"-like posture, is commonly preferentially selected by older adults in order to reduce the computational cost of dealing with the multiple degrees of freedom present during performance of a multisegmental dynamic postural task – in an attempt to mitigate against the less efficient information processing system
- Moreover, it has been suggested that since age-related declines in coordinated behaviour are a function of both cognitive and afferent information processing problems, these are highly task dependent (Serrien et al., J Gerontol B Psychol Sci Soc Sci 2000)
- Therefore, central integration limitations associated with aging are more profoundly manifested when the postural system is dynamically challenged by self-imposed perturbations, which induce higher requirements for inter-segment coordination in order to maintain balance

19.3.4.4 Overall Factors Governing the Ability to Maintain Quiet Stance

- "Proper" body alignment and mechanical axis
- Maintenance of basic muscle tone
- Low-grade activation of anti-gravity muscles
- Role of stretch reflexes doubted by many
- Proper functioning of the basic components, as just described

19.3.4.5 Relative Contribution of Different Components and Inputs

- With slow perturbations and in usual postural sways in quiet stance; all inputs are of importance – sensorimotor, vision, vestibular
- With quick or larger perturbations, the body predominantly relies on sensorimotor input. In general, sensorimotor input works better at in-

forming the central nervous system when and where to react to postural perturbations (also the time lag between input and response is twice as quick with sensorimotor input than with, say, visual input)
- Vision is not absolutely essential for postural control. For instance, one can stand with eyes closed, or can still walk in a darkened room, but visual cues are important in children learning how to walk or if somehow there is diminished sensorimotor input, as in walking on a foamy surface, or in the face of proprioceptive loss

19.3.4.6 Quiet Stance Represents Continuous Sways
- This refers to the fact that no person can in fact stand absolutely still (not even the guards in front of Windsor Castle)
- Laboratory analysis of force platforms (Fig. 19.3) showed that quiet stance involves continuous sways of the body, mainly in the antero-posterior direction. With more perturbations, our central nervous system tends to adopt different strategies for adaptation

19.3.5 Strategies with Small and Larger Postural Perturbations
- Researchers found that our central nervous system harbours some types of muscle strategies to handle motion perturbations. They are:
  – Ankle strategy
  – Hip strategy
  – Stepping strategy

19.3.5.1 Ankle Strategy
- To put it simply, the ankle strategy is such that the central nervous system adjusts the body sways with reference to the ankle joint
- For instance, if the body sways forwards, this will trigger firing of ankle plantar flexors, hamstrings, paraspinals, etc.

19.3.5.2 Hip Strategy
- The hip type of strategy tends to be used more often with larger postural perturbations, or during standing on a soft surface, or when the area available for base of support is small
- There is some evidence to suggest also that vestibular input is needed for a hip strategy. Preferential use of a hip strategy is common in the elderly

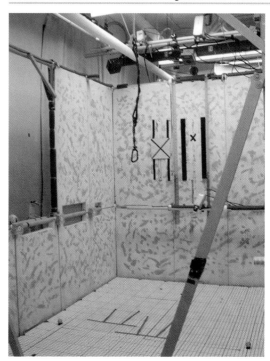

Fig. 19.3. Example of a "moving platform" for the study of falls in the elderly, this type of platform is used in Sunnybrook – where many famous papers on this subject originated

19.3.5.3 Stepping Strategy

■ The stepping strategy is usually employed in the face of large perturbations that displace the COM (centre of mass) outside the boundaries of the lower limb base of support

19.3.6   Age-Related Changes in the Use of Muscle Strategies

■ Research revealed that many elderly people have adopted the use of hip strategy rather than the ankle strategy in the face of motion perturbations. In other words, previous studies showed age-related redistribution of joint torques from ankle joint plantar flexion to hip joint extension in gait

19.3.7   More on Hip Strategy

▪ Thus, a hip strategy was used to maintain stability when the inertia of movement increased; the thigh muscles were activated before those of the leg. Even frequent running does not prevent this shift. Active elderly people may increase this redistribution to compensate for muscle function reduction (Hans et al., Gait Posture 2006)

▪ This underlines the importance of proper rehabilitation of the hip after hip fracture in an attempt to prevent further falls

19.3.8   Effect of Hamstring Activation in Falls in the Elderly

▪ Recent research has suggested that a decrease in the hamstring activation rate among the elderly is responsible for a higher horizontal heel contact velocity and increased likelihood of slip-induced falls compared with their younger counterparts who tend to have a higher hamstring activation rate than older adults. This results in heel contact velocity in younger adults being sufficiently reduced before the heel contact phase of the gait cycle. Notice hamstrings are important and act as a decelerator in the initial heel contact in gait (see Chap. 8; (Lockhart et al., Gait Posture 2005)

19.3.9   A Word on the Less Used Ankle Strategy

▪ Brownlee et al. suggested that older fallers frequently have proprioceptive dysfunction leading to unstable balance control. Thus, it appears that factors like proprioceptive dysfunction may well also contribute (at least) to a decrease in the use of the ankle strategy. This may result in the so-called reversal of the firing pattern of the lower limb, which will be discussed next

19.3.10   Reversal of the Lower Limb Muscular Firing Pattern in the Elderly

▪ Postural activation in young individuals usually proceeds in a distal to proximal direction and the ankle strategy is often used in motion perturbations. This sequence tends to be disrupted in elderly individuals. This implies that more proximal muscles may be activated first in the elderly, e.g. the first muscle event can be activation of the contralateral quadriceps. Moreover, for young individuals, soleus inhibition is only present for the ipsilateral muscle, whereas inhibition is present for both muscles (i.e. ipsilateral and contralateral) in elderly individuals. This asymmetric, anticipatory sequence is specific to the forthcoming (unilateral) movement in young but not in elderly individuals. The latter perform the rapid movement with less stability, as reported by Mankowski et al., and a hip strategy is used to maintain stability when the inertia of movement increases, with the thigh muscles commonly activated before those of the leg

19.3.11 Concept of Steady-State Gait Pattern

▨ Altered ankle and hip joint movement patterns and muscle activation patterns in the elderly have just been described. Additionally, Kerrigan et al. noted that the altered ankle and hip joint movement patterns tend to persist in the elderly regardless of walking speed. This steady state gait pattern is dependent on the behaviour of the ankle and hip

19.3.12 Central Nervous System Capacity for Change

▨ It should be noted that the different strategies used by the central nervous system are not mutually exclusive. There is room for fine tuning, especially if similar perturbations are repeatedly applied, resulting in a process of "learning"

▨ In healthy individuals, the central nervous system anticipates spontaneous change in body position during quiet stance and continuously modulates ankle extensor muscle activity to compensate for the change. Recent studies by Masani investigated whether velocity feedback contributes by modulating ankle extensor activities in an anticipatory fashion, facilitating effective control of quiet stance

▨ The findings agree with previously published studies in which it was shown that the lateral gastrocnemius muscle is actively modulated in anticipation of the body's COM position change

▨ These findings further suggest that the actual postural control system during quiet stance adopts a control strategy that relies notably on velocity information, and that such a controller can modulate muscle activity in an anticipatory manner without using a feed-forward mechanism (Masani, Neurophysiology 2003)

19.3.13 Changed Neural Control in the Elderly

▨ In the elderly, recent research suggests that the effects of speed of central processing and attentional capacities may affect postural sways, recalling that sensory information is processed centrally by various areas of the human brain. This information processing is sometimes perturbed in the elderly and more so in elderly fallers

19.3.14 Summarising Common Postural Changes in Elderly Fallers

- Fallers demonstrate significantly greater amounts of sway in the antero-posterior (AP) direction and need greater muscle activity during quiet standing compared with younger individuals, which can be due to altered ankle strategy, or as suggested in other studies, due to decreased ability to detect small motions in the most distal joints
- Even elderly non-fallers demonstrated significantly greater muscle activation and co-activation compared with the younger individuals
- No significant differences were found between elderly fallers and elderly non-fallers in measures of postural sway or muscle activity. However, greater postural sway in both the AP and medio-lateral (ML) directions and trends of greater muscle activity were found in those older adults who demonstrated lower scores on clinical measures of balance
- In fact, relatively high levels of muscle activity are a characteristic of age-related declines in postural stability and such activity is correlated with short-term postural sway
- It is, however, unclear whether increases in muscle activity preclude greater postural instability or vice versa, i.e. increased muscle activity is a compensatory response to increases in postural sway. In either case, such increased muscle activities may also predispose to easy fatigue among the elderly. This forms one of the many rationales for muscle retraining after falls and/or hip fractures in the elderly. However, the overall body of evidence suggests that central processing factors frequently act as an important limitation to postural stability in the elderly – in that a close relationship between central processing activity and attentional capacities plus postural stability was demonstrated

19.4   Science Behind Altered Gait in Elderly Fallers and Non-Fallers – What Have We Learnt from Gait Analysis?

19.4.1   Introduction

■ As far as stability in gait is concerned, two very fundamental requirements of effective gait are to sustain progression and maintain balance to prevent falling

■ Balance during walking can be compromised commonly when initiating gait, while maintaining progression (either forward or backward) and, when terminating gait (Sparrow Gait Posture 2005). In all these tasks, balance is particularly challenged during the transition from one (either statically stable or dynamically stable movement pattern) to another

19.4.2   Normal Controls of Human Walking

■ Traditional teachings have it that the main determinants of gait include:
  – Stability in stance (foot and ankle)
  – Clearance (of foot) in swing
  – Pre-positioning of foot (terminal swing)
  – Adequate step length
  – Energy-efficient fashion (normal energy expended 2.5 kcal/min, less than twice that used in just standing or sitting). This requires the presence of efficient phase shifts (see Chap. 8)

■ But gait is much more than traditional teachings, in fact we can see from the above teachings that not one word is mentioned about the need for the integrity of long-term gait parameters like control of stride-stride variations. In fact, as we will show shortly, gait in healthy individuals does obey long-term fluctuational analysis (as does the inter-beat variability of the human heart, circadian rhythm, and even the branching of trees that we see in nature) and is far from an erratic, totally random undertaking or "white noise". Even normal postural sways in quiet stance (which we talked about in the last section), also obey long-term fluctuational analyses (Stambolieva K et al, Acta Physiol Pharmacol Bulg. 2001). It is high time therefore to think seriously about revising the traditional definition of gait before further discussion

19.4.3   Traditional Definition of Gait

■ A repetitive sequence of limb movements to safely advance the body forwards with minimum energy expenditure

19.4.4   What is Missing in the Definition?

■ The above definition of gait commonly found in most textbooks holds too simplistic a view of this complex, yet seemingly simple neuromuscular task

19.4.5   New Revised Definition

■ A repetitive sequence of limb movements to safely advance the human body forwards with minimum energy expenditure, which requires higher cognitive neural function and a functioning neuromuscular system for its proper execution. It is far from being a simple automated task

19.4.6   Qualifier

■ In fact, it should be pointed out that not only does human gait involve higher cognitive neural function, but also recent evidence from basic science studies of fractal dynamics such as those of Hausdorff from Harvard revealed that some gait parameters obey definite patterns of long-range fluctuations in the same way that many other normal bodily physiological functions obey long-range fluctuational patterns like heart rate

19.4.7   Long-Range Physiological Controls

■ We will begin by talking in more detail about the long-range physiological controls of human walking, as well as showing the reader similar examples from other human body systems such as the cardiovascular and pulmonary systems, as well as examples in nature such as branching of trees

■ One needs to understand these very basic control mechanisms and possible perturbations before one can design:
  – A good fall prevention programme
  – A sound hip fracture rehabilitation programme

19.4.8 Important New Discoveries in Fine Physiological Controls of the Human Body

▪ Research in recent years has clearly shown that the traditional, very simplistic model of "homeostasis" does not always apply in all of the physiological controls of all biologic systems in the human body

▪ Examples are abundant: as in the control of heart rate, control of breathing, circadian rhythms, and of relevance here, the control of the act of human walking

19.4.9 What Is the Evidence for the Theory of "Long-Term Fluctuations"?

▪ Step-to-step fluctuations in walking rhythm, that is, the duration of the gait cycle, also referred to as the stride interval (Fig. 19.4), in normal healthy human gait (not walking on a treadmill) was found to demonstrate long range fluctuations

▪ The stride interval is analogous to the cardiac inter-beat interval, and, like the heartbeat, it was traditionally and originally thought to be quite regular under healthy conditions. The reader is strongly advised to view the illustrations contained in the article published by Goldberger et al. available from the official website of *Proceedings of the National Academy of Sciences in USA*, which, for copyright reasons, are difficult to reproduce here. The relevant web address is: www.pnas.org (pnas reference 012579499)

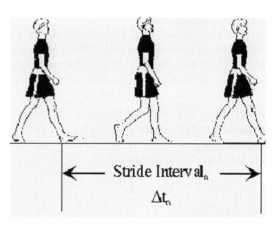

$$\longleftarrow \text{Stride Interval}_n \longrightarrow$$
$$\Delta t_n$$

Fig. 19.4. Stride interval, courtesy of *www.physionet.org*

■ However, subtle and complex fluctuations are apparent in the duration of the stride interval, just like the inter-beat interval of the heart on more careful analysis by researchers like Hausdorff

■ In fact, it was found that the fluctuations in the stride interval exhibit the type of long-range correlations seen in the healthy human heart beat for example, as well as other scale-free, fractal phenomena

■ The stride interval, at any instant, depends in a statistical sense on the intervals at relatively remote times, and this dependence has sometimes been called the "memory effect"

19.4.10   More Elaboration

■ In other words, fractal dynamics were recently detected in the apparently "noisy" variations in the stride interval of human walking

■ Dynamic analysis of these step-to-step fluctuations revealed a self-similar pattern: fluctuations on one time scale are statistically similar to those on multiple other time scales, at least over hundreds of steps, with healthy individuals walking at their normal rate (Hausdorff et al., J Appl Physiol 1996)

■ Furthermore, Hausdorff found that this fractal property of neural output may be related to the higher nervous centres responsible for the control of walking rhythm. However, during metronomically paced walking (as on treadmills), these long-range correlations disappear; variations in the stride interval then become random (uncorrelated) and non-fractal

19.4.11   What Exactly Does the Word "Fractal" Mean?

■ The concept of a fractal is most often associated with geometrical objects satisfying two criteria: *self-similarity* and *fractional dimensionality*. Self-similarity means that an object is composed of sub-units and sub-sub-units on multiple levels that (statistically) resemble the structure of the whole object. Mathematically, this property should hold on all scales. However, in the real world, there are necessarily lower and upper bounds over which such self-similar behaviour applies. The second criterion for a fractal object is that it has to have a fractional dimension. This requirement distinguishes fractals from Euclidean objects, which have integer dimensions. As a simple example, a solid cube is self-similar since it can be divided into sub-units of eight smaller solid cubes that resemble the large cube, and so on. However, the cube (despite its self-similarity) is not a fractal because it has a third dimension. The concept of a fractal structure, which lacks a characteristic length scale, can be extended to the analysis of complex temporal processes, be it stride-stride variability, inter-beat variability of the heart beat, etc. (according to data from Physionet, at www.physionet.org)

19.4.12   Does the Fractal Gait Rhythm Exist Only During Walking at One's Normal Pace, or Does It Occur at Slower and Faster Walking Rates as Well?

- Recent studies indicated that the fractal dynamics of walking rhythm are normally quite robust and appear to be intrinsic to the locomotor system with different walking rates (after Hausdorff)

19.4.13   How Do Scientists Analyse These Complex Noise-Like Long-Range Fluctuations, Be It Heart Beat or Stride Variations?

- Detrended fluctuation analysis (DFA) is a scaling analysis method used to estimate long-range power-law correlation exponents in noisy signals. Recent studies showed that the DFA result of noise with a trend can be exactly determined by the superposition of the separate results of the DFA on the noise and on the trend, assuming that the noise and the trend are not correlated. If this superposition rule is not followed, this is an indication that the noise and the superposed trend are not independent, so that removing the trend could lead to changes in the correlation properties of the noise (Kun Hu et al., Phys Rev 2001)

19.4.14   Clues to the Presence of Higher Neural Controls in Gait

- The breakdown of fractal, long-range correlations during metronomically-paced walking demonstrates that influences above the spinal cord (a metronome) can override the normally present long-range correlations. This finding is of interest because it demonstrates that supra-spinal nervous system control is critical in generating the robust, fractal pattern in normal human gait

19.4.15   Effects of Aging

- Fractal gait dynamics depend on central nervous system function, as mentioned. In addition, it was found that the stride interval fluctuations are more random (less correlated) for the elderly than for the younger individual

▨ Even among healthy elderly adults who have otherwise normal measures of gait and lower extremity function, the fractal scaling pattern is significantly altered compared with young adults

19.4.16   Effects of Dual Task in the Elderly

▨ Dual tasking does not affect the gait variability of elderly non-fallers or young adults. In contrast, dual tasking destabilises the gait of idiopathic elderly fallers, an effect that appears to be mediated in part by a decline in Executive Function (Springer et al., Mov Disord 2006)

19.4.17   How Does This Research on Fractal Dynamics Concern Orthopaedists?

▨ Since there is evidence that degradation of short and longer range correlation properties may be associated with the loss of integrated physiologic responsiveness in some elderly patients (thereby increasing susceptibility to injury and fragility fractures), it is essential to develop a user-friendly mathematical model for calculation of fractal dynamics to allow early detection of elderly people at risk of falls (Fig. 19.5)

▨ This does not mean that traditional assessment of standard "risk factors" are no use, but the new tool will potentially add a new objective dimension to our analysis of falls in the elderly

▨ In particular, the study of gait variability, the stride-to-stride fluctuations in walking, offers an important way of quantifying locomotion and its changes with aging and disease as well as a means of monitoring the effects of therapeutic interventions and rehabilitation (Hausdorff, J Neuroeng Rehabil 2005)

▨ Another beauty of this new tool is that for the first time, there is an objective measure for differentiating changes due to aging from changes due to the disease process causing a high level of gait disorders in frequent fallers (the term "disease" here means there comes a point in some elderly people's life when the central nervous system can no longer compensate and initiates more adaptive response to prevent falls)

▨ Overall, fractal analysis may offer promising insights into the control mechanisms of the neuromuscular system during gait

▨ As for prediction, it was found that scaling exponents can be used as prognostic indicators. Furthermore, detection of more subtle degradation of scaling properties may provide a novel early warning system in subjects with a variety of pathologies including those elderly people at high risk of falling (Peng, Physica A 1998)

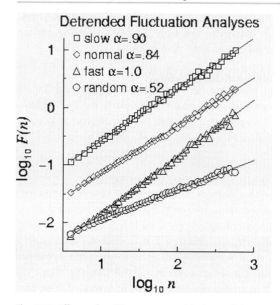

Fig. 19.5. Effects of walking rate on stride interval dynamics. Fluctuation analysis confirmed the presence of long-range correlations at all three (slow, normal, fast) walking speeds and their absence after random shuffling of data points (courtesy of physionet.org; picture originated from Hausdorff's famous article in J Appl Physiol 1996)

19.4.18   What Are the Latest Developments in the Practical Clinical Use of Fractal Dynamics?

■ Recently, the first studies of gait variability in animal models of neurodegenerative disease have been described, as well as a mathematical model of human walking that characterises certain complex (multifractal) features of the motor control's pattern generator (data from physionet.org)

19.4.19   How About Gait Parameters Other Than Stride-to-Stride Fluctuations?

■ Research on gait about to be discussed suggests that measures of gait variability may be more closely related to falls, rather than measures based on the mean values of other walking parameters

■ That said, some researchers observed that increased step variability is a hallmark of fallers in a study investigating step length variability at gait initiation in elderly fallers and non-fallers, and in young adults (Mbourou et al., Gerontology 2003)

19.4.20 What About Other Investigations Like the Sensory Organisation Test?

■ Patients with repeated falls have been subjected to assessment by expensive machines that perform the Sensory Organisation Test (SOT) or "Balance Masters" in the author's hospital and in many other centres (Fig. 19.6)

■ While these are useful in detecting anomalies in postural controls, it does not look at the much more dynamic act of walking. Notice that most elderly fall during the act of walking. Newer tools such as fractal analysis nicely compliment the results obtained by SOT or related machines

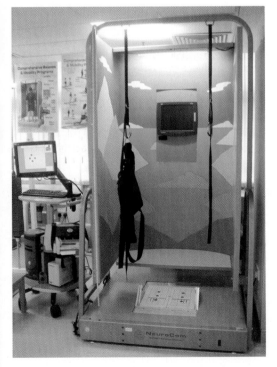

Fig. 19.6. Machine with capabilities for performing the Sensory Organisation Test (SOT)

19.4.21   Key Concept

▨ Recall from our previous discussions that many elderly with gait dysfunction have affection of higher executive function. The extra-pyramidal system, frontal lobe and limbic systems are apparently likely to be the key players involved in a "multisystem neurodegenerative syndrome" that is clearly different from usual "aging" among many elderly fallers and those elderly with a high-level of gait deviations detectable by the use of fractal analysis techniques

▨ Documenting extra-pyramidal and frontal lobe signs are essential in assessing fallers or elderly with gait problems

19.4.22   What Are the Other Areas of Fall Analysis?

▨ Gait analyses comparing young and elderly gait, as well as comparing healthy elderly with elderly who fall frequently, will throw light on this subject besides standard clinical assessment (e.g. Tinetti gait and balance score, 6-min walk test), and assessment by SOT or the use of fractals, as just discussed

19.4.23   The Importance of "Subtask" Analysis

▨ In order to ease analysis of frequent fallers, researchers have resorted to the use of "subtask" analysis, or in other words breaking down the complex situations whereby the elderly fall into several events to ease investigation and research

19.4.23.1   What Are the Components of the "Subtask Analysis" of Gait?

▨ Subtask analysis mainly involves the investigation of:
 – Gait initiation
 – Negotiating obstacles
 – Turning
 – Gait terminations

▨ However, we will also look at some other relevant factors such as effects of poor lighting, implications of elderly walking with a fearful gait, etc.

19.4.23.1.1 On Gait Initiation

▨ Not uncommonly, falls can occur during gait initiation

▨ The elderly display several striking differences compared with the younger individuals during gait initiation:

- Weight-bearing during initial standing is considerably more unequal and reaction time 46% longer
- A gradually decreasing anticipatory activation of ankle muscles is part of the compensatory strategy in the preparatory postural adjustment in elderly people
- Swing leg peak posterior force tends to be smaller, but the increase in vertical force larger
- Older adults appear to initiate walking with less TA (tendo Achilles) anticipation
- There is evidence in the literature that deficient TA anticipation is accompanied by less anticipatory backward displacement of the centre of foot pressure

One way to circumvent this would be to initiate walking by swaying forward. This type of compensatory modification is in line with previous observations by researchers revealing that older adults often develop an anterior shift of the centre of gravity within the base of support, thereby improving stability. In practice, this anterior shift of the CG in the elderly is predisposed by the frequently stooped posture that they adopt with an element of thoracic kyphosis and with hips partially flexed

Possibility of Decreased Spinal Motor Neuron Excitability

In addition to the deficient TA anticipation, the older adults apparently deviate with regard to activation of the LG (lateral gastrocnemius) in the stance leg as well. The function of this muscle during gait initiation does not seem merely to be to "push-off" from the ground, but helps also to control the forward movement of the body in preparation for the swing leg leaving the ground

Recent data have revealed that the function of the LG tends to be missing in a minority of the younger individuals, but missing in the majority (59%) of the elderly individuals, due to the lack of LG activation in the stance leg until the swing leg has already left the ground. Lower peak forces in all directions in the stance leg accompanied this delayed LG and TA activation in the elderly individuals

In contrast to the deviation in anticipatory TA muscle activity, delayed LG activation was present both when the starting leg was chosen freely and predetermined. This finding, together with the reported age-related differences in the H-reflex during gait initiation, is suggestive of possible decreased spinal motor neuron excitability

However, gait initiation changed significantly when the starting leg was predetermined. In fact, in this case, the deficiency in TA anticipation was no longer apparent. In the stance leg all forces were smaller, LG was recruited later, and unlike the younger individuals, it was generally recruited after the swing leg had left the ground (Henriksson et al., Gait Posture 2005)

Muscle Activity at Initiation of Gait

Recent EMG data provide a clear indication of the patterns of phasic muscle activity for normal elderly people during gait initiation. EMG testing revealed a less reliable expression in the elderly of tibialis anterior and the medial gastrocnemius at the onset of gait. A proportion of individuals who lacked swing leg gluteus medius activity in the release phase was observed in young or elderly people

It is interesting to note that the tendency is for muscle activity to be more variable in the preparatory phase than in the stepping phase, which suggests that the preparatory phase may be a particular source of difficulty in patients with high level gait disorders (Mickelborough, Gait Posture 2004)

19.4.23.1.2 On Negotiating Obstacles

- In general, the elderly tend to adopt a swing hip flexion strategy to achieve a higher leading toe clearance than younger persons
- With increasing obstacle height, the older group increased linearly the leading toe clearance by changing fewer joint angular components than the younger group, allowing the maintenance of the necessary stability of the body with minimum control effort
- When the trailing limb was crossing, the older people showed no significant difference in the trailing toe clearance compared with the younger individuals
- Overall, the older group seemed to use a more conservative strategy for obstacle-crossing. Failure to implement this strategy during obstacle negotiation may (paradoxically) increase the risk of falls owing to an inability to recover from unexpected tripping or stumbling
- But increased leading toe clearance would thus require increased muscular demands on the swing limb. If these demands were not met – for instance as a result of age-related muscle weakness – the elderly might not be able to recover from tripping over the obstacle and the risk of falling would also increase (Lu et al., Gait Posture 2006)

Increased Demand on Muscles
of Normal Healthy Elderly People Negotiating Obstacles

- In general, studies found that older adults demonstrated greater relative activation levels compared with young adults. Gluteus medius activity, in particular, was significantly increased in the elderly compared with the young during periods of double-support (weight transfer)

- Increase in obstacle height resulted in greater relative activation in all muscles, confirming the increased challenge to the musculoskeletal system. While healthy elderly adults were found to be able to successfully negotiate obstacles of different heights during walking, their muscular strength capacity was significantly lower than young adults, resulting in relatively higher muscular demands. The resulting potential for muscular fatigue during locomotion may place individuals at higher risk of trips and/or falls

Medio-Lateral Motion of COM in Crossing Obstacles

- Medio-lateral (M/L) COM motion during obstructed walking may be a better parameter to identify persons at greater risk of imbalance. Examining the motion of the whole body COM may be a valuable tool in clinical evaluations of patients with balance disorders. Information about an individual's ability to control their COM trajectory during obstacle crossing allows us to identify individuals at risk of imbalance and falls, which may provide early detection, allowing preventative intervention before falls actually occur (Chou, Gait Posture 2003)

- Elderly patients with balance disorders demonstrated significantly greater and faster lateral motion of the COM when crossing over obstacles. These measurements distinguish elderly patients with imbalance from the healthy elderly individuals. Furthermore, the increased M-L motion of the COM during obstacle crossing showed a positive correlation with an increased M-L range of motion of the swing foot trajectory. This increase in M-L motion is suggestive of a compensatory adjustment in the swing foot trajectory to land the swing foot at an appropriate location that would establish a new base of support to counter the balance disturbance in the frontal plane

19.4.23.1.3 On the Act of "Turning" During Walking

- The act of turning tends to carry with it an increased risk of injury due to a decrease in stability. Many falls in the elderly occur during turning

▨ The most pronounced differences were demonstrated in the M/L ground reaction force impulse, i.e. in straight walking, the impulses tended to shift the body towards the contralateral limb. In turning, the IN and OUT impulses shifted the body towards the ipsilateral and contralateral limbs respectively. Knee flexion during stance was increased on the IN limb, while ankle plantar flexion increased on the OUT limb consistent with body lean during turning; differences in joint kinetics during turning were negligible, however

▨ Notice that a non-uniform centre of mass trajectory was found, even upon turning at very slow speeds

▨ In summary, turning appears to be a complex set of changes in ground reaction impulses, joint kinematics and kinetics, which alters both the COM trajectory and trunk orientation. Increased M/L impulses seem the most likely cause of the turn, with compensatory alterations in rotational moments at the hip, knee and ankle and a decrease in stride and limb length (Orendurff et al., Gait Posture 2006)

▨ Older adults also tend to slow their step velocity when turning. These changes were accompanied by corresponding step length and width modifications (Fuller et al., Canada)

▨ Even the physically active and well-adapted elderly women in one study showed differences in the kinematics of 180° turn execution

▨ Hence, frail elderly people would be expected to exhibit even more caution in their turning strategies. Despite being more cautious, the minimum foot separation distance and maximum pelvic rotational velocity of the elderly frequently reflects greater average variability than in younger persons. Increased step variability is a common finding of fallers, as alluded to earlier, further underlying the difficulty when it comes to turning

19.4.23.1.4 Patterns of Gait Termination and Clinical Significance

▨ Gait termination is a challenge to stability and the process by which the centre of mass is maintained within the base of support is common to other gait tasks in which the walker is destabilised either by obstructions or changes in direction. Another general phenomenon of interest is the realisation of how quantitative changes in one parameter (such as walking speed or stimulus delay), may precipitate qualitatively different responses, either one short or long step or two steps prior to termination. The short-step response in termination is a particularly interesting feature of human gait that is infrequently reported in traditional accounts of symmetrical phases of the stride cycle (Sparrow et al., Gait Posture 2005)

The Process of Gait Termination in Real Life

- In general, stopping at a preferred or comfortable speed is expected to be relatively efficient compared with suddenly stopping when walking faster or accelerating, such as in real life when running to catch a bus or to cross the road
- This led some researchers to ask whether laboratory studies of the various gait tasks or "subtasks" that we have cited here, such as initiation, turning and obstacle crossing, can be shown to properly represent performance in the everyday environment, since gait tasks undertaken in the real world when there may be less opportunity to preplan the response may be undertaken very differently from those in the laboratory. Further discussion on this point will be given later

19.4.23.1.5 Descent of Stairs

- Descent of stairs involves controlled lowering and eccentric muscle work of the lower extremity. Studies involving healthy older adult volunteers show that they tend to perform descent of stairs at a slower speed and with greater motion outside the plane of progression than young adults, as reported in *Gait Posture*. There was also observed increases in hip and pelvis motion

Stairs Training for the Elderly

- We know that descent of stairs mainly involves eccentric exercise instead of concentric strength. A recent study found that training using eccentric ergometers improved stair descent speed in frail older adults whilst training using conventional resistance machines did not (Lastayo et al., J Gerontol A: Biol Sci Med Sci 2003)
- Resistance training of frontal and transverse plane hip muscles may be key factors in improving negotiation of stairs
- The implication here is that merely prescribing exercises involving relatively lightweight elastic resistance bands targeting the hip abductors and external rotators produces inadequate muscle loading to induce significant strength improvements in these muscles – one further reason for higher intensity muscle strengthening exercises in frequent

fallers and after hip fractures. Furthermore, performing exercises whilst changing levels such as with the use of a stepping box may be more beneficial for future stair negotiation

- The aerobic component of our training programme (part of circuit training, which will be discussed later) should also include exercises designed to challenge dynamic balance maintenance

19.4.23.1.6 Head Movement During Gait in the Elderly

- During gait, our head (which contains the gravity sensors – the vestibular system and the visual system), must be stabilised in space to provide a steady frame of reference
- Also, during walking, our head needs to be free to move to allow the scanning of surrounding objects and steering of locomotion. Much literature in the past concentrated on the lower limb, but the head – and in particular eye movements and scanning – are important. Investigation of the effects of eye movements by the use of optical tracking devices in gait is under way in Sunnybrook Hospital in Toronto, Canada (Fig. 19.7)
- In a recent study reported in *Gait Posture*, it was found that head, trunk and pelvic movements are coordinated in a task-dependent

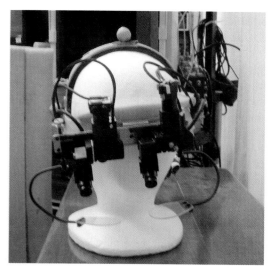

Fig. 19.7. Optical tracking device used in some research laboratories for investigation of falls

manner such that their movement amplitudes induced by rapid voluntary head motions are larger in walking than in standing. This task-dependent movement coordination is again affected by aging: elderly individuals tend to use a different balance strategy, compared with younger individuals, by limiting their head movement velocity and upper body movement amplitude. This strategy is likely being used to prevent the destabilising effect of rapid head motion on upright posture (Paquette et al., Gait Posture 2006). Manoeuvres like sudden head rotation during gait can have a destabilising effect on the gait of the elderly, and should be avoided if feasible, just like performing dual-tasking during walking, as mentioned already

19.4.23.1.7 The Trunk Segment

- It has been demonstrated in recent studies that the trunk segment plays an important role in stabilising the anterior–posterior motion of the head during walking, but plays only a minor role in attenuating trunk to head accelerations in the vertical direction
- The statistically significant differences in head and trunk accelerations between young and elderly individuals were mainly restricted to the anterior–posterior direction and are probably motivated by the need to maximise dynamic stability in critical parts of the gait cycle

19.4.23.1.8 Fear of Falling in the Elderly

- Giladi found that older adults with a disturbed gait of unknown origin appear to share common characteristics. They tend to walk more slowly than "healthy" controls with increased unsteadiness and with excessive fear of falling (Giladi, J Neurol 2005)
- Tinetti et al. reported that fear of falling in older adults contributes to changes in the gait characteristics in community-dwelling older adults. Tinetti felt that the older adults tend to walk slower to ensure a safer gait and many have higher levels of anxiety and depression compared with normal adults with little fear of falling

What Significance Do We Attach to Elderly People with a Fearful Gait; Does It Only Suggest Aging?

- In a study of individuals with high-level gait disorders, only the fractal index was significantly different between fallers and non-fallers. These findings underscore the idea that the gait changes in older adults who walk with fear may after all be an appropriate response to unsteadiness, are likely a marker of underlying pathology, and are not simply a physiological or psychological consequence of normal aging (Hermana et al., Gait Posture 2004)

That having been said, the fear of falling may have a downside in that it could cause problems with balance control, due to an increase in muscle stiffness

Other Relevant Findings in Research

In this and other studies on gait changes among elderly with a high level of gait disorder (HLGD), one finds that:

- Gait variability is markedly increased among older adults with an HLGD and fear of falling compared with control subjects of similar age, as mentioned
- Physical factors (e.g. muscle strength, balance disturbances) are not associated with the level of gait variability among the older adults with an HLGD. Instead, neuropsychological factors, especially fear of falling, and depression are significantly related to stride-to-stride variability
- Among the older adults with an HLGD, fall history was not related to fear of falling, gait speed or other clinical measures. The fractal scaling index was in fact the only measure that was related to fall history

Clinical Implications

We have talked about the pros and cons of fear of falling. Fear of falling and gait unsteadiness are closely related. Alterations in frontal lobe and extra-pyramidal function are likely causes of the unsteady gait, as well as changes in higher executive function

Since fear of falling plays such an important role in elderly gait disorder, neuropsychological interventions should also be considered

19.4.23.1.9 Studies on the Effect of Reduced Lighting on Gait

Studies revealed that a number of elderly people fall at night due to insufficient lighting

Whereas both healthy older controls and patients with a higher-level gait disorder walk more slowly in reduced lighting, only the latter's stride variability increases (Hamel et al., Gait Posture 2005)

19.4.23.1.10 Why Is There Not Much Research on "Fall Recovery"?

- The reason here is more than obvious; such types of research are unlikely to have approval by the ethical committees of most hospitals

19.4.23.1.11 Can the Above Results Be Extrapolated to Real-Life Situations?

- Gait tasks undertaken in the real world when there may be less opportunity to pre-plan the response may, for example, be undertaken very differently from those in the laboratory. Such considerations have particular importance for older adults or those with gait pathologies. One suggestion is that gait research might be usefully supplemented by measurements of gait characteristics in real-world environments in order to validate our laboratory simulations of everyday gait tasks (Sparrow et al., Gait Posture 2005)

19.4.23.1.12 What Is the Evidence That Human Walking Is a Cognitive Task Requiring Executive Function?

- Studies on the effects of dual tasks suggest that the regulation of the stride-to-stride fluctuations in stride width and stride time may be influenced by attention loading and may require cognitive function (Hausdorff, Exp Brain Res 2005)
- An example would be performance of a cognitive task (like repeating random digits) while walking

19.4.23.1.13 Patients with Dementia

- Studies on the effect of dementia on gait found that divided attention markedly impairs the ability of patients with Alzheimer's disease to regulate the stride-to-stride variations in gait timing. This susceptibility to distraction and its effect on stride time variability, a measure of gait unsteadiness, may partially explain the predilection for falling observed in patients with dementia
- The results also support the concept that persons with dementia have significant impairments in the cognitive domain of attention and gait can be very much affected, since, as was pointed out earlier, locomotor function relies upon cognitive, especially executive, function (Sheridan, J Am Geriatr Soc 2003)

19.5   The Actual Act of Falling in the Elderly –
Analysing the "Cascade of Falling"

19.5.1   The Cascade of the Act of Falling Leading
to Hip Fractures: Introduction

■ The cascade of falling is described here in accordance with the model put forward by Cummings. The act of falling can be visualised and broken down into a series of events or cascade, just like researchers resort to the use of subtask analysis of gait, as described in the previous section

19.5.2   Cascade of Falling (According to Cummings)

■ Not all falls result in hip fracture in the elderly, but a model of the cascade from the act of falling leading to hip fracture consists of the following (Fig. 19.8):

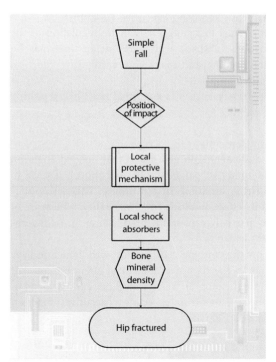

Fig. 19.8. The "cascade" or sequence of events leading to a fall and hip fracture (originally published in Chap. 12 of the author's companion volume *Orthopedic Traumatology – A Resident's Guide*)

- Position of impact
- Local protective response
- Local protective soft tissue structures
- Bone mineral density
- Other factors, e.g. local geometry of the femur

19.5.2.1   Position of Impact

▨ Notice that owing to the difference in the body's response to a fall, the effect of the position of impact is such that a hip fracture is much more likely to occur after a fall in a patient in their 80 s rather than one in their 60 s

19.5.2.1.1   Distribution of Contact Force During Impact to the Hip

▨ Recent research has found that during a fall on the hip, two pathways exist for energy absorption and force generation at contact:
- A compressive load path directly in line with the hip
- A flexural load path due to deformation of muscles and ligaments peripheral to the hip
▨ The result suggested that only 15% of total impact force is distributed to structures peripheral to the hip and that peak forces directly applied to the hip are well within the fracture range of the elderly femur. It was also found that impacting with the trunk upright significantly increases peak force applied to the hip (Robinovitch et al., Ann Biomed Eng 1997)
▨ Another study found a 38% reduction in the trunk angle at impact, and a 7% reduction in hip impact velocity for relaxed vs muscle-active falls; thus, presence of protective muscle reflex activation during a fall may have a bearing on the final results (Van den Kroonenberg et al., J Biomech 1996). Another study (also in J Biomech) showed that active responses reduce the impact forces experienced at the hip and shoulder in falls to the side. Decreased effectiveness of protective responses, due to increases in reaction time and decreases in strength with age, may help explain why so many hip fractures occur in the elderly, but so few occur in younger people (Sabick et al., J Biomech 1999)

19.5.2.2   Local Protective Response

▨ The therapist looking after a patient after hip fracture can help by teaching the patient better protective mechanisms in case of an impending fall

■ Home modification, training with the use of aids and upper and lower limb muscle strengthening are also important. Community Nursing Service (CNS) nurses can help to reinforce those techniques learned during the hospital stay after the patient has been discharged from the hospital

19.5.2.2.1 Importance of Strategies to Reduce Impact on the Hip During Falls

■ Realisation that during a fall, hip fracture risk increases 30-fold if there is direct impact to the hip is probably the best reason for find ways to break a fall, and lessen the impact on the hip (according to Robinovitch). In fact, research is already under way regarding and exploring new ways to break especially a sideways fall using modified techniques borrowed from martial arts

19.5.2.2.2 Strategies in Preventing the Brunt of Falling on the Hip

■ In a recent study, it was found that only two out of the six individuals were able to break the fall with their arm or hand (J Biomech 1996). Newer studies have taught us techniques to lessen the impact on the hip of a sideways fall. A recent study by Robinovitch revealed that, during a sideways fall, individuals can avoid impact to the hip and thereby lower the risk of hip fracture by rotating forward or backward during descent. These seemingly simple yet very effective safe-landing strategies should be considered when designing exercise-based hip fracture prevention programmes, and therapists are highly advised to read the original article by Robinovitch et al. (J Bone Miner Res 2003)

■ Recently, incorporation of martial arts (MA) techniques was found to be useful in breaking the brunt of falling. It was found that the reduction in hip impact force was associated with a lower impact velocity and less vertical trunk orientation. Rolling after impact, which is characteristic of MA falls, is likely to contribute to the reduction of impact forces as well. Using the arm to break the fall was not essential for the MA technique to reduce hip impact force. These findings provided support for the incorporation of MA fall techniques in fall prevention programmes for the elderly (Groen et al., J Biomech 2006)

19.5.2.3   Local Protective Soft Tissue Structures

- The adequacy of the soft tissue envelope around the hip, and the bulk and tone of the musculature around the hips of the elderly are important to damp down the energy of impact (e.g. training gluteus maximus, gluteus medius and minimus, vastus lateralis)
- In general, an emaciated and thin patient in their 80 s with atrophied hip muscle is more likely to have a hip fracture after a fall. The CNS nurses can help teach and supervise the elderly wearing, say, hip protectors (if the family had purchased one). Advice on nutrition can also be provided

19.5.2.3.1   Research on the Use of Hip Protectors

- In a meta-analysis, hip protectors reduced hip fractures in *groups* of patients at a high risk of falls (Van Schoor et al., JAMA 2003)
- Research also found that compliance is a major issue when it comes to the wearing of hip protectors in the elderly. In one study, although approximately 50% of elderly rest home residents who are mentally able would wear hip protectors in order to prevent hip fractures; however, long-term compliance drops to only about 30%. Compliance could be increased substantially if the pads and undergarments were modified to enhance their fit and to reduce the discomfort associated with their use (Villar et al., Age Aging 1998)
- In the recent Cochrane Database Systematic Review performed in 2005, reviewing pooled data from 11 trials conducted in nursing or residential care settings, including six cluster-randomised studies, the result showed evidence of a marginally statistically significant reduction in hip fracture incidence only. The authors concluded that accumulated evidence seems to cast doubt on the effectiveness of the provision of hip protectors in reducing the incidence of hip fracture in older people. Acceptance and adherence by users of the protectors remain poor due to discomfort and practicality (Parker et al., Cochrane Database Systematic Review 2005, CD001255). Better design of hip protectors to improve their acceptability to older people and improve the level of compliance is certainly eagerly awaited. Two of the newer designs of hip protectors are shown in Figs. 19.9 and 19.10

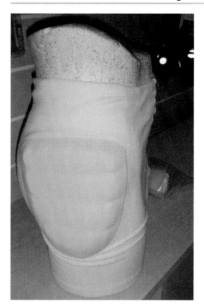

Fig. 19.9. Hip protector sometimes used in nursing homes in an attempt to prevent hip fracture during a fall

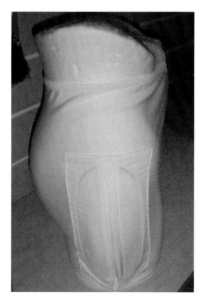

Fig. 19.10. Another hip protector design with inter-changeable pads

19.5.2.4   Bone Mineral Density

■ Patients with osteoporosis (bone mineral density [BMD] – 2.5 SD) are more prone to hip fractures. Prevention and management of osteoporosis is most important. This was discussed in detail in the companion volume of this book

■ CNS or community-based nurses can also see whether elderly patients have difficulty in taking medications and help ensure proper administration of medication, e.g. of bisphosphonates. Dietary calcium and vitamin D as supplements are often needed, especially in institutionalised elderly people living in nursing homes. Previous studies by Massachusetts General Hospital (MGH) reviewed that silent osteomalacia is not uncommon and should be ruled out, particularly in institutionalised older people

■ Although intervention thresholds for osteoporosis should be based on absolute fracture risk, there is a large variation in hip fracture incidence among different regions of the world. A recent study examined the heterogeneity of hip fracture probability in different regions from recent estimates of hip fracture incidence and mortality to adjust intervention thresholds. Ten-year probabilities of hip fracture were computed in men and women at 10-year intervals from the age of 50 years and lifetime risks at the age of 50 years from the hazard functions of hip fracture and death (Kanis, J Bone Miner Res 2001)

Table 19.2. Ten-year hip fracture probabilities with relative and absolute risks, corresponding T-score values and age

Age	T-score	Relative risk	Absolute risk (%)
50	0	1	0.2
	–1	2	0.4
	–2	4	1.1
60	0	1	0.4
	–1	2	1
	–2	4	2.7
70	0	1	0.7
	–1	2	1.9
	–2	4	5.3

(Kanis et al., J Bone Miner Res 2001)

- The table depicts the 10-year hip fracture probabilities with the relative and absolute risks and the corresponding T-score values and age (Table 19.2)

19.6   Incorporation of Results of Gait Analysis in the Elderly into Rehabilitation after Acute Hip Fracture

19.6.1   Principle of Retraining the Ankle Strategy

- Studies have shown that elderly people tend to adopt a hip strategy rather than ankle strategy as an adaptive or anticipatory response to either postural perturbations or when anticipating potential gait instability during gait, like crossing an obstacle, as was discussed previously. Even if an ankle strategy was selected, the activation is significantly slower than that in younger individuals (Mackey, Gait Posture 2006)
- But since the hip may still be painful and stiff after hip fracture, and studies have found that persistent pain in the hip is not uncommon, even after hip fracture surgery (Herrick, J Am Geriatr Soc 2004), relearning the use of the ankle strategy to prevent falls and improve balance will assume an even more important role and needs to be incorporated into the new rehabilitation programme
- The implication from the above is that the resident in charge of the patient should carefully document and test the status of both ankle and foot units of the hip fracture patient. This includes checking for sores and corns (especially if painful), ROM, malalignment and any diminished sensation (may need to rule out any neuropathy, especially in diabetics)

19.6.2   Retraining the Hip Strategy

- Recall that commonly observed changes in kinematics include reversal of the normal firing and muscle activation pattern of the lower limb, relative lack of swing leg gluteus medius activity, increased muscle demand around the hip in crossing obstacles, affected trunk–pelvic coordination, abnormal hamstring activation pattern during initial heel contact of gait. Furthermore, the strength of hip abductors may be further compromised by surgery itself or inadequately treated postoperative pain around the hip wound causing muscle shutdown. This situation should be corrected promptly since most elderly people rely more on a hip strategy rather than an ankle strategy to counteract motion perturbation and persistently affected hip strategy after the fracture may predispose to further falls, either in hospital or at home. This underlies the importance of muscle strengthening and restoration of a proper hip strategy, as well as resistance training of frontal and transverse plane hip muscles maybe being key factors in improving stair negotiation, as stair walking is a very demanding task for the elderly. Improving trunk–pelvic muscle coordination, as well as core stability, should also be our aim

19.7 Incorporation of Other Principles and Techniques Learned in Rehabilitating Acute Hip Fracture

19.7.1 Layout of the Discussion That Follows

- Preoperative assessment and concept that rehabilitation should start in the preoperative phase: importance of documentation of frontal lobe (cognitive) function and extra-pyramidal functions
- Optimisation of surgical results, particularly for pertrochanteric fractures
- Realistic weight-bearing postoperative protocol
- Role of closed circuit training and muscle resistance training
- Role of sensorimotor training, balance and proprioceptive training
- Role of osteoporosis treatment, and preventive issues

19.7.2 General Assessment

- Assess fall risk
- Intrinsic and extrinsic factors of fall need to be looked into
- Vision and hearing
- Review the use of drugs especially of sedatives, narcotics, etc.
- Osteoporosis risk (BMD testing with dual-energy X-ray absorptiometry). Refer to the paper by Kanis concerning the relative risk in different countries discussed previously
- Cognitive assessment

19.7.3   Relevant Questions on the Fall Event

■ What were you doing at the time of your fall (e.g. walking, standing still, getting up from a chair)?
■ Were you feeling well before you fell?
■ Did you notice any symptoms (e.g. dizziness, palpitations, chest pain, visual disturbance) prior to or following your fall?
■ Did you black out or lose consciousness when you fell?

19.7.4   Osteoporosis Risk

■ Historical risk factors besides age:
  - Low body mass index
  - Current smoking/alcoholism
  - Maternal history of hip fracture
  - Chronic disease: renal, hepatic, malabsorption, auto-immune, etc.
  - Surgical history: gastric bypass, gastrectomy, colectomy, total abdominal hysterectomy bilateral salpingo-oophorectomy
  - Medication use: glucocorticoids, thyroid supplement, dilantin, phenobarbital, Depo-Provera, gonadotropin-releasing hormone agonists, aromatase inhibitors, heparin

19.7.5   Physical Examination

■ Special attention should be paid to the cardiovascular, neurologic and musculoskeletal systems

19.7.5.1 Faller-Specific Factors

■ Pulse rate and rhythm
■ Supine and standing BP
■ Mental status
■ Visual acuity and visual fields
■ Muscle power, especially in lower limbs
■ Neck movements
■ Knee joint stability
■ Foot deformities, proprioception, sensation
■ Romberg test
■ Timed up and go test, 6-min walk, elderly mobility score

19.7.5.2 Sensory Organisation Test

■ The SOT may be especially important when we examine and interview persons who are afraid to disclose that they fall frequently. Tinetti suggested that falling in the elderly of the community is related to long-term care admissions, and some older people may be afraid that if they are honest about their fall, they may not be able to live where they want

▓ The use of the SOT is also important as there is the potential that patients will be unable to recall a fall; therefore, under-reporting occurs (Whitney et al., Arch Phys Med Rehabil 2006)

19.7.5.3 Management
▓ Intervention with regard to reversible medical factors
▓ Environmental assessment and modifications
▓ Gait assessment and retraining
▓ Safety alarm and transfer training
▓ Hip protectors (discussed in Sect. 19.5.2.3.1)
▓ Rehabilitation

19.7.6 Restoring Strength and Balance Through Exercise
▓ Mechanical loading to the skeleton helps maintain BMD
▓ High loads of low frequency are deemed best
▓ Strengthening, proprioceptive and balance exercises
▓ Back extension exercises shown to improve gait, well-being, reduce falls, and maintain height in osteoporotic women
▓ Ambulation and transfer training
▓ Tai chi for balance (see Sect. 19.13.4 onwards)

19.7.7 Role of Postural Retraining Early in Hip Fracture Rehabilitation
▓ We know that for a person to have stable posture, there must be proper body alignment, as well as proper sensorimotor, visual and vestibular input
▓ Checking and documenting vision, vestibular function, body's frontal/sagittal plane alignment, sensation and proprioception are important

19.7.8 General Rule
▓ If one or more of these inputs or cues are defective, other inputs should be optimised
▓ Example: a common scenario will be a patient with DM and hip fracture, with a peripheral sensory neuropathy affecting both the sensori-

motor lower limb input as well as the ankle strategy type of central nervous system adaptation to motion perturbation. He will also have pain from the hip from the fracture itself and surgery, which may affect the use of the hip strategy for posture stability

19.7.9   Solution
■ In such a scenario, we need to:
- Give adequate pain relief, train up the hip abductors to prevent hip weakness as the ankles are already at fault (neuropathy takes time to recover)
- Have the neuropathy treated by physicians, and proper DM control
- Check any deficiency of other input – especially vision and vestibular function and have these cues corrected as soon as possible

19.7.10 Partial Weight-Bearing After Surgery for Fractures of the Lower Extremity: Is It Achievable?
■ In a recent paper by Vasarhelyi in Gait Posture 2006, the author found partial weight-bearing starting from 200 N and a stepwise increase in the load level until full weight-bearing was not feasible or practical with regard to measured load levels. The clinical consequence is that a more individualised postoperative loading regime controlled by dynamic measurements such as plantar pressure measurements for only those patients with critical stability of their osteosynthesis might be appropriate
■ Recall that in the face of an aging population, one expects to see more and more trochanteric hip fractures. And, as such, research into new implants and surgical techniques in managing these fracture patterns is imperative. Details of surgical optimisation in trochanteric hip fractures can be found in the companion book *Orthopedic Traumatology – A Resident's Guide*

19.8   High-Intensity Muscle Strength Training and the Role of Proper Nutrition

19.8.1   Rationale for High-Intensity Muscle Strength Training
■ Lamoureux et al. had shown a strong association between lower extremity isometric strength and the ability of elderly individuals to negotiate obstacles. This, combined with the additional findings of other

related studies, add emphasis to the need for muscle strengthening as a preventative intervention to provide improved function in the ambulatory tasks of daily living, as well as performance of instrumental activities of daily living and social re-integration (Lamoureux et al., J Am Geriatr Soc 2002)

■ Slipping events are in fact very explosive and ballistic; therefore, in order to control or recover from a slipping event, rapid force productions of lower-extremity muscles are required. This is the second main reason for properly administered high-intensity muscle strengthening exercises after a hip fracture

19.8.2 Heavy Resistance Training

■ The impact of heavy resistance training in the elderly on maximum voluntary contraction and rate of force development have been investigated in the past, and promising clinical results were reported from researchers at the Hospital for Special Surgery, New York (Peterson et al., Top Geriatr Rehabil 2004)

■ Furthermore, the findings of gait changes in the elderly such as the increased demand on the gluteus medius compared with those in young adults. Gluteus medius activity was significantly greater in the elderly than in the young during periods of double-support and further demand and activation in most muscles on negotiating obstacles, confirming the increased challenge to the musculoskeletal system. The resulting potential for muscular fatigue during locomotion enhances fall risk (Hahn et al., Gait Posture)

19.8.3 Use of Circuit Training in High-Intensity Muscle Strengthening

■ The modern trend for using regimens like "circuit resistance training" that de-emphasise the traditional, very brief intervals of heavy muscle strengthening in standard resistance training protocols is gaining in popularity. This is because this form of training provides a more general conditioning, with demonstrated improvements in body composition, muscle endurance and strength, as well as cardiovascular fitness (Petersen et al., Can J Sports Sci 1989)

19.8.4 Number of Stations Can Be Individualised

■ Typical stations include:
- The stationary bicycle
- Use of free weights (resistance level at 60% of 1 RM)
- Therapeutic ball
- Upper body ergometer
- Cardiovascular conditioning/treadmill
- Isokinetic exercises
- Isotonic exercises

19.8.5 Importance of Adjunctive Sensorimotor Training

■ Sensorimotor training as an adjunct to high intensity muscle exercise was reported by Granacher et al. (Gait Posture 2006) to result in a decrease in onset latency, an enhanced reflex activity in the prime mover, as well as a decrease in maximal angular velocity of the ankle joint complex during motion perturbation impulses induced during treadmill training. No significant changes were observed in the group with high resistance muscle training only or in the control group. The results clearly indicate that sensorimotor training has an impact on spinal motor control mechanisms in the elderly. Training-induced improvements in perception and procession of afferent information could be a possible reason for the increase in reflex contraction. Due to these adaptive processes, sensorimotor training could also be a well-suited method for fall prevention programmes for elderly people

19.8.6 Role of Neuromuscular Coordination and Joint Torques

■ For an intervention to be effective in maintaining or restoring gait performance, however, improving muscle strength only would not be sufficient. Functional performance is determined by appropriate balance of forces generated by multiple muscles. Therefore, not only is the maximum force generated by a muscle relevant, but also optimal muscle length, muscle fibre composition, relative strength of agonists and antagonists and neuromuscular coordination. However, these have been mentioned in Chap. 9 and will not be repeated here

19.8.7 Any Prospect of Altering the Built-in Steady-State Muscle Firing Pattern in Elderly Gait Patterns?

■ One study indicated that correlated fluctuations in the joint kinematics from one gait cycle to the next may influence the selection of a steady state gait pattern and the authors suggested that the different steady state gait patterns observed in the elderly may be due to an altered neuromuscular memory of prior joint behaviour

■ Further scientific research in the future should address whether correlated joint fluctuations in aging can be altered by a change in passive dynamic biomechanical factors found in the viscoelastic properties of the musculoskeletal system or by training, say, biofeedback (Kurz et al., Gait Posture 2006)

19.8.8 A Brief Word on Proper Nutrition for Hip Fracture Patients

■ Previous studies from MGH as well as a study from Japan by Sato (Bone 2002) revealed a 20% incidence of vitamin D deficiency and proper assessment and supplementation is important. Another study by Patterson (J Bone Joint Surg Am 1992) revealed that up to half of hip fracture patients admitted to one hospital in New York had evidence of significant protein malnutrition, bringing our attention to the fact that dietary factors are important and should be incorporated into a proper hip fracture rehabilitation protocol. This is especially so since particularly in the first few weeks after a hip fracture in an elderly person, there is evidence of significant negative nitrogen balance. The second implication of the important finding of negative nitrogen balance in the initial around 6–8 weeks after hip fractures imply that the above-mentioned high-intensity exercise training is best started as from 2–3 months after the index fracture.

19.9   Administration of an Outreaching Community-Based Secondary Fall Prevention Programme Upon Completion of Acute Rehabilitation – Started by the Author and Co-Workers

19.9.1   The Post-Discharge Fall Prevention Pilot Programme

- The programme was started in the cluster of hospitals where the author works in 2004, the aim of the programme includes:
  - Decreasing fall accidents in the home setting
  - Reducing hospital re-admission of high-risk patients
  - Identifying the chief cause(s) of the fall and provide advice on preventive measures
  - Explore the feasibility of extending the period of the next orthopaedic follow-up

19.9.2   Setting up a Panel for Fall Prevention

- Rehabilitation specialist
- Traumatologist
- Director of allied health
- Physiotherapist
- Occupational therapist
- Patient relations officer

19.9.3   Inclusion Criteria

- Age ≥65
- Non-institutionalised patient with a telephone at home living within the catchment area served by the author's regional hospital
- Current admission being caused by fall with or without hip fracture

19.9.4   Protocol

- A case manager will be assigned to the patient according to home address
- Comprehensive assessment and health education advice including fall prevention techniques, need for home modification, etc.
- The first home visit by a community nurse will be provided within 3 days of discharge, then followed by weekly telephone follow-up, paying additional visits as needed. Final home visit will be provided just prior to next clinic follow-up with serial documentation of subjective and objective patient parameters

■ The case manager is empowered with the channels to refer patients to a special fall prevention clinic, occupational therapists, physiotherapist, or non-government organisations, particularly those that run fall prevention and muscle strengthening programmes, as necessary

19.10   Reporting the Result of the Pilot Programme of Community-Based Fall Prevention

19.10.1   Relevant Data of the Pilot Programme

■ A total of 73 patients entered the pilot programme, the vast majority being referred by clinicians. Around 66% of all the patients had fractures, 7% from osteoporotic vertebral collapse after the fall; the remaining 27% of patients suffered persistent diffuse musculoskeletal joint pain after the fall. The average timed up and go result was 33 s and Elderly Mobility Scale score was 9.2/20 during the first home visit assessment. Fifty-nine patients were agreeable to detailed reassessment at the end of the programme. The mean age of the 73 patients was 79

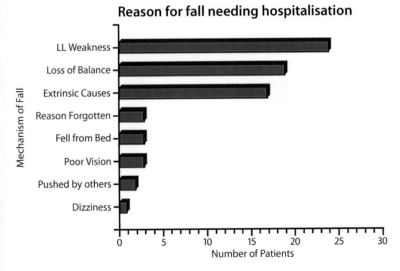

Fig. 19.11. Notice that if more effort is invested, the real cause of the fall can be found in the majority of cases. Intrinsic factors tend to dominate as the main cause when someone reaches their 80 s

■ The rest of the findings are now presented as graphs for easier visualisation

19.10.2   Breakdown of the Causes of a Fall Leading to Initial Hospitalisation

■ It can be seen that the main reasons for a fall include intrinsic factors in this group of patients with a mean age of around 80 (Fig. 19.11)

■ This phenomenon is predicted by the author's original study on double hip fracture presented earlier in this chapter (Sect. 19.2)

19.10.3   Consequence of a Fall Leading to Initial Hospitalisation

■ It can be seen that the brunt of the impact falls on the hip causing the hip either to fracture or persistent hip pain (Fig. 19.12)

■ This further underlines the importance of previous discussions of the need to teach methods of lessening the brunt of the impact of falling on the hip (Sect. 19.5.2.2.2)

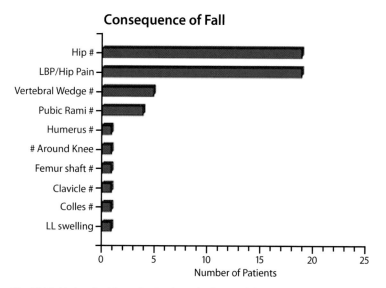

Fig. 19.12. Notice the hip and spine bear the brunt of the impact forces of a fall, particularly the former

19.10.4   Falls Detected After Hospital Discharge

■ It can be seen that although there was a total of 11 falls among the 73 patients after hospital discharge, only one patient required admission due to the fall, or around 1%. This underlines again the importance of teaching patients how to mitigate against the consequences of a fall, should a fall occur after discharge by our therapist or CNS nurses (Figs. 19.13, 19.14)

19.10.5   Hospital Re-Admissions Post-Discharge

■ It will be seen that by far the majority of hospital re-admissions were from medical causes, or consequences of immobility. Only one hip fracture occurred during the pilot period and this was in the one person requiring hospital re-admission who was mentioned in Sect. 19.10.4 (Figs. 19.15, 19.16)

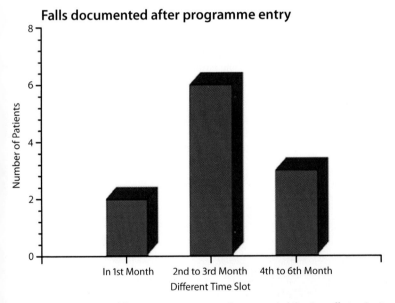

Fig. 19.13. Notice that falls continue to occur after our rehabilitative efforts. As it takes time to completely retrain muscular strength, teaching ways to mitigate the consequences of a fall is important

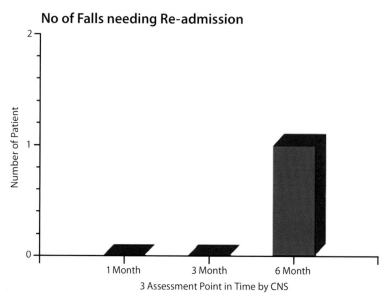

Fig. 19.14. Proper teaching of ways to mitigate the impact of a potential fall resulted in a minority of fall patients requiring hospital re-admission

Reason for re-admission within 3 months

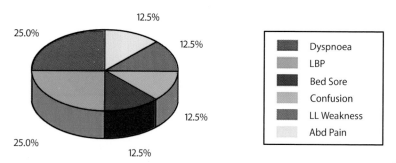

Fig. 19.15. Most recorded re-admissions were due to medical causes

Re-admission Reason (4th to 6th Months)

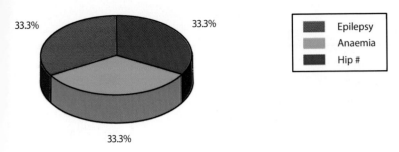

Fig. 19.16. Nearly half a year after discharge, there is a chance that muscle strength may weaken again; this underlines the importance of referral to proper agencies for continuous care, and muscle strengthening

19.10.6   Referral to Other Agencies for Continuous or Enhanced Care

■ The chart reveals clearly that not uncommonly, referral to physiotherapy for further strength training is required of these older people, either as outpatient physiotherapy or to physiotherapists in private non-government organisations (NGO). Those with extrinsic factors identified during home visits by community nurses are referred to occupational therapists. An occasional patient at very high risk of falling, despite previous training, will be referred back to fall prevention clinics (Fig. 19.17)

19.11   Potential Important New Role of Non-Government Organisations (NGO) in Administering High-Intensity Muscle Strengthening Exercises

19.11.1   Timing of Intervention and the Role of NGO

■ We have alluded to the important role of high-intensity muscle strength retraining throughout this chapter. We have also alluded to the key point that the timing of such intervention is important. In fact, the early phase of a fracture hip rehabilitation programme

Cross Referrals by CNS Nurses

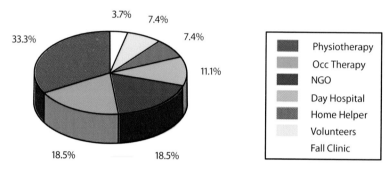

Fig. 19.17. Continuous liaison and mutual referrals between our community nurses and other members of the multidisciplinary team are important and always encouraged

should focus more on posture and balance retraining, training of transfer and ambulation, education regarding techniques of fall prevention for the patient and carer, and other measures such as home modification as required, attention to nutrition and osteoporosis treatment

- Although not yet proven beyond doubt, the evidence to date including research in highly-regarded institutions, like the Hospital for Special Surgery in New York, tend to support a more delayed initiation of really high-intensity muscle retraining for older people, and especially after the phase of negative nitrogen balance is over
- However, in the US, most payer and health rebate systems emphasise the early postoperative period and do not tolerate any delayed rehabilitation efforts. Even in other countries, most insurance payments only cover the perioperative period. This brings to light the future extremely important role of other commercial private non-government and charitable organisations, which are equipped with the necessary instruments to undertake high-intensity muscle strength retraining at a time that is most fruitful and cost effective. In the author's opinion, this timely intervention of suitable therapy is much better than half-hearted exercises for a few weeks only. There is a pressing need for

us to design prospective randomised clinical trials to ascertain the best time at which to initiate these high-intensity exercises in elderly patients

■ In the final analysis, let us not forget the principle that the potential to strengthen muscle with a training programme designed for the elderly is the same as for that for younger individuals – even though we need to begin the programme with lower intensity training and slowly step this up as time passes

19.12   Setting Up Fall Prevention Clinics

19.12.1   Aim of Fall Prevention Clinics

■ To have a channel of referral for difficult cases of falls with multiple causes, i.e. truly multifactorial situations, such as high-risk individuals or patients being detected by our community nursing service

■ Mobilisation of resources and relevant referrals can be made to tackle problems like: urological problems, neurological problems and/or arrange nerve conduction testing

■ Arrange an appointment for fall assessment by special machines made for assessment of balance

■ Initiate referrals for gait analysis as required

■ Management of more challenging cases of osteoporosis such as resistance to bisphosphonates, initiation of newer therapies such as pulsatile PTH (parathyroid hormone) therapy and/or osteomalacia management

19.13   Primary Prevention of Hip Fracture

19.13.1   Aims of Primary Prevention of Falls

■ Primary prevention involves mainly the following and can be performed by the primary care physician or community nurses:
  - General fall risk assessment
  - Environmental modification, especially for those with cognitive impairment
  - Physical fitness retraining
  - Limiting osteoporosis
  - Maintaining cognitive function

19.13.2   Role of Community Nurses

■ In the author's hospital, we have empowered our home-reaching community nurses to initiate fall prevention. The work-flow or protocol is depicted in Fig. 19.18. As with our programme of secondary fall prevention, it will be overlooked by the Panel on Fall Prevention

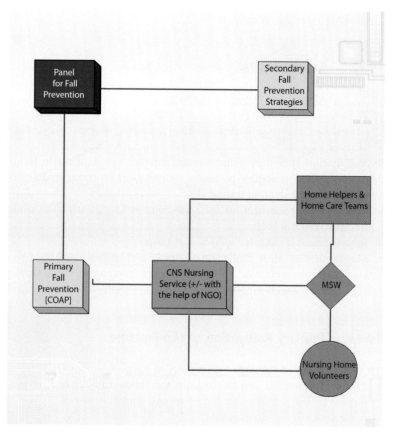

Fig. 19.18. Close liaison between our community nursing service and not only the Panel for Fall Prevention, but also the various other non-government as well as voluntary agencies. Such a scheme works both for primary and secondary fall prevention. *COAP* Community Orthopaedic Ambulatory Programme, *CNS* Community Nursing Service, *NGO* non-government organisation, *MSW* medical social worker

■ If our community nurses pick up individuals who are at very high risk of falls, there is a mechanism for referring these semi-urgently to our Fall Prevention Clinics

19.13.3   Role of Using Fractal Dynamics in Early Detection of Potential Fallers

■ As was previously mentioned in Sect. 19.4.13, detection of more subtle degradation of long-range fluctuations in gait parameters, such as stride-stride variability, may provide a novel early warning system in individuals with a variety of pathologies, including those elderly people at a high risk of falling (Peng, Physica A 1998)

■ The recent development of a mathematical model of human walking that characterises certain complex (multifractal) features of the motor control's pattern generator is a major step forward. The interested reader is referred to the very informative Physionet website, which is funded by the National Institutes of Health

19.13.4   Role of Tai Chi Exercises in Primary Fall Prevention

■ The role of Tai Chi exercises as a measure for both primary and secondary fall prevention has attracted interest both in the USA and recently in Europe, besides in its place of origin in Asia. Details of Tai Chi exercises and their possible efficacy will be talked about in the coming section

19.14   Role of Tai Chi Exercises

19.14.1   Rationale of the Use of Tai Chi in Fall Prevention

■ Reduction in the fear of falling (Sattin et al., J Am Geriatr Soc 2005)

■ Improved lower extremity muscle strength, flexibility and physical fitness (Choi et al., J Adv Nurs 2005)

■ Improved functional balance (e.g. as measured by Berg balance scale) and reduction in the number of falls (Li et al., Med Sci Sports Exerc 2004; Judge, Am J Prev Med 2003)

■ May be of benefit to cardiorespiratory function, immune capacity, mental control, besides flexibility, and balance control (Li et al., Br J Sports Med 2001)

■ Improvement in single-stance postural sway (Judge et al., Phys Ther 1993)

- General sense of well-being and in fact many patients who belonged to the Tai Chi treatment arm in the famous FISCIT study (see below) was found to be still practicing Tai Chi as long as 1–2 years after the study had finished
- May improve psychosocial indices of frailty, besides favourable effects upon the occurrence of falls (Wolf et al., J Am Geriatr Soc 1996)

19.14.2   Components of Tai Chi Exercise

- Tai Chi exercises feature the following:
  - Series of concomitant coordinated upper plus lower limb movement proceeding from simple to more complex manoeuvres
  - Stress on manoeuvres that shift the centre of support from one leg to the other, frequently with concomitant truncal rotational movement
  - Stress on mind–body interaction
  - As complexity of exercise proceeds, progresses from using double leg stance to single leg stance
  - The base of support progressing from wide base of support to a progressively smaller base of support, and eventually to single leg stance
  - Other advantages include low cost, no need to purchase expensive computerised balance-training equipment, and can be taught in groups, unlike machines like the Balance Master, which can only train one person at a time

19.14.3   The FISCIT Study

- Wolf et al. designed the important FISCIT study (The Atlanta Frailty and Injuries: Cooperative Studies and Intervention Techniques), which is a prospective, randomised, controlled clinical trial with three arms, including Tai Chi, computer-based balance training and education only. Intervention length was 15 weeks, with primary outcomes measured before and after intervention and at 4-month follow-up. Falls were monitored continuously throughout the study
- Wolf et al. found that the fear of falling responses and intrusiveness responses were reduced after Tai Chi intervention compared with the education only group. After adjusting for fall risk factors, Tai Chi was found to reduce the risk of multiple falls by 47.5%. The authors went on to conclude that a moderate Tai Chi intervention can impact fa-

vourably on defined biomedical and psychosocial indices of frailty. This intervention can also have favourable effects upon the occurrence of falls. Tai Chi warrants further study as an exercise treatment to improve the health of older people (Wolf et al., J Am Geriatr Soc 2003)

19.14.4   Possible Mechanism of Action

▨ Although experts like Wolf expressed the viewpoint that the mechanism by which Tai Chi exercise works in improving balance and preventing falls in the elderly is largely unknown, recent studies conducted at Queen Elizabeth Hospitals using high-quality video devices of the manoeuvres of the Tai Chi masters seem to indicate that at least some of the Tai Chi manoeuvres are not unlike the training of balance and proprioception given to the patient by therapists. Further detailed research is eagerly awaited with three possible treatment arms including the use of prospective randomised controlled trials comparing Tai Chi vs conventional exercise programme vs computer-based balance training protocols like those used in the FISCIT study in the USA

▨ One prospective trial on Tai Chi was recently started in the Netherlands, which is the first trial in Europe on Tai Chi and fall prevention (Zeeuwe et al., BMC Geriatr 2006)

19.15   Recapitulating and The Future

▨ In this thesis the author has referred to and discussed a number of new ideas in the arena of hip fracture rehabilitation and fall prevention. The latter is deemed inextricably linked to the former

▨ The following recapitulates the key points:
  – According to the author's study on double hip fragility fracture, which will be published shortly by the *Journal of Orthopaedic Surgery* (in press), it is expected that with an aging population, the number of double hip fractures and trochanteric fractures will rise
  – As pointed out in the same study, the part played by intrinsic factors such as the main cause of the fall rises quickly as one ages, particularly when someone reaches their 80 s. Therefore, faced with an aging population, the role of new scientific techniques like the calculation of the fractal index as an early predictor of potential

fallers is a valuable tool. The fact that many biological systems in the body like inter-beat variation in our heart rate, as well as many things in nature itself (like branching of trees) obey similar laws is no longer science fiction, and was recently reported in the highly regarded journal *Nature*. The coming of age of a mathematical model for the calculation of fractal dynamics will definitely be a leap forward in our understanding of the nature of the control of gait, as well as other physiological systems of the human body

- As emphasised throughout this chapter, the concept of secondary fall prevention as well as osteoporosis assessment and treatment being inextricably linked in any decent hip fracture protocol is of extreme importance. The dramatic event of a hip fracture creates a golden opportunity for the orthopaedist to intervene and the patient's compliance is also likely to be better. We have discussed the result of our pilot programme of fall prevention, which showed that fall prevention education, including techniques to mitigate the impact on the hip, and exercises tend not only to reduce falls, but also reduce the chance of re-fracture, particularly of the hip if the fall does recur. As such, the hospital re-admission rates will also be likely to fall. The role of Tai Chi in both primary and secondary fall prevention appears promising and we await the results of prospective randomised trials in this area

- As far as osteoporosis management is concerned, it is worthwhile noting the recent AAOS (American Academy of Orthopaedic Surgeon) Position Statement stressing the need not only to enhance the care of patients with hip and fragility fractures, but the importance of prevention as well, which is very much an obligation of orthopaedic surgeons. There is also a move towards possibly making the important topic of osteoporosis evaluation and treatment a potential medico-legal requirement in the future (http://www.aaos.org/wordhtml/papers/position/1159.htm)

■ Recent developments worthy of being incorporated into a new evidence-based hip fracture rehabilitation protocol include:
  - That one should seriously consider the retraining of the use of the ankle and hip strategies, particularly in hip fracture patients who are frequent fallers
  - The importance of a multidisciplinary team in managing and retraining the patient after a hip fracture is important. In a meta-

analysis and review for the Cochrane Library in 2002, Cameron suggested a trend towards improved outcome when multidisciplinary programmes are utilised. It must never be forgotten that the psychosocial aspects and tackling the frequent depression in fallers are important in preventing social isolation. There is a general move towards early discharge back to the community and the use of rehabilitation day hospitals for further training after discharge from hospital is the way to go

- The role of high-intensity muscle strength retraining including circuit training and also of introducing this type of training at a key point in time when the phase of negative nitrogen balance after a hip fracture is over is important. Since recent research seemed to suggest that the optimal time may be many weeks if not months after the initial fracture (remember the effect of hip fracture on an elderly person is not totally unlike that of high-energy trauma on a younger person), the role of non-government organisations in picking up this important part of rehabilitation in the future cannot be over emphasised

- It is the hope of the author that the above has given the reader a new, fresh, and more holistic look at fracture hip rehabilitation in the geriatric population. The author wishes to take this opportunity to thank the community nurse department of his hospital particularly Anna without whose support the massive fall prevention program would not come into reality

General Bibliography and Key References

Ip D (2006) Orthopedic Traumatology – A Resident's Guide. Springer, Berlin Heidelberg New York

Ip D (2005) Orthopedic Principles – A Resident's Guide. Springer, Berlin Heidelberg New York

Onslow L (2005) Prevention and Management of Hip Fractures. Whurr, West Sussex

Winter DA (1991) The Biomechanics and Motor Control of Human Gait: Normal, Elderly, and Pathological. University of Waterloo Press, Ontario

Goldberger AL, Amaral LAN, Glass L, Hausdorff JM, Ivanov PC, Mark RG, Mietus JE, Moody GB, Peng C-K, Stanley HE (2000) PhysioBank, PhysioToolkit, and PhysioNet: Components of a New Research Resource for Complex Physiologic Signals. Circulation 101(23):e215–e220 [Circulation Electronic Pages; *http://circ.ahajournals. org/cgi/content/full/101/23/e215*]

Ip D (2006) Do elderly with double hip fragility fractures form a unique sub-group among geriatric hip fracture patients? J Orthop Surg (Hong Kong) (December 2006 issue)

Goldberger AL, Hausdorff JM et al. (2002) Fractal dynamics in physiology: alterations with disease and aging. Relevant web-source: *www.pnas.org/cgl/dol/10.1073/pnas.012579499*

(PNAS Feb 19 2002; 99: Suppl 1: 2466–2472)

Selected Bibliography of Journal Articles

1. Sattin R (1992) Falls among older persons: a public health perspective. Review of Public Health 13:489–508

2. Patterson C, Torresin W (1989) Falls in the elderly – keep your patient's feet on the ground. Geriatrics April 15

3. Lu TW, Chen HL et al. (2006) Comparisons of the lower limb kinematics between young and older adults when crossing obstacles of different heights. Gait Posture 23(4):471–479

4. Savelberg HH, Verdijk LB et al. (2006) The robustness of age-related gait adaptations: can running counterbalance the consequences of ageing? Gait Posture (in press, available online doi:10.1016/j.gaitpost.2006.04.006)

5. Mian OS, Thom JM et al. (2006) Kinematics of stair descent in young and older adults and the impact of exercise training. Gait Posture (in press, available on line doi:10.1016/j.gaitpost.2005.12.014)

6. Granacher U, Gollhofer A et al. (2006) Training induced adaptations in characteristics of postural reflexes in elderly men. Gait Posture (in press, available on line doi:10.1016/j.gaitpost.2005.12.007)

7. Vasarhelyi A, Baumert T et al. (2006) Partial weight bearing after surgery for fractures of the lower extremity – is it achievable? Gait Posture 23(1):99–105

8. Hahn ME, Lee HJ et al. (2005) Increased muscular challenge in older adults during obstructed gait. Gait Posture 22(4):356–361

9. Sparrow WA, Tirosh O (2005) Gait termination: a review of experimental methods and the effects of ageing and gait pathologies. Gait Posture 22(4):362–371

10. Paquette C, Paquet N et al. (2006) Aging affects coordination of rapid head motions with trunk and pelvis movements during standing and walking. Gait Posture 24(1):62–69

11. Hausdorff JM, Yogev G et al. (2005) Walking is more like catching than tapping: gait in the elderly as a complex cognitive task. Gait Posture 21(1) [Suppl 1]:S7

12. Hadar-Frumer M, Giladi N et al. (2005) Idiopathic "cautious" gait disorder of the elderly: more than fear of falling. Gait Posture 21 [Suppl 1]:S115

13. Henriksson M, Hirschfeld H (2005) Physically active older adults display alterations in gait initiation. Gait Posture 21(3):289–296

14. Brunt D, Santos V et al. (2005) Initiation of movement from quiet stance: comparison of gait and stepping in elderly subjects of different levels of functional ability. Gait Posture 21(3):297–302

15. Herman T, Giladi N et al. (2005) Gait instability and fractal dynamics of older adults with a "cautious" gait: why do certain older adults walk fearfully? Gait Posture 21(2):178–185

16. Mickelborough J, van der Linden ML (2004) Muscle activity during gait initiation in normal elderly people. Gait Posture 19(1):50–57

17. Chou LS, Kaufman KR et al. (2003) Medio-lateral motion of the center of mass during obstacle crossing distinguishes elderly individuals with imbalance. Gait Posture 18(3):125–133

18. Chou LS, Kaufman KR et al. (2001) Motion of the whole body's center of mass when stepping over obstacles of different heights. Gait Posture 13(1):17–26

19. Okada S, Hirakawa Y et al. (2001) Age-related differences in postural control in humans in response to a sudden deceleration generated by postural disturbance. Eur J Appl Physiol 85:10–18

20. Woollacott M (1993) Age-related changes in posture and movement. J Gerontol 48:56–60

21. Winter DA, Patla AE (1990) Biomechanical walking pattern changes in the fit and healthy elderly. Phys Ther 70:340–347

22. Judge JO, Davis RB et al. (1996) Step length reductions in advanced age: the role of ankle and hip kinetics. J Gerontol 51A(6):303–312

23. Wallman HW (2001) Comparison of elderly nonfallers and fallers on performance measures of functional reach, sensory organization, and limits of stability. J Gerontol A Biol Sci Med Sci 56:M580–M583

24. Wolfson L, Judge J et al. (1995) Strength is a major factor in balance, gait, and the occurrence of falls. J Gerontol A Biol Sci Med Sci 50:Spec No:64–67

25. Caggiano E, Emrey T et al. (1994) Effects of electrical stimulation or voluntary contraction for strengthening the quadriceps femoris muscle in an aged male population. J Orthop Sports Phys Ther 20(1):22–28

26. Magaziner J, Simonsick EM et al. (1990) Predictors of functional recovery one year following hospital discharge for hip fracture: a prospective study. J Gerontol 45(3):M101–M107

27. Cotton DWK (1994) Are hip fractures caused by falling and breaking or breaking and falling? Photoelastic stress analysis. Forensic Sci Int 65:105–112

28. Riley PO, DellaCroce U et al. (2001) Effect of age on lower extremity joint moment contributions to gait speed. Gait Posture 14(2):79–84

29. Winter DA, Patla AE et al. (1998) Stiffness control of balance in quiet standing. J Neurophysiol 80(3):1211–1221

30. Hatzitaki V, Amiridis IG et al. (2005) Aging effects on postural responses to self-imposed balance perturbations. Gait Posture 22(3):250–257

31. Perrin PP, Jeandel C et al. (1997) Influence of visual control, conduction, and central integration on static and dynamic balance in healthy older adults. Gerontology 43(4):223–231

32. Hay L, Bard C et al. (1996) Availability of visual and proprioception afferent messages and postural control in elderly adults. Exp Brain Res 108(1):129–139

33. Serrien DJ, Swinnen SP et al. (2000) Age-related deterioration of coordinated interlimb behavior. J Gerontol B Psychol Sci Soc Sci 55(5):P295–P303

34. Thurmon E, Lockhart TF (2006) Relationship between hamstring activation rate and heel contact velocity: factors influencing age-related slip-induced falls. Gait Posture 24(1):23–34

35. Masani K, Popovic MR et al. (2003) Importance of body sway velocity information in controlling ankle extensor activities during quiet stance. J Neurophysiol 90(6):3774–3782

36. Hausdorff JM, Purdon PL et al. (1996) Fractal dynamics of human gait: stability of long-range correlations in stride interval fluctuations. J Appl Physiol 80(5):1448–1457

37. Chen Z, Hu K et al. (2002) Effect of non-stationarities on detrended fluctuation analysis. Phys Rev E 4(1):041107

38. Springer S, Giladi N et al. (2006) Dual-tasking effects on gait variability: The role of aging, falls, and executive function. Mov Disord 21(7):950–957

39. Hausdorff JM (2005) Gait variability: methods, modeling, and meaning. J Neuroeng Rehabil 2:19

40. Peng CK, Hausdorff JM et al. (1998) Multiple time scales analysis of physiological time series under neural control. Physica A, 249:491–500

41. Ivanov P, Peng CK (1998) Scaling and universality of heart rate variability distributions. Physica A 273:587–593

42. Mbourou GA, Lajoie Y et al. (2003) Step length variability at gait initiation in elderly fallers, non-fallers, and young adults. Gerontology 49(1):21–26

43. Orendurff MS, Segal AD et al. (2006) The kinematics and kinetics of turning: limb asymmetries associated with walking a circular path. Gait Posture 23(1):106–111

44. LaStayo PC, Ewy GA et al. (2003) The positive effects of negative work: increased muscle strength and decreased fall risk in a frail elderly population. J Gerontol A Biol Sci Med Sci 58(5):M419–M424

45. Giladi N, Herman T et al. (2005) Clinical characteristics of elderly patients with a cautious gait. J Neurol 252(3):300–306

46. Hamel KA, Okita N et al. (2005) Foot clearance during stairs descent: effects of age and illumination. Gait Posture 21:135–140

47. Sheridan PL, Solomont J et al. (2003) Influence of executive function on locomotor function: divided attention increases gait variability in Alzheimer's disease. J Am Geriatr Soc 51(11):1633–1637

48. Robinovitch SN, Hayes WC et al. (1997) Distribution of contact force during impact to the hip. Ann Biomed Eng 25(3):499–508

49. Van den Kroonenberg AJ, Hayes WC et al. (1996) Hip impact velocities and body configurations for voluntary falls from standing height. J Biomech 29(6):807–811

50. Sabick MB, Hay JG et al. (1999) Active responses decrease impact forces at the hip and shoulder in falls to the side. J Biomech 32(9):993–998

51. Robinovitch SN, Inkster L et al. (2003) Strategies for avoiding hip impact during sideways falls. J Bone Miner Res 18(7):1267–1273

52. Groen BE, Weerdesteyn V et al. (2006) Martial arts fall techniques decrease the impact forces at the hip during sideways falling. J Biomech (in press, available online doi:10.1016/j.jbiomech.2005.12.04)

53. Van Schoor NM, Smit JH et al. (2003) Prevention of hip fractures by external protectors: a randomized controlled trial. JAMA 289(15):1957–1962

54. Villar MT, Hill P et al. (1998) Will elderly rest home residents wear hip protectors? Age Aging 27(2):195–198

55. Parker MJ, Gillespie WJ et al. (2005) Hip protectors for preventing hip fractures in older people. Cochrane Database Systematic Review (3):CD001255

56. Kanis JA, Johnell O et al. (2002) International variations in hip fracture probabilities: implications for risk assessment. J Bone Miner Res 17(7):1237–1244

57. Mackey DC, Robinovitch SN (2006) Mechanisms underlying age-related differences in ability to recover balance with the ankle strategy. Gait Posture 23(1):59–68

58. Herrick C, Steger-May K et al. (2004) Persistent pain in frail older adults after hip fracture repair. J Am Geriatr Soc 52(12):2062–2068

59. Whitney SL, Marchetti GF et al. (2006) The relationships between fall history and computerized dynamic posturography in persons with balance disorders and vestibular disorders. Arch Phys Med Rehabil 87(3):402–407

60. Lamoureux EL, Sparrow WA et al. (2002) The relationship between lower body strength and obstructed gait in community dwelling older adults. J Am Geriatr Soc 50(3):468–473

61. Peterson GE, Ganz SB et al. (2004) High intensity exercise training following hip fracture. Top Geriatr Rehabil 20(4):273–284

62. Petersen SR, Haennel RG et al. (1989) The influence of high velocity circuit resistance training on VO$_2$max and cardiac output. Can J Sport Sci 14(3):158–163

63. Kurz MJ, Stergiou N (2006) Original investigation correlated joint fluctuations can influence the selection of steady state gait patterns in the elderly. Gait Posture (in press, available online doi:10.1016/j.gaitpost.2005.09.010)

64. Sato Y, Inose M et al. (2002) Changes in the supporting muscles of the fractured hip in elderly women. Bone 30:325–330

65. Patterson BM, Cornell CN et al. (1992) Protein depletion and metabolic stress in elderly patients who have a fracture of the hip. J Bone Joint Surg Am 74A:251–259

66. Sattin RW, Easley KA et al. (2005) Reduction in fear of falling through intense Tai Chi exercise training in older, transitionally frail adults. J Am Geriatr Soc 53(7)1168–1178

67. Choi JH, Moon JS et al. (2005) Effects of sun-style Tai Chi exercise on physical fitness and fall prevention in fall prone older adults. J Adv Nurs 51(2):150–157

68. Li F, Fisher KJ et al. (2004) Tai Chi: improving functional balance and predicting subsequent falls in older persons. Med Sci Sports Exerc 36(12):2046–2052

69. Judge JO (2003) Balance training to maintain mobility and prevent disability. Am J Prev Med 25(3):150–156

70. Li JX, Hong Y et al. (2001) Tai Chi: physiological characteristics and beneficial effects on health. Br J Sports Med 35(3):148–156

71. Judge JO, Lindsey C et al. (1993) Balance improvements in older women: effects of exercise training. Phys Ther 73:254–262

72. Wolf SL, Barnhart HX et al. (1996) Reducing frailty and falls in older persons: an investigation of Tai Chi and computerized balance training. Atlanta FICSIT Group. J Am Geriatr Soc 44(5): 489–497

73. Zeeuwe PE, Verhagen AP et al. (2006) The effect of Tai Chi Chuan in reducing falls among elderly people: design of a randomized clinical trial in the Netherlands. BMC Geriatr 6(1):6

74. Cameron ID, Handoll HH et al. (2001) Co-ordinated multi-disciplinary approaches for in-patient rehabilitation of older patients with proximal femoral fractures. Cochrane Database Syst Rev (3):CD000106

Subject Index